Manual of
Dysphagia Assessment
in Adults

Dysphagia Series

Series Editor

John C. Rosenbek, Ph.D.

Dysphagia Assessment and Treatment Planning: A Team Approach

Rebecca Leonard, Ph.D., and Katherine Kendall, M.D.

The Neuroscientific Principles of Swallowing and Dysphagia

Arthur J. Miller, Ph.D.

Management of Adult Neurogenic Dysphagia

Maggie Lee Huckabee, M.A., and Cathy A. Pelletier, M.S.

The Swallowing Management of Cancer Patients

Paula A. Sullivan, M.S., and Arthur M. Guilford, Ph.D.

Manual of Dysphagia Assessment in Adults

Joseph T. Murray, M.A.

Manual of Dysphagia Assessment in Adults

Joseph Murray, M.A., CCC-SLP

Veteran's Affairs Medical Center
Ann Arbor, Michigan

SINGULAR

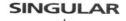

™

THOMSON LEARNING

Africa • Australia • Canada • Denmark • Japan • Mexico • New Zealand • Philippines
Puerto Rico • Singapore • Spain • United Kingdom • United States

COPYRIGHT © 1999 Delmar. Singular Publishing Group is an imprint of Delmar, a division of Thomson Learning. Thomson Learning™ is a trademark used herein under license.

5 6 7   XXX 03

For more information, contact Singular Publishing Group, 401 West "A" Street, Suite 325 San Diego, CA 92101-7904; or find us on the World Wide Web at http://www.singpub.com

Library of Congress Cataloging-in-Publication Data

Murray, Joseph, act8—
    Manual of dysphagia assessment in adults / by Joseph Murray.
        p. cm. — (Dysphagia series)
      Includes bibliographical references and index.
      ISBN 1-56593-871-2 (softcover : alk. paper)
      1. Deglutition disorders — Diagnosis-Handbooks, manuals, etc.
    I. Series.
      [DNLM: 1. Deglutition Disorders—diagnosis. WI 250M982m 1999]
    RC815.2.M87 1999
    616.3'1—dc21
    DNLM/DLC   98-41268
    for Library of Congress   CIP

Contents

Foreword

Scientific and clinical activities in dysphagia are among the fastest growing in healthcare. Speech-language pathologists, physicians, surgeons, nurses, dietitians, dentists, occupational and physical therapists, physiologists, and social workers are among the professionals doing the work. Singular Publishing Group's new series, **Dysphagia**, is designed to support and motivate the best of this research and clinical activity. Like dysphagia as a field of knowledge, **Dysphagia**, the series, is multidisciplinary. The highest levels of research and clinical productivity in dysphagia require responsible scholarship, the ability to cope with ambiguity, and a recognition that dysphagia's effects on people extend well beyond mealtime. Books in the series also are shaped by that scholarship, tolerance for ambiguity, and sensitivity. Authors are contemporary experts and masterly practitioners.

One of the best such practitioners of the clinical art and science is Joseph Murray, author of *Manual of Dysphagia Assessment in Adults*. Joe is a scholar-clinician with long experience in bedside, clinical, and instrumental evaluation of dysphagic men and women. His scholarship and clinical acumen shine from each of this book's pages. He has outlined the specifics of chart review, taking a history, and completing the clinical and a variety of popular, useful instrumental examinations. Better yet, he has written extensively and wisely about conceptual and physiologic underpinnings of each, about their strengths and weaknesses, and about the criteria for their selection and interpretation.

Joe wanted to write a helpful book. He has done so. He wanted the content to be the best extant. He has succeeded. He wanted it to be straightforward enough to help the student and beginning clinician and sufficiently conceptual and databased to inform the most experienced practitioner. He was successful. He wanted to highlight the challenges and dangers of each evaluative technique without paralyzing the reader. He has. He wanted the book to be fun and it is. Buy it for the quotes and quirky turns of phrase and then wear it out with multiple readings for the content.

Too seldom do we see the writer-clinician behind the words of a professional book. This book is an exception. I would send my grandmother to Joe Murray for evaluation. I can see that he would serve her wisely and well.

John C. Rosenbek, Ph.D.
Series Editor

Preface

The dysphagic patient presents himself to the clinician for assessment in many forms. At times the individual appears as an informed self-advocate, with well-defined symptoms, easily identified signs, and the ability to follow the prescribed treatment devised from clearcut instrumental imaging. More often, the symptoms are unreported, the signs are masked by co-occurring medical problems, and the patient is found to be unable to participate in the identification and amelioration of the impairment or disability.

In this book, I have attempted to render a guide for the clinician who is commissioned to assess and formulate treatment for the dysphagic patient. The guide has been drafted to provide assistance to those clinicians, both recent graduates and seasoned veterans, who are newly challenged by this commission. As in any field of study, dysphagia assessment induces confusion in both the neophyte and the practiced professional who, as they seek to conceive a method for systematically approaching each unique patient, are confounded by the mixture of conventional wisdom, art, and applied and basic science that commonly is offered. Although there is much in the way of good, unabashed basic science in the study of dysphagia, it is more difficult to separate the chaff from the seed when attempting to gain advantage from the body of applied scientific research.

It is my hope that this book will assist the needy professional by guiding him or her through the process of assessment from the initial chart review to the final report of findings. The book starts with a means for developing a detailed survey of the patient's medical history. The reader then will be provided with a guide for performing an interview to develop further the patient's health history by systematically probing for information salient to the patient's swallowing problem. A protocol for performing the clinical swallowing examination is provided with descriptions for administrating each step and for judging the patient's performance. The two most common instrumental assessment procedures for dysphagia, fluoroscopy and flexible laryngoscopy (FEES), are then described. Protocols are provided, and step-by-step administration and interpretation of the examinations detailed. Finally, the clinician is guided through methods for reporting the findings of the assessment.

I hope that readers will find this text useful as both an initial guide and as a continuous reference as they carry out the task of providing assessment services to dysphagic patients.

Acknowledgments

This book would not be possible without the constant and unfaltering patience of my loving wife Maureen, who, during much of the preparation of this text, was carrying the first human addition to our household. I would also like to apologize to the non-human members of the household, Eastern Margaret in particular, who missed many walks as a result of my attention to the text and my inattention to her needs. I would like to give special thanks to my mentor Susan Langmore for providing guidance and advice throughout my career and to all of the people, Barbara Higman, Stacy, Montana, and Jessie, who read my awful first drafts. Special acknowledgment is extended to Ken Schatz and Irene Balmer who provided the foundation for understanding the puzzling physiology and to Liz Callaway who continues to teach me the intricacies of assessment and proper patient care. Dorinda Jacob and other wonderful students, who in turn helped me learn to teach are thanked. Another special acknowlegement goes to Liza Dominguez, D.M.D., M.S., for her patient review of things dental and for the contributed figure. I thank Robert McClurkin and George Dellas at Kay Elemetrics and Nick Tsaclas at Pentax for supplying the excellent imaging equipment. To Dan Cutler (a real artist) for his honest appraisal and gentle critique of the figures I have created for this book. To Scott for his quick and professional response to requests for photographic and digital details. Special thanks go to Jay Rosenbek for providing his insight, great humor, and for the opportunity to write this text. To Marie Linvill and Kristen Banach, first for realizing the minutia of details of which I never could have conceived, and second for directing the execution of same. Without them this would be the book that never got done. And finally, given that I have been provided this unencumbered public forum for expression, I would like to thank my mother and father for their presumed (and cautiously suspected) unwavering faith and for their important (and very tangible) support during my shaky path from child to adult. For my child's sake, may I be half as patient and forgiving.

CHAPTER 1

Medical Record Review and Patient Interview

*"A good historian must know the physiologic bases
for symptoms in order to ask the proper questions."*
Anonymous

or

*"The best history taker is he who can best interpret
the answer to a leading question."*
Paul H. Wood (1907–1962)

INTRODUCTION

Without a well-developed history, the picture provided by clinical symptoms or even instrumental assessment often is not complete enough to make recommendations related to treatment. The initial patient interaction should include a session devoted to the gathering of information that will act as a guide for seeking out physical findings either clinically or instrumentally. The history-taking session should illuminate the patient as a dynamic entity, often with diverging components, and will shape the decision-making process and, ultimately, the outcome of intervention. To secure as complete a picture of the patient as possible, certain goals for the history-taking session must be constructed and examined. The goals are intended to assist in establishing priorities for the assessment process. They also will help us determine how the whole per-

son lives and compensates for the presence of the dysphagia.

Table 1–1 summarizes the goals of the history-taking session. At the close of the history-taking section, you should have achieved goals 1 through 3. Careful inspection and integration of the first three goals should yield a preliminary determination of the scope of the assessment.

THE INTERVIEW PROCESS

Achieving the goals of the interview portion of the assessment in an orderly fashion is highly desirable, but unlikely. In an ideal world, the patient, or the patient's designated informant, comes to the initial meeting with an armful of up-to-date records and well-developed, unambiguous clinical signs and symptoms. The cli-

Table 1–1. Goals of the history-taking session.

1. To determine if there is a swallowing problem and, if so, the nature and extent of the dysphagia.

2. To determine any causal factors that may contribute to the dysphagia.

3 To determine the patient's functional abilities and disabilities, with attention to adaptations and compensations that exist to make up for an impairment.

4. To provide a basis for determining the scope of the assessment.

nician dashes off questions from a finely honed checklist and the patient provides chronologically ordered, information-rich responses. In the real world, the historical data gathering session may be the least ordered of any patient contact. Quite often, patients will have an unclear picture of the assessment process or may deny the existence of a swallowing problem. Many patients may anticipate and fear an unfavorable outcome from the examination and withdraw in response to questions. Alternately, the patient can present the clinician with a great flood of information, much of it superfluous to the task at hand. At times the clinician and a well-meaning but unfocused patient or surrogate simply are not speaking the same language.

Example:

Clinician: "Could you tell me why you have come to see me today?"

Wife: "He can't get anything down."

Patient: "The food, it won't go down."

Clinician: "How long has this been going on?"

Patient: "About 2 months."

Clinician: "Have you lost any weight?"

Patient: "No."

Wife: "He could stand to lose some weight."

Clinician: "You haven't eaten anything in 2 months and yet you haven't lost any weight?"

Wife: "I didn't say he didn't eat, he eats all day, but he has trouble with it sticking in his throat, nothing goes down the way it should."

Patient: "It takes me all day."

SETTING UP THE INITIAL INTERVIEW

The interview process must begin before the patient actually enters the office. It is essential to have as clear a picture of the patient's problem as possible. Initiating the interview by discussing information gleaned from the permanent record will give the patient a positive signal that you knew something about the problem before he or she arrived.

MEDICAL RECORD REVIEW

Constructing the framework for understanding a patient's condition is much easier when one can rely on the works of others. Patients frequently will present with an accumulation of medical problems that have been examined and treated over a number of years—sometimes by a great number of health care professionals—before the onset of dysphagia. If the patient has been closely followed, the medical record can provide the clinician with a bounty of data that will enhance the initial interview.

Memory impairment or dementia can greatly affect the accuracy of information obtained during the interview and, even in the absence of these impairments, patient recall bias can substantially affect clinical assessment and diagnosis of chronic disease (Boyer et al., 1995). For this reason the medical record review is absolutely essential in gaining the "big picture" of the patient. The collection and filtering of what is sometimes a huge amount of information accumulated from previous writings can appear to be an overwhelming task, but an organized search should shorten the process significantly. The contents of a typical medical record are listed in Table 1–2.

The dysphagia clinician will attempt to narrow the focus while reviewing the medical record. Special consideration should be placed on gathering information regarding medical conditions that contribute to the presence of dysphagia, reviewing results of previous dysphagia assessments, and reviewing reports related to the physical condition of the patient (Table 1–3).

In addition to the items listed in Table 1–3, a well-maintained medical record would supply the clinician with some sense of how the patient either copes with or is disabled by a disease process. In particular, the clinician's review should focus on determining whether an impairment or grouping of impairments is present that has the potential to affect negatively the maintenance of hydration, nutrition, pulmonary status, or quality of life. Form 1–1 provides a sample data sheet for entry of pertinent medical information.

❶ DISEASE PROCESSES

Enter the patient's record of disease processes as gathered from the record review. Entry should be in the form of a brief list. Order the list from earliest record to latest. For reference, Table 1–4 provides a sample entry.

Discussion

The clinician should determine the disease process or combination of contributing factors that are related to the presence of the dysphagia. The course of recovery or progressive decline found in the diseases and surgical procedures linked to dysphagia will vary widely. Once a specific disease process has been identified, the clinician should attempt to determine the patient's position in the span of expected recovery or deterioration. Making this determination allows the clinician some latitude later in the assessment process when decisions regarding efficacious intervention arise.

Table 1–2. Contents of the medical record.

The patient's medical history

Findings from the physical examination performed by the physician

Reports of laboratory tests

Findings and conclusions from special examinations

Findings and diagnoses from consultants

The diagnoses from the responsible physician

Notes on treatment, including medication, surgical operations, and radiation

Progress notes by physicians, nurses, and other care specialists

Table 1–3. Narrowing the focus of the chart review.

Review reports that provide information regarding medical conditions that contribute to the presence of dysphagia

Review results of previous dysphagia assessments or treatments

Review reports that provide information related to the physical condition of the patient that may be affected by the presence of dysphagia

Medical History Data Sheet

❶ DISEASE PROCESSES

Diagnosis	Date Identified	Resolution
_____	_____	_____
_____	_____	_____
_____	_____	_____
_____	_____	_____

❷ SURGICAL PROCEDURES

Procedure	Date Performed	Resolution
_____	_____	_____
_____	_____	_____
_____	_____	_____
_____	_____	_____

❸ AIRWAY STATUS

A. Artificial Airway

Type	Duration
_____	_____

B. Ventilation

Type	Duration
_____	_____

❹ PULMONARY STATUS

A. Pneumonia

Date Identified	Course/Resolution
_____	_____

B. Radiographic Findings

Date Identified	Course/Resolution
_____	_____

❺ Nutrition

A. Oral Intake

% Oral _____

Diet type _____

Supplements _____

(continued)

B. 24-hour Diet Recall

Breakfast _____

Lunch _____

Dinner _____

Other _____

C. Enteral Intake

Route/type: _____

Current % Enteral _____

	Date 1	Date 2	Date 3	Date 4
Type	_____	_____	_____	_____
Start	_____	_____	_____	_____
Stop	_____	_____	_____	_____

D. Parenteral Nutrition

	Date 1	Date 2	Date 3	Date 4
Type	_____	_____	_____	_____
Start	_____	_____	_____	_____
Stop	_____	_____	_____	_____

E. Weight Change

Current weight _____

Usual weight _____

% weight change _____

Duration of change _____

Patient perception of change _____

F. Lab Values/Blood Parameters

	Date 1	Date 2	Date 3	Date 4
Albumin level	_____	_____	_____	_____

❻ **Hydration**

Hydration Measures

	Date 1	Date 2	Date 3	Date 4
A. Fluid in/out	_____	_____	_____	_____

	Date 1	Date 2	Date 3	Date 4
B. Lab Values				
C. Serum sodium	_____	_____	_____	_____
D. Serum Osmolality	_____	_____	_____	_____

Table 1–4. Example Entry: Disease processes.

Diagnosis	Date Identified	Resolution
Hypertension	9/89	Controlled by meds
COPD	2/75	Good control/inhalers until mid 80s now with O_2. Frequent exacerbations requiring hospitalization 4/87 recently 5/94 and 1/98. Now inpatient on ward

It is important to remember that identifying only the primary disease may not describe a patient's condition thoroughly. All components of the disease, including treatments such as radiation for tumor reduction, should be accounted for.

The following sections contain a limited listing of some of the more frequently encountered disease processes associated with dysphagia. A brief summary of the disease processes and some key characteristics of the associated dysphagia will be discussed.

Vascular Disorders

Regardless of cause or localization, a cerebrovascular accident (CVA) is sudden and the resulting onset of dysphagic symptoms that sometimes accompany the event is just as sudden. The rapid onset of dysphagia in this population often will trigger an emergent request for the assessment of swallowing function by the patient care team. Dysphagia with aspiration is common in the early period following acute stroke (Kidd, Lawson, Nesbitt, & MacMahon, 1993). The prevalence of dysphagia in patients with acute nonhemorrhagic stroke has been found to be 28% to 45% (Barer, 1989; Gordon, Hewer, & Wade, 1987; Odderson, Keaton, & McKenna, 1995). The acute period lasts approximately 6 weeks, during which time some function may return (Teasell, Bach, & McRae, 1994). Odderson, Keaton, and McKenna, (1995) found that 21% of patients with dysphagia during the acute period of stroke had normal swallow function at discharge. Barer (1989) found that 45% of his patients with initial poststroke dysphagia had a resolution of symptoms within 1 week.

Unresolved dysphagia in patients with stroke, on the other hand, is associated with a number of negative health outcomes, including chest infection, malnutrition, dehydration, and death (Gordon et al., 1987; Smithard, O'Neill, Parks, & Morris, 1996). Dysphagia also is associated with lower functional index scores on admission to an acute care unit (Odderson et al., 1995)

Imaging studies (computer assisted tomography or magnetic resonance imaging) of the brain or brain stem generally will determine the presence, site, and extent of a stroke or brain injury and will be recorded in the patient's medical record. Some research suggests that the localization of a stroke may cue the clinician to potential findings during the instrumental assessment. Robbins and Levin (1988), in a study of dysphagia in unilateral stroke patients, found that subjects with left CVA demonstrated more oral stage difficulties and displayed more difficulty in initiating coordinated movement than patients with right CVAs. In the left CVA group, the presence of oral or verbal apraxia was correlated with the severity of the dysphagia. Subjects with right CVAs more frequently appeared to demonstrate involvement of the pharyngeal stage of the swallow with reduced pharyngeal peristalsis and increased incidence of aspiration. In a later study, Robbins, Levin, Maser, Rosenbek, and Kempster (1993) looked at patients with first middle cerebral artery (MCA) stroke and found differences in the patterns of dysphagia that were related to the site of lesion. In this study, the patients in the right hemisphere subgroup demonstrated swallowing patterns characterized by higher incidence of laryngeal penetration and aspiration of liquid.

Hamdy and colleagues (1996) performed cortical mapping of the hemispheres of dysphagic and nondysphagic subjects. In their study, it was found that the muscles involved in swallowing appear to be bilaterally, but asymmetrically, represented on the precentral cortex and are independent of handedness. Further, it was found that dysphagic subjects had a much smaller area of pharyngeal representation on the intact hemisphere than the nondysphagic subjects did. The authors suggested that the production of dysphagia was a consequence of damage to the dominant hemisphere for swallowing motor output. Perhaps most interesting, it was observed that swallowing recovery was associated with an increase in the area of representation of pharyngeal motor output on the intact hemisphere and not on the affected hemisphere.

Daniels and colleagues (1998), hypothesized that focal lesions of the anterior insular cortex contribute to oral and pharyngeal dysmotility by disrupting connections to crucial cortical, subcortical, and brainstem sites associated with deglutition. In another study (Daniels & Foundas, 1997), it was suggested that a lesion in the anterior insula may reduce the magnitude of sensory input and increase the threshold for triggering a pharyngeal swallow resulting in a delay in the elicitation of the swallow.

It should be noted that some focal brainstem lesions may result in dysphagia as the only clinical presentation and are so small that they may not be detected via imaging studies such as MRI (Alberts, Bertels, & Dawson, 1990). In some cases, a rapid onset of dysphagia may not be observed if a number of small bilateral periventricular infarcts accumulate, in which cases, the dysphagia may be slowly progressive (Buchholz, 1994).

Degenerative Disorders

Parkinson's Disease. Multiple prepharyngeal, pharyngeal, and esophageal abnormalities are found in the majority of patients with Parkinson's disease (Leopold & Kagel, 1997). The severity of the dysphagia generally correlates well with the severity of the Parkinson's disease (Eadie & Tyrere, 1965; Edwards, Pfeiffer, Quigley, Hofman, & Balluff, 1991). In the later stages of the disease, virtually all patients have some form of pharyngeal or esophageal dysphagia (Kirshner, 1989). The time it takes to consume a meal may be prolonged greatly in a patient with advanced Parkinson's due to the synergistic effect of a prolonged oral stage and impaired pharyngeal and upper esophageal stages of the swallow (Born, Harned, Rikkers, Pfeiffer, & Quigley, 1996).

The timing of the assessment may be critical in the maintenance of independence of the patient with Parkinson's. Early assessment may identify an impairment in a timely manner and allow the clinician to advise the patient about the use of compensatory strategies that may prevent, or postpone, disability. Patients with Parkinson's disease may not report swallowing difficulties during the initial interview (Bird, Woodward, Gibson, Phyland, & Fonda,1994; Robbins, Logemann, & Kirshner, 1986).

Neuromuscular Disorders

Motor Neuron Disease. Gradual progression of symptoms over several months or even years is typical of patients with forms of motor neuron disease such as amyotrophic lateral sclerosis (ALS). In psuedobulbar forms of ALS, there may be a report of difficulty in voluntarily initiating a swallow, whereas reflexive swallowing may be triggered in the normal fashion. A general weakness and wasting of muscles is found in the bulbar forms of ALS. When the disease presents with dysphagia as the predominant complaint, a mixture of bulbar and pseudobulbar palsy often is found.

When comparing normals to patients with motor neuron disease (MND), Hughes and Wiles (1996) found that patients were significantly more likely than normal subjects to complain of a number of symptoms that lasted longer than 1 month. The most significant of these symptoms were the presence of coughing episodes when eating, problems with excessive saliva, "things going down the wrong way," and food sticking in the throat after swallowing. There also may be reports of more swallows per mouthful of food and more time needed to finish a meal.

Strand, Miller, Yorkston, and Hillel (1996) suggested that, as respiratory capacity and speech intelligibility decline in the patient with ALS, swallowing function also declines. Coughing when attempting to swallow thin liquids is an early complaint and is an indicator of a relentless progression of dysphagic symptoms that ultimately requires the placement of an enteral feeding tube and includes the eventual loss of ability to swallow oropharyngeal secretions.

Inflammatory Myopathy. Inclusion body myositis, polymyositis, dermatomyositis, and sarcoid myopathy are inflammatory myopathies that result in diffuse proximal muscle weakness. Patients generally will complain of limb impairment before dysphagia (Bucholtz, 1994); however, some patients with inflammatory myopathy will present with gradually progressive dysphagia as the only symptom (Shapiro, Martin, DeGirolami, & Goyal, 1996). These patients may complain of solid food sticking in the throat and multiple swallows to clear a bolus. They also may have altered their diets to compensate for their difficulties.

Neurological Side Effects Due to Medication

Some cases of dysphagia can result from medications administered to the patient during treatment. Medication can induce central nervous system or peripheral nervous system effects that result in oropharyngeal dysphagia.

In a review of iatrogenic dysphagia related to neurological dysfunction, Bucholz (1995) cited the frequent administration of sedatives to patients who are difficult to manage due to behavioral problems such as combativeness or agitation. The administration of sedatives produces lethargy and/or depressed sensorium. The clinician should review the dates of initiation of orders, or changes in dose, of CNS depressants such as hypnotic agents, anticonvulsants, antihistamines, neuroleptics, barbiturates, and other antiseizure medications. Patients with underlying neurologic disease and dysphagia are at a greater risk for exacerbation of dysphagia with the administration of sedatives or other CNS-depressant medications.

Movement disorders that can result from the administration of neuroleptics also used to treat the agitated behavior seen in some patients with neurological disorders can have a negative impact on posture and the coordination of the oral and pharyngeal stages of the swallow.

Peripheral nervous system side effects can include pharyngeal weakness from myopathies related to corticosteroids and L-tryptophan. Disturbances of salivation can be related to anticholinergic agents and lead to dry mouth (xerostomia). These changes can reduce the volume and increase the viscosity of the oropharyngeal secretions. Reduced bolus formation and changes in the patient's ability to initiate a swallow are typical of patients with xerostomia (Loesche et al., 1995).

Progressive Anatomic Change

Cervical Osteophytes. Anterior cervical osteophytes most often are seen in middle-aged and elderly males and can cause a slowly progressing dysphagia. Patients with cervical osteophytes usually complain of dysphagia with more difficulty swallowing solids than liquids. Often there is a concomitant history of arthritis and the patient may experience pain with lateral neck movements.

Zenker's Diverticulum. Zenker's diverticulum is a herniation or outpouching of tissue in the striated portion of the upper esophagus resulting from reduced upper esophageal sphincter opening with normal pharyngeal propulsion and bolus flow (Shaw et al., 1996).

Patients with documented Zenker's diverticulum may be referred for dysphagia assessment due to worsening symptoms or for recurrence of symptoms following pouch removal or myotomy. Previous radiograms or fluoroscopic studies should be examined for location and size of the defect.

❷ SURGICAL PROCEDURES

List surgical procedures in chronological order. List the date performed and resolution or chronicity of the principle problem leading to the surgery. See Table 1–5 for an example of an entry.

DISCUSSION

Dysphagia is frequently a side effect resulting from surgical procedures. Surgery also can be performed to enhance swallow function. Following is a short sampling of several surgical procedures, both causative and palliative, related to dysphagia.

Anterior Cervical Spine Surgery

Surgical treatment of degenerative diseases such as spondylosis, ossification of the poste-

Table 1–5. Example entry: Surgical procedures.

Procedure	Date Performed	Resolution
Colonectomy	2/93	Chemo and radiation, no recurrence
Tracheostomy	4/95	For vent support. Removed and closed 5/95
Carotid endarterectomy	2/98	CVA during procedure, ensuing dysphagia

rior longitudinal ligament, or traumatic fractures usually requires an anterior approach for access to the anterior aspect of the spinal cord and nerve roots (Herkowitz, Kurz, & Overholt, 1990). The dysphagia associated with this surgery can affect oral and pharyngeal biomechanics and present itself as transient or persistent in duration. Bucholz (1995), found persistent dysphagia in postoperative anterior cervical fusion patients. Fluoroscopic assessment demonstrated localized pharyngeal paresis near the level of the surgery that was speculated to be caused by mechanical disruption of motor innervation to the pharyngeal constrictor muscles, resulting in persistent dysphagia.

Carotid Endarterectomy

Cranial nerve damage following carotid endarterectomy has been reported in 5% to 50% of cases (Evans, Mendelowitz, Liapis, Wolfe, & Florence, 1982; Theodotou & Mahaley, 1985). Impairment can be so severe as to warrant feeding gastrostomy placement and tracheostomy (AbuRahma & Lim, 1996). Damage to the cranial nerves is thought to result from inclusion of the nerve in arterial clamps, diathermy burn in the vicinity of the nerve, and damage sustained from self-retaining retractors (Aldoori & Baird, 1988). Dysphonias of swift onset following the surgery likely will be noted in the medical record.

Esophageal Cancer Surgery

Pharyngeal dysphagia frequently follows esophagectomy (Bucholz, 1995; Hambraeus, Ekberg, & Fletcher, 1987). Damage to the recurrent laryngeal nerve (Heitmiller & Jones, 1991) or nerve fibers in the pharyngeal plexus (Bucholz, 1995) during resection contribute to the pharyngeal dysphagia. Mechanical tethering of the laryngeal complex following neck anastamosis and damage to the recurrent laryngeal nerve may combine and produce a synergistic effect that results in the frequently reported diffuse bilateral pharyngeal involvement seen immediately postsurgery in these patients.

Head and Neck Resection

Resection of the head and neck invariably will compromise swallow function. Discrete tissue resection and reconstruction often results in predictable difficulties in mastication and swallowing. Many surgical interventions will, however, involve adjacent anatomic structures and make it difficult to predict the nature and extent of deglutitive impairment.

Oral Cavity Surgery. Resection of the oral cavity will have obvious effects on oral stage function, and reconstruction may result in pharyngeal stage problems as well. Anterior tongue mobility is important in controlling the placement of the bolus during mastication of solid foods. Patients with resections that prevent oral manipulation of solids often resort to consuming foods that do not require mastication, such as purees and liquids, while maintaining adequate nutrition (Hirano et al., 1992). It is estimated that one third to one half of the mobile portion of the tongue may be removed before serious disability results.

When primary cancers of the tongue involve adjacent structures, disability may become more apparent after resection. Floor-of-mouth resection often accompanies partial glossectomy and the reconstructive process to repair the resulting defect can have variable effects on swallowing ability (McConnel, Mendelsohn, & Logemann, 1987). The use of tissue flaps to fill the missing floor of mouth results in the construction of a "dead space" of adynamic, insensate tissue in the oral cavity (Kronenberger & Meyers, 1994). Residue in the floor of the mouth following a swallow is a typical finding for these patients (Panchal, Potterton, Scanlon, & MacLean, 1996; Pauloski et al., 1993).

Total glossectomy will have predicted deleterious effects on the oral stage of the swallow. Significant portions of the suprahyoid musculature that provides laryngeal support and elevation during the swallow typically are removed (Kronenberger & Meyers, 1994), resulting in pharyngeal stage problems and, subsequently, increased risk for aspiration (Weber, Johnson, & Myers, 1993).

In a study conducted by Pauloski et al. (1994), it was determined that postsurgical swallowing function in oral cancer patients generally remains unchanged between 1 and 12 months postsurgery. This is important to remember when the oral cancer patient who is more than 1 year postsurgery presents with complaints of worsening dysphagia as recurrence of the cancer may be suspected.

Partial Laryngectomy. The supraglottic laryngectomy and hemilaryngectomy procedures preserve portions of the larynx and are intended to avoid a permanent tracheal stoma. The varied anatomic changes that occur as the result of these procedures invariably challenge the patient to protect the altered airway during deglutition. A temporary tracheostomy tube is placed during surgical healing, as is a nasogastric tube for nutritional support. Initiation of oral feeding is attempted postoperatively within 14 days (Kronenberger & Meyers, 1994).

Total Laryngectomy. The total laryngectomy procedure involves the complete removal of all laryngeal structures with a closing of the anterior wall of the hypopharynx, resulting in a complete and permanent separation of the airway and alimentary tract. Although this precludes lower airway aspiration of food, liquid, and oropharyngeal secretions, bolus propulsion from the oropharynx to the esophagus

and stomach remains a common difficulty. Reduced tongue propulsion and a narrowing of the neopharynx combine to inhibit the free transit of the bolus (McConnel, Mendelsohn, & Logemann, 1986). Nasogastric feeding tubes are placed immediately following surgery and oral intake trials are initiated within the first 1 to 4 weeks after surgery when post-surgical edema is somewhat reduced.

Radiotherapy

External beam radiation, in combination with chemotherapy, is widely employed as the primary treatment of head and neck cancers. Although often successful in achieving the desired effect of inhibiting the growth of cancer cells and preserving organ function, it has the unfortunate side effect of causing tissue fibrosis in the areas that are irradiated (Chandler, 1979). The larynx is at particularly high risk for an adverse response to high dose radiation due to the amount of poorly vascularized cartilage that makes up its framework (Berger, Freeman, Briant, Berry, & Noyek, 1984; McGuirt, 1997). Tissue fibrosis has been shown to contribute to the sluggish movement of anatomic structures. Specifically, reduced tongue base retraction and reduced laryngeal elevation during the swallow have been reported (Lazarus et al., 1996).

When radiation is used in concert with surgical procedures, the effects of fibrosis may be masked by the dysphagia resulting from reconstruction. Swallowing function may appear to degrade or improve during the postsurgical healing process as the positive effects of reduction in edema and increased muscle function are overcome or equalized by the negative effects of tissue fibrosis.

❸ AIRWAY STATUS

List the salient details and presence or absence of documented upper airway obstruction, artificial airways, and ventilatory support. A sample entry is provided in Table 1–6.

Discussion

Attention should be directed to information regarding the integrity of the upper airway and, in particular, the larynx. Protection of the lower airway from the entry of foreign objects,

Table 1–6. Example entry: Airway status.

Artificial Airway	Type	Duration
	#8 plastic, cuff inflated	placed 2-5-98

Ventilation Course

Patient placed on ventilator emergently after desaturation 2-1-98.
Oral endotracheal tube replaced with cuffed trach on 2-5-98.
Trial of vent weaning throughout this week. Pt. on blow by mask
for 2 hours per day.

food, liquid, gastric contents, and oropharyngeal secretions is the primary function of the larynx. This function of the laryngeal airway may be impaired due to anatomical changes such as tumor or edema or can result from surgery or trauma or from paresis due to neuromuscular disease, stroke, or brain injury.

Anatomic Changes

Because the left recurrent laryngeal nerve traverses lower into the viscera than does the pathway of the right recurrent laryngeal nerve, the chance of left recurrent laryngeal nerve paralysis is more likely in the postoperative cardiac patient. Outright severing of the nerve is possible during chest surgery, resulting in permanent damage and paralysis. Bruising may occur as a result of pressure applied during clamping and bracing which may present as a paralysis immediately postoperatively but resolve as the nerve heals. Compression of the recurrent laryngeal nerve can occur as a result of tumor development along its path. During the interview process, these patients may present with a severe dysphonia suggestive of inadequate adduction.

A. Artificial Airways

Artificial airways are established when the natural airway no longer can provide the body with an adequate means for exchanging gases (Table 1–7).

Although the establishment of an artificial airway generally is performed in an emergent fashion, there are instances of elective placement. The decision to extubate, decannulate, or generally reduce the degree of artificial airway intervention is made when the indications for the support are no longer present. De

Larminat, Montravers, Dureuil, and Desmonts (1995) found that patients with primary pulmonary problems but without neurological disease who had undergone endotracheal intubation for longer than 24 hours were more likely to demonstrate significantly greater latencies in the onset of the pharyngeal swallow when compared with nonintubated patients. The authors suggested that alterations in local sensory receptors related to mucosal inflammation secondary to the endotracheal intubation contributed to the swallowing delay. It was found that swallowing function had essentially normalized 2 days postextubation.

The synergistic interplay of acute sickness, associated weakness, edema, disruption of pharyngeal and laryngeal biomechanics, muscle atrophy, and confused proprioception following the introduction of an artificial airway has been well documented (Bonnano, 1971; Cameron, Reynolds, & Zuidema, 1973; Dettelbach, Gross, Mahlmann, & Eibling, 1995; Felman, Deal, & Urquhart 1966; Nash, 1988). The effect of an artificial airway on the biomechanics of the swallow will be discussed in greater detail in the following chapters. The clinician should record the type of artificial airway and variations in the use of peripheral devices.

The patient on ventilatory support is particularly susceptible to dehydration and malnutrition (Driver & Lebrun, 1980). The ventilated patient often is immobile and unable to communicate hunger or thirst and, as a result, may suffer from malnutrition, which in turn deleteriously affects breathing function. Malnourishment is associated with poor bacterial clearance from the lungs (Green, Jakab, Low, & Davis 1977) as well as lowered vital capacity, inspiratory flow, and ventilatory drives (Branson & Hurst 1988; Doekel, Zwillich, & Scoggin, 1978; Weissman et al., 1983; Zwillich,

Sahn, & Weil, 1977). When the nutritional status of malnourished ventilated patients improves, there is an improvement in respiratory function. Basilli and Deitel (1981) found that successful weaning from the ventilator was directly related to the nutritional status of the ventilated patient.

❹ PULMONARY STATUS

List the pertinent information relating pulmonary status in the space provided on Form 1–1. Also list the findings of radiographs and the date the radiograph was performed. See Table 1–8 for a sample entry.

Discussion

A. Pneumonia

Suspicion of aspiration pneumonia may be the trigger for the initial consult to assess swallow function. The diagnosis of aspiration pneumonia is not always a straightforward process and is dependent on a combination of clinical findings. The most common clinical findings in patients with pneumonia are cough, fever, abnormal and focal lung findings, tachycardia, and respiratory rates above 20 per minute (Niederman & Fein, 1991). Many investigators have found that fever and respiratory complaints are not always present and that as many as 40% of patients with pneumonia are afebrile (Venkatesan et al., 1990). The confusing clinical presentation is prevalent especially in the elderly population (Finkelstein, Petkun, Greedman, & Antopol, 1983). Even with the most sophisticated assessment using bronchoalveolar lavage and specimen culture (Fagon et al., 1990), it is difficult to tell aspiration pneumonia from community acquired or nosocomial pneumonias unrelated to events of aspiration. Some physicians will find it necessary to make a determination of aspiration pneumonia based upon the clinical history. Others may omit the moniker "aspiration" from the record.

The determination of aspiration pneumonia should include a suspicion of dysphagia or aspiration of gastric contents in the clinical history. The presence of a new infiltrate demonstrated via radiograph, elevated white blood cell count (12,000 or above), and a fever (oral temperature >100.5° F) are addi-

tional findings that give weight to the clinical impression of aspiration pneumonia.

A patient with a history of multiple aspiration pneumonias should be closely examined for risk factors other than aspiration. Patients who currently are smoking with chronic obstructive pulmonary disease (COPD) have a twofold risk for pneumonia hospitalization (Bently & Mylotte, 1991).

OTHER PULMONARY SEQUELAE. Other pulmonary sequelae to aspiration can be identified during the interview session. These may include upper/lower respiratory infection, ex-

Table 1–7. Indicators for the establishment of an artificial airway.

Relief of upper airway obstruction due to
  Soft tissue obstruction
  Neoplasm in upper airway
Lack of airway protective reflexes
  pharyngeal, laryngeal, tracheal and/or carinal reflexes inhibited or absent
Facilitation of suctioning
Support of ventilation

Table 1–8. Example entry: Pulmonary status.

Pneumonia

Date Identified	Course/Resolution
2-1-98	Pt. with elevated white blood count, fever, and sputum production. Broad spectrum antibiotics administered. Now on day 10 of antibiotics. Fever reduced, continues with sputum production.

Radiographic Findings

2-1-98	Consolidation in right middle and lower lobes.

acerbation of chronic upper or lower airway obstruction (COPD), and acute bronchitis.

B. Radiographs

The most common imaging procedure used to enhance the differential diagnosis of pneumonia is the plain chest film. This image is captured via X ray with the patient positioned in the posteroanterior and lateral projections while he or she suspends respiration, preferably at the point of full inspiration.

With the chest film, the radiologist is able to inspect the two basic areas of the lungs, namely, the proximal and terminal airways. The proximal airways such as the bronchi, bronchioles, and respiratory bronchioles act to conduct gases to the more distal tissues of the terminal airways. The terminal airways are active in the exchange of gases during respiration and include the respiratory bronchioles, alveolar ducts, and alveolar sacs.

The radiographic image is scanned by the radiologist for evidence of abnormal shadows in the terminal airways. A shadow, referred to as a "consolidation," suggests that fluid or solid material has replaced or displaced gases in that area of the lung. The most common cause of consolidation is the acute inflammation of tissue and resulting collection of exudate that is associated with pneumonia (Rubens, 1993).

For many years, it was believed that a right lower lobe consolidation was more likely to be related to an event of aspiration. It was thought that aspiration was more likely to occur along the right mainstem bronchi because of the relatively straighter course of conduction to the terminal airways. It now is thought that the site of consolidation is related to the patient's position at the moment of aspiration.

❺ NUTRITION

A. Oral Intake

Mark the information as indicated in the record if available in Table 1–9. During the face-to-face interview, a 24-hour diet recall should be elicited from the patient and recorded in this section.

Discussion

Measures of oral intake should include information related to the amount and consistencies of food that the patient typically prefers. The clinician should request a 24-hour diet recall during the interview process. In addition, the use of nutritional supplements should be explored: How often are they consumed? Do they function as supplements or do they make up the majority of calories consumed?

B. 24-Hour Dietary Recall

A dietary assessment can be performed by having the patient report the amount and types of foods consumed during the previous 24 hours. This generally will provide a representative sample of the patient's typical dietary intake in the absence of an acute illness with sudden onset.

The clinician will need to rely on the patient's ability to report accurately all of the foods consumed in the previous 24 hours. The accuracy of the report may be enhanced by

Table 1–9. Example entry: Oral intake.

Percentage Oral Diet	30%
Diet	Puree with liquids thickend to nectar
Supplements	Two 8-oz. formula pudding containers
24-hr Diet Recall: Breakfast	3-oz oatmeal with thick milk
Lunch	Nothing
Dinner	4-oz mashed potatoes/8-oz soup
Other	8-oz pudding

providing the patient with a variety of food containers, beverage containers and a ruler to assist in determining portion sizes (Yuhas, Boland, & Boland, 1989). Underreporting in recall records is attributed to memory limitations and the skill of the interviewer in probing for foods consumed (Buzzardet et al., 1996). Dubois and Boivin (1990) found that reading the completed 24-hour recall back to the patient prompted the report of additional items that were consumed, and that those additional items accounted for 28% of the total intake.

Enteral/Parenteral Intake

Determine if enteral or parenteral nutrition is presently being administered. Make note of intermittent use and record the dates when initiated and discontinued. See Table 1–10 for a sample entry.

C. Enteral Intake

Enteral feeding is a method of delivering nutrition directly to the gastrointestinal tract via a tube. It is initiated when a patient cannot consume an adequate amount of food orally. Indications for the initiation of enteral feedings are outlined in Table 1–11.

The most popular method for delivering enteral feedings is by introducing a tube either transnasally or through the wall of the abdomen with the distal tube placed in the stomach, jejunum, or duodenum. Entry via pharyngostomy or esophagostomy is used less frequently for enteral nutrition.

Nasogastric Tubes. Feeding NG tubes generally are used when the need for nutritional support is expected to be of a short duration. Feeding tubes are introduced transnasally and passed through the upper esophageal sphincter into the esophagus and terminate in either the stomach, duodenum, or jejunum. Nasogastric tubes also can be used to suction material from the GI tract following surgery or GI bleed. Because the tube generally is placed blindly without the assistance of fluorography, inadvertent placement within the tracheobronchial tree may occur.

Misplacement of the NG tube puts the patient at risk for pneumothorax and pneumonia. To determine the likelihood of misplacement, air is introduced into the tube via syringe and the stomach monitored via auscultation to grossly determine appropriate placement. The location of the distal end of the tube then is verified via radiograph and the tube is secured to the patient's nose with tape or, in extreme cases when the risk of self-extubation is high, with sutures.

NG tubes generally are not left in for periods longer than 5 to 6 weeks because of the amount of attention necessary for the maintenance of proper function. NG tubes tend to migrate after placement for a number of reasons. Patients inadvertently or intentionally pull on the tube, requiring replacement or repositioning. The smaller tubes also are more likely to clog after repeated use or when med-

Table 1–10. Example entry: enteral /Parenteral intake.

Enteral Intake

Route/type: PEG tube

Current % Enteral 75%

	Date 1	Date 2	Date 3	Date 4
Type	dobhoff	PEG		
Start	12/2/97	12/15/98		
Stop	12/17/97			

Parenteral Nutrition

	Date 1	Date 2	Date 3	Date 4
Type	TPN			
Start	11/8/97			
Stop	12/2/97			

Table 1-11. Indications for initiating enteral feedings.

Consistent aspiration of food or liquids

Oral and/ or pharyngeal weakness resulting in fatigue before adequate intake is achieved

Asthenia

Anorexia

Reduced consciousness or comatose state

Pharyngeal obstruction preventing oral intake

Obstruction of the esophagus

Obstruction of the stomach or lower gut

Malabsorption of food in the gastrointestinal tract

---

ications that have been passed through the tube have not been crushed adequately. If the tube is not cleared appropriately, it must be replaced. With each replacement, the patient must go through the discomfort of swallowing the tube and be subjected to additional radiographs. NG tubes also are considered by patients to be uncomfortable and visually unappealing.

Gastrostomy and Jejunostomy Tubes.

For longer term enteral feeding, gastrostomy tubes (G-tubes) or jejunostomy tubes (J-tubes) are considered more reliable (Kirkland, 1989). These tubes can be introduced through direct surgical procedures or through endoscopic placement. The percutaneous endoscopically placed feeding tube has become increasingly popular and can be placed in the stomach (PEG) or jejunum (PEJ).

The larger bore of these tubes allows more reliable delivery of crushed medications and a greater variety of nutritional preparations than the smaller bore NG tubes. Patients may choose to blenderize regular foodstuffs and pass them through the tube rather than using commercial formulas. Although they become clogged less frequently, gastrostomy and jejunostomy tubes do have complications. Skin breakdown and infection around the stoma are not uncommon, and tubes can become dislodged. A retracted feeding tube must be replaced within 16–24 hours to avoid closing of the stoma.

D. Parenteral Nutrition

Nutrition can be delivered directly to the bloodstream of a patient who does not have an intact gastrointestinal tract or is at risk for complications resulting from the placement of an enteral feeding tube. Nutrients are delivered directly to the circulating blood and bypass the alimentary tract and the first circulatory pass through the liver. Parenteral nutrition can meet the total nutritional needs of the patient (total parenteral nutrition—TPN), or can supplement tube or oral feeding. The site of entry of the nutritional solution is either a central venous site, such as the suclavian vein, or a peripheral vein.

Patients who are nutritionally maintained via TPN often have a difficult time during the transition to oral feeding (Lenssen, 1989). The high concentrations of glucose and amino acids in TPN solutions has been linked to depression of appetite (Hansen, DeSomery, Hagedorn, & Kanasy, 1977). Also, through disuse during TPN, the gastrointestinal system initially may not tolerate the introduction of food or formula; patients may experience nausea, vomiting delayed gastric emptying, or diarrhea during the transition to enteral or oral feeding. The length of time the patient was maintained on TPN feedings and any side effects during the transition to enteral or oral feeding should be examined and recorded in this section.

ANTHROPOMETRIC MEASURES

Anthropometric measures involve measurement of the body or specific body parts. There are a number of measures described in the literature that are used to monitor changes that reflect malnutrition. Measurements of tricep skinfolds and mid-upper arm muscle circumference have been used in the past with some success, but require very specific training to ensure reproducible results (Blackburn, Bistrian, & Maini, 1977). Other readily available measures usually are more useful to the clinician. The single most useful measure is the determination of changes in weight.

E. Weight Change

Record fluctuations in weight. Determine the change in weight by first obtaining current and usual weights. Calculating the percentage of change by using the equation provided in Table 1–12. If possible, the patient's perception of the weight loss should be elicited during the interview session. Acquire an actual weight on the day of the visit.

Table 1–13 provides a sample weight change entry.

Discussion: Weight Loss

Unintentional loss of weight is an indicator for depletion of nutritional stores. Social, psychological, medical, and age-related issues should be taken into account when exploring the genesis of weight loss.

Social Issues. Particular attention should be given to the frail, homebound elderly patients who are unlikely to initiate the process of accessing the support systems available in the community. An elderly patient with an early dementing process may find the process of obtaining assistance too baffling to penetrate. Alternately, some individuals may struggle heroically to maintain a sense of independence. It is wise never to assume that some other discipline has attended to the needs of the single elderly patient. The historical data intake may serve to reveal problems that would otherwise remain obscured.

Psychiatric Issues. Older persons are more likely to have a loss of weight when suffering from depression than younger patients (Fitten, Morley, Gross, Petry, & Cole, 1989). Morley and Silver (1995) determined that depression was the cause of weight loss in 35% of elderly outpatients.

Patients with dementia may forget to consume enough calories to maintain proper nutrition. Miller, Morley, Rubenstein, and Pietruszka (1991) found that 26% of underweight individuals demonstrated inappropriate attitudes toward eating. Some of these attitudes included "liking their stomach to be empty," feeling terrified of being overweight, feelings that food controlled their life, and avoidance of certain food additives.

Medical Causes. Weight loss can be due not only to inadequate food consumption, but also to a number of disease processes and even the therapies designed to control those diseases (Bidlack & Wang, 1995).

Movement Disorders. Elevated metabolic rate resulting from movement disorders such as Parkinsonism and tardive dyskinesias that increase muscular activity can lead to weight loss.

Medication. A great number of drugs can cause nausea and vomiting; drugs with these

Table 1–12. Weight change calculation.

$$\% \text{ Weight Change} = \frac{(\text{Usual weight} - \text{Actual weight})}{(\text{Usual weight})} \times 100$$

Table 1–13. Example entry: Weight change.

Current weight	165
Usual weight	198
Weight change	17%
Duration of change	Approx. 6 months
Patient's perception	Unpleasant food in nursing home. Avoids meals and supplements. Denies dysphagia.

side effects can compromise food intake, resulting in nutrient depletion and subsequent weight loss. Reviewing the medication list and enlisting the assistance of the prescribing physician or pharmacist may help in identifying the offending drug. A simple adjustment in dose may alleviate nausea, or an alternate drug may be available.

Patients with constipation may overuse laxatives, resulting in loss of nutrients due to malabsorption. This in turn leads to malnutrition and weight loss. Also, some bulk-forming preparations using dietary fiber can result in a decrease in appetite with an accompanying reduction in food consumption because of the feeling of fullness (Smith, 1995).

Injury/Surgery. When a body is traumatized as a result of an injury, surgery, or because of infection, a loss of body protein occurs (Ziegler, Szeszycki, Estivariz, Puckett, & Leader, 1996). The loss of body protein is directly related to an increase in the metabolic process triggered by the immune response. There is often a shift to the catabolic state following major surgeries. The patient with surgery to the gut such as gastrectomy likely will be required to remain NPO for several days following the operative procedure. This patient will experience a double jeopardy as the shift to the catabolic state coincides with a reduction of oral intake.

Cancer. A malignancy often affects a patient's intake of food negatively to the point where anorexia and weight loss are the warning sign leading to the original diagnosis (DeWys, 1977, 1979). Anorexia and cachexia are present in 50% of advanced cancer patients and in 80% of terminally ill cancer patients (Maltoni et al., 1997). Alterations in the patient's metabolic processes and in his or her nutritional intake can result from the cancer itself or from a combination of the malignancy and the treatment for the malignancy.

Cachexia and Asthenia. Cachexia is a condition that is characterized by a complex of symptoms and is considered to be different from simple starvation. The symptoms include anorexia, tissue wasting, weakness, impaired organ function, apathy, water and electrolyte imbalances, and decreased resistance to infection (DeWys,

1977). The genesis of cachexia-associated weight loss is linked to a combination of alterations in taste, food aversions, increased energy expenditure, and metabolic alterations (Giacosa, Frascia, Sukkar, & Roncella, 1996). Much of the change in metabolic function is linked to the changes caused by the tumor itself. Initially, the body produces an immune response to defend against the tumor. Cytokines are substances secreted by immune cells during the immune response and are intended to antagonize the tumor (Giacosa et al., 1996). When the immune response is unable to kill a rapidly growing tumor, the cytokines continue to be produced, causing widespread effects such as anorexia, metabolic abnormalities, and wasting syndrome. Cytokines such as cachectin (tumor necrosis factor-alpha), Interleukin-1, Interleukin-6, and Interferon have been shown to induce anorexia with resulting weight loss (Albrecht & Canada, 1996). Figure 1–1 illustrates the pathophysiology of cachexia.

Nausea and Vomiting. Nausea and vomiting also are observed frequently in the cancer patient undergoing chemotherapy or radio-

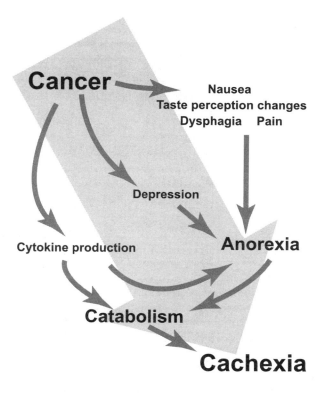

Figure 1–1. Pathophysiology of cachexia.

therapy and have a negative effect on food intake (Fainsinger et al., 1991; Lichter, 1996). Maltoni et al. (1997) identified a direct correlation between the weight loss, anorexia syndrome, and nausea. He further suggested that the presence of nausea had a greater impact on nutritional status and weight loss than the serum level of cytokines such as tumor necrosis factor-alpha and Interluken-6.

Asthenia. Asthenia is a term used to describe a state of reduced strength consisting of a complex of three symptoms: fatigue, mental fatigue, and weakness. Asthenia typically accompanies cachexia in patients with advanced cancer and is thought to be caused by the same metabolic abnormalities responsible for cachexia. When a patient is severely weakened, fatigue may set in before a meal is completely consumed, further reducing the amount of food and number of calories consumed.

Duration of Weight Loss. The temporal duration of the weight loss is especially important and is considered to have a great impact on the clinical course of the patient. The relationship between weight loss and temporal duration is summarized in Table 1–14. The patient's usual weight prior to the weight loss first should be determined. The percent-age of change then should be compared to the table to determine the severity level. Attention should be directed to distinguishing weight losses due to fluid loss associated with dehydration and malnutrition due to muscle wasting.

F. Lab Values/Blood Parameters

There are a number of measures derived from blood and urine that reflect the over all nutritional status of the individual. Nitrogen balance, blood-urea nitrogen, serum albumin, serum prealbumin, and serum transferrin all provide markers for protein energy malnutrition. The most commonly referenced and clinically useful measure is that of serum albumin. Protein energy malnutrition can be tracked over time. See Table 1–15 for an example entry.

Discussion

Albumin is a plasma protein produced by the liver when proteins are metabolized. Albumin is critical to the maintenance of fluid balance, blood pressure, and normal circulation. Serum albumin concentration is a direct indication of visceral protein stores and generally is a very

Table 1–14. Evaluation of weight change and nutritional status.

Nutritional Status	Mildly Compromised	Moderately Compromised	Severely Compromised
Time			
1 week		<2	≥2
1 month		<5	≥5
3 months		<7.5	≥7.5
6 months	<10	10–15	>15

Source: From *Nutrition status classification scheme.* Department of Veteran's Affairs VHA Handbook. (1994). Washington, DC: Veteran's Health Administration, Dietetic Service.

Table 1–15. Example entry: Lab values/blood parameters.

	Date 1	Date 2	Date 3	Date 4
	2/2/98	2/9/98	2/15/98	3/1/98
Albumin level	3.2	2.9	2.0	3.7

sensitive marker for malnutrition in the hypoalbuminemia and mixed marasmus state malnutrition syndromes. In healthy subjects, albumin concentrations in the blood are found at levels between 4.1 and 5.5. Patients in a recumbent position for an extended period of time will have serum albumin levels that are approximately 0.5 g/dl lower than levels for ambulatory patients. This difference is due to the effect of recumbency on the distribution of cellular fluids (Watts, Morris, Khan, & Polak, 1988). In patients with severe edema or liver failure serum, albumin levels may be inaccurate due to the extra fluids found in their system. Refer to Table 1–16 for serum standards.

EXPANDED DISCUSSION: NUTRITION

Often overlooked, particularly in the frail elderly, the most dramatic yet insidious sequelae of dysphagia is malnutrition. Very few severely malnourished patients are documented as such in the medical record (Burns & Jensen, 1996). When probing for signs of malnutrition, one study found that 47% of all stroke patients were malnourished when admitted to a rehabilitation service (Finestone, Greene-Finestone, Wilson, & Teasell, 1995). The proportion of acute stroke patients with malnourishment was found to increase as the hospitalization continued (Davalos et al., 1996). In this study, malnutrition was found in 16.3% of the patients on admission, 26.4% after the first week, and 35% after the second week. The authors also found that malnutrition was associated with higher frequency of respiratory and urinary tract infections, bedsores, increased length of stay, and greater mortality. In addition, patients with dysphagia had a sixfold increase in their risk for poor outcome. Malnutrition also has been found to be significantly related to increased length of stay in rehab settings (Finestone, Greene-Finestone, Wilson, & Teasell, 1996).

Metabolic Processes

Proper nutrition requires a constant replenishment of energy, structural materials, and regulatory substances. The transition from a well-nourished condition to malnourished one is caused by a disruption in the equilibrium of nutrient intake and other bodily needs. This balance is disrupted and malnourishment occurs if this need is not met when (1) the intake of nutrients is decreased, (2) the body requires a greater amount of nutrients, and (3) the body's utilization of the nutrients is altered (Jeejeebhoy, 1994).

The body expends energy at a rate of about 1,800 kilocalories/day. Glucose is the primary energy source for the much of the body. The maintenance of basic brain, blood, and muscle function requires 180 g of glucose a day. The brain alone metabolizes 100 to 150 g of glucose each day (Ferrendelli, 1974). Once new nutrients cease to be introduced to the patient via PO feeding or parenteral feeding, the body's nutritional stores are tapped to provide this energy. This process is referred to as the hypermetabolic response. In a well-nourished individual, glucose is produced by the anabolism, or synthesis, of carbohydrates in the liver. In the absence of new carbohydrates entering the digestive tract, the liver will attempt to produce glucose in a process known as gluconeogenesis. The body uses adipose tissue (fat tissue) as a source of glycerol and muscle tissue as a source of protein (amino acids). The glycerol and protein are synthesized in the liver to produce glucose, which is then used by the body for energy. When gluconeogenesis occurs, the body is no longer using an anabolic process to produce the energy necessary for survival and is considered to be in a catabolic state.

Protein is the primary solid matter of all muscles and organs and makes up a major portion of the bones, teeth, skin, nails, hair,

Table 1–16. Serum standards for nutrition assessment.

Severity	Normal	Mild	Moderate	Severe
Albumin (g/dl)	3.5–4.0	3.5–3.2	3.2–2.8	<2.8

blood, and serum (Robinson & Lawler, 1982). As protein becomes less plentiful, the body prioritizes its use and directs available protein stores to the tasks that are most likely to sustain life, specifically, maintaining brain and organ function. The use of protein for the repair of skin tissue becomes a low priority, and skin lesions, such as patchy dermatitis, are seen. Because of the redirection of protein, the malnourished postsurgical patient or patient with decubitis ulcers will experience greater difficulty in the healing of wounds.

As the stores of fat and protein continue to be tapped, body weight is reduced. In states of prolonged starvation, the metabolic rate and total energy expenditure decrease and are accompanied by decreased activity, increased sleep, and lowered body temperature. Muscle wasting may proceed to the point where the intercostal muscles are no longer able to function to sustain adequate gas exchange during respiration and the patient may die of respiratory failure.

Malnutrition Syndromes

Malnutrition, specifically protein-energy undernutrition, is divided into three types: Marasmus, Kwashiorkor, and mixed Marasmus Kwashiorkor (Fogt et al., 1995). The term "marasmus" is derived from the Greek term for "withering." Marasmus, or nonedematous protein energy malnutrition, results when a patient is unable to consume or biologically convert an adequate supply of calories. The body consumes muscle, fat, and glycogen for nutrition in the absence of new calories. Somatic protein (skeletal muscle) and adipose tissue are depleted, whereas visceral protein (protein contained in the blood and organs) remains intact. A "skin-and-bones" presentation typifies the marasmic patient as a result of muscle wasting. Marasmic patients frequently have 60% or less of their expected body weight. The skin is dry and does not display an elastic return in form when wrinkled. The hair may fall out and appear dry. The metabolism is slowed and body temperature is below normal. Common complications include acute gastroenteritis, dehydration, respiratory infections, and eye lesions (Torun & Chew, 1994).

"Kwashiorkor" is derived from the Ghanaian term for "the displaced child" and describes the malnourished condition of a child who has been weaned from the mother's breast milk upon the arrival of a new sibling. The weaned child typically will then consume a calorie-rich but protein-poor diet. An alternate term for this type of malnutrition is "hypoalbuminemia," a term that accurately describes a decrease in serum albumin concentrations associated with reduction in visceral protein stores. In hypoalbuminemia, somatic protein and adipose tissue remain intact. Body weight may be normal or even above normal due to swelling. The swelling is related to the depleted plasma albumin, which leads to reduced oncotic blood pressure. Plasma water is decreased as it accumulates in extracellular tissues, resulting in the characteristic edema of the hands, legs, feet, and abdomen associated with this condition (Torun & Chew, 1994).

In the third malnutrition syndrome, the patient is described as being in a "mixed marasmic kwashiorkor state." Edema of kwashiorkor and wasting of muscle in marasmus are observed. During early treatment the edema may subside, revealing the "skin-and-bones" presentation common to marasmic malnutrition.

⑥ HYDRATION

There are a number of ways to monitor dehydration, ranging from common blood lab values to the physical measurement of fluid input and output. An example of entries for fluid in/out and lab values related to hydration is provided in Table 1–17.

Discussion

A. Fluid In/Urine Out Monitor

This method simply compares the intake of fluids to the output of urine. Fluid intake and output in urine are generally equal. The normal output of urine (see Table 1–18) usually indicates that there is no active dehydrating process if renal and cardiac functions are normal. Fluid output less than 500 ml would indicate that the kidneys are not excreting enough fluid to expel the obligatory wastes and that a dehydrating process is occurring. Reduced output is likely due to reduced oral intake, again barring other complicating factors such as cardiac or renal problems.

Table 1–17. Example entry: Hydration measures.

Fluid In/out	Date 1	Date 2	Date 3	Date 4
	2-1-98	2-12-98		
	780/449	1000/650	____	____
Lab Values	**Date 1**	**Date 2**	**Date 3**	**Date 4**
Serum sodium	155mmol/L	141mmol/L	____	____
Serum Osmolality	320mmmol/kg	290 mmmol/kg	____	____

Table 1–18. Normal daily losses of water.

Source	ml of Loss
Feces	100–200
Urine	1000–1500
Lungs	250–400
Perspiration	400–10,000

Source: From *Normal and Therapeutic Nutrition,* by R. H. Robinson and M. R. Lawler (Eds.), 1982, 16th ed., p. 163, New York: Macmillan Publishing. Reprinted with permission.

Fluid intake can be altered for several reasons. Any patient with a precautionary diet restriction that excludes thin liquid intake should be monitored for dehydration. For instance, patients who require thickened liquids often reduce their intake of fluids if they find the consistency unappealing.

Incontinence in the elderly will reduce the accuracy of the liquid intake and urine output monitor. Urinary incontinence affects 5% to 10% of the noninstitutionalized elderly population and as many as 50% of the elderly in institutions (Williams & Pannill, 1982). At times, the elderly may restrict their fluid intake in an effort to decrease the frequency of urination or to reduce the possibility of incontinence, putting them at further risk for dehydration.

It often is presumed that the placement of a feeding tube alleviates a patient's nutrition and hydration needs. However, careful attention is not always paid to providing adequate nutrient solution, and free water may not be included as an adjunct to the nutrition regimen (Chernoff, 1995). Adding free water is especially important with high osmolality enteral feeding solutions.

B. Serum Sodium

Serum sodium levels are a measure of the amount of sodium in the bloodstream. As previously discussed, when water is not available to flush the system of excess sodium, the concentration of the serum increases and the dehydrating process begins.

C. Osmolality

Osmolality describes the concentration of particles in a solute. Serum osmolality levels are derived by determining the concentrations of sodium, urea and glucose in the blood serum. An increase in the number of particles in the solute relates to a reduction in the amount of water contributing to the weight of the serum (Table 1–19).

Water serves numerous critical functions in the body. Among its many functions, water carries both nutrients and waste through the body, gives form to the body's cells, and acts as the mediator of body temperature. Although it is impossible to identify one function as being more important than another, one very important function of water is that of regulating the complex distribution of solutions in the body. Of particular interest is the distribution of electrolytes in the blood solu-

Table 1–19. Dehydration types and lab values.

Lab Value	Hypertonic	Normal	Hypotonic
Serum sodium levels	>145 mmol/L	140 mmol/L	<135 mmol/L
Serum osmolality	>300 mmol/kg	285–295 mmol/kg	<280 mmol/kg

tion. Of those electrolytes, sodium will garner most of our attention as it makes up 90% of the positively charged electrolytes in the blood. It is an essential element for the control of fluid distribution in the body and also is essential in transmitting nerve and muscle impulses. For this reason, a sodium deficit results in muscle weakness.

Sodium and water concentrations in the blood are balanced by complex kidney and hormonal mechanisms, which generally are maintained in equilibrium in the healthy individual. As sodium levels rise, the body reacts by retaining enough fluid to distribute the sodium in the solution and maintain equilibrium.

As a rule of thumb, the daily intake of fluids must equal the total loss of fluids from the body during that day. The kidney is obliged to excrete approximately 600 ml of fluid, in normal circumstances, just to dissolve wastes. The kidney will excrete an additional 400–900 ml of fluid during the day, the amount of which is dependent on intake. Water also is flushed from the system in a number of other ways via the production of urine, water loss through the excretion of feces, through the lungs during respiration, and through perspiration, regardless of fluid intake. All of these obligatory losses of fluid account for an additional 750–11,000 ml of output.

When fluid intake is decreased, the blood solution becomes concentrated with electrolytes and other wastes. The kidneys are obligated to expel these wastes and obtain fluid for excretion from the body's stores. As body water is tapped, the serum concentration of the electrolytes increases, at which time dehydration and its associated problems occur. Some of the many effects of dehydration include hypotension, elevated body temperature, constipation, nausea, vomiting, and mucosal dryness (Chernoff, 1995). Dehydration increases the risk of mortality from infec-

tion and, if left untreated, the mortality risk may exceed 50% (Mahowald & Himmelstein, 1981).

There are a number of causes for dehydration. It is common following surgery due to fluid losses from vomiting, hemorrhage, diuresis, and fever. Confusion and dementia, depression, immobility due to restraints, and feeding dependence all contribute to dehydration (Weinberg & Minaker, 1995).

The elderly are particularly susceptible to dehydration for a number of reasons (Lavizzo-Mourey, Johnson, & Stolley, 1988). The elderly have a lower amount of total body water than the young and thus are more susceptible to rapid dehydration (Schoeller, 1989). In the elderly, there is a reduction in thirst perception resulting from a decrease in the number of osmoreceptors, cells that monitor the concentration of electrolytes in the blood. With reduced thirst perception, there is a predictable and well-documented reduction in the intake of fluids (Fish et al., 1985; Miller et al., 1982; Phillips et al., 1984). The institutionalized elderly are more likely to experience arthritis, paresis, and the placement of restraints, all of which reduce one's ability to freely obtain fluids. Table 1–20 outlines some of the risk factors associated with reduced fluid intake.

The contributing event or combination of events will define the specific variations of dehydration. *Isotonic dehydration* occurs when water and sodium are lost from the body at equal rates. This is seen in cases in which vomiting and diarrhea are present. Hypertonic dehydration occurs when the loss of water is greater than the loss of sodium from the body. This condition is known as *hypernatremia*. The most common cause of this type of dehydration is the presence of fever, which leaches water from the lungs (increased respiratory rate) and skin (increased perspiration). The patient with fever is less likely to initiate a

Table 1–20. Risk factors for reduced oral intake of fluids.

Risk Factor	Related Triggers
Confusion	Dementing process, reduced consciousness, fever, drug-induced changes to level of alertness
Restraints	Confusion, combativeness
Immobility	Paresis, coma
Reduced thirst	Decrease in osmotic receptors
Incontinence	Prostate surgery, dementia, advanced age
Liquid restrictions	Dysphagia, thin liquid restriction
Tube Feeding	Dysphagia, oral intubation, head and neck or gut surgery

search for fluids due either to incapacitation or altered mental status that further exacerbates the dehydration. When elderly nursing home residents with fever were screened for dehydration, it was found that 60% were dehydrated (Pals et al., 1995). In the same study, it was found that 41% of nursing home seniors with dehydration and fever were hypernatremic. *Hypotonic dehydration* occurs when sodium is lost from the body at a rate greater than the loss of water. This reduction in sodium is observed in patients who overuse diuretics.

CONSIDERATIONS FOR A SUCCESSFUL INTERVIEW

USE OF QUESTIONNAIRES AND SURROGATE INFORMANTS

Questionnaires

If you allow a patient to talk all day he will eventually tell you everything you need to know. Few of us, however, have a great deal of time to spend on history-taking. In an attempt to shorten the amount of patient contact time, many clinicians forego lengthy face-to-face question and answer sessions by utilizing a questionnaire. A good set of questions can be a time-saver in acquiring some important information but will not reliably provide the clinician with a well-developed or accurate historical record. The clinician and patient usually can share responsibility for inaccura-

cies found in both face-to-face questioning and self-completed questionnaires. Collen and colleagues (1969) demonstrated that there are significant inconsistencies in patient responses when the same question is asked a second time in an identical fashion on a subsequent visit. On the average, one of five patients answering "yes" to a question changes the answer to "no" on a second test. The data collector often will contribute to inaccuracies by interpreting the patients, responses to questions on the questionnaire and recording an entry that the interviewer feels more accurately reflects what the patient meant to say (Grossman, Barnett, McGuire, & Swedlow, 1971). To avoid these problems, the scope and purpose of an ordered list of questions for an interview or a self-administered questionnaire should be inspected closely prior to its use. If a questionnaire is to be employed, it is best used to provide information regarding age, gender, address, and phone numbers.

Surrogate Informants

A large number of patients presenting with dysphagia as the result of neurologic impairment will be unable to respond to the interviewer's questions due to receptive or expressive communication problems or cognitive deficits and may be accompanied by a surrogate. The surrogate's role in the interview may be to fill in the details not revealed by the patient or to act as the primary informant throughout the interview process. Surrogates have been found to provide high levels of agreement for questions related to medical history and demographics in patients with stroke, dementia, and Alzheimer's disease (Rocca et al., 1986; Weiss, Fletcher, Palmer, Nicholl, & Bulpitt, 1996). Surrogates may, at times, provide a greater amount of information than the patient would readily volunteer if he or she was able to communicate. With few exceptions, proxies were more likely than subjects to report the presence of a condition, symptom, or functional problem (Magaziner, Bassett, Hebel, & Gruber-Baldini, 1996).

CONDUCTING THE INTERVIEW

On arrival, secure a private, quiet area to review the patient's history. Many patients do not want to reveal their personal medical problems in a crowded waiting area or in the hallway outside of the radiology suite. The clinician should be armed with a writing implement and be ready to jot down information as it presents itself. It would be wise to have the data sheet present with the information already gleaned from the medical record.

A poorly conducted historical data collecting session can misdirect the entire assessment process before it begins. It is unwise to proceed with a lengthy set of "canned" questions once the verbal exchange of information is initiated with a patient. The patient may feel that the questions are unrelated to his or her health experience or that the interviewer is drawing inaccurate conclusions from short responses.

The professional conducting the interview often is guilty of limiting the amount of uninterrupted time the patient is allotted for expressing his or her concerns. The patient should be given the chance to complete a response once it is elicited. Bertakis, Roter, and Putnam (1991), found that patients were less satisfied with the initial interview when the interviewer dominated the session by controlling the conversation. Physicians were found to interrupt patients an average of 18 seconds into the patient's description of the presenting problem (Frankel & Beckman, 1989). By directing the conversation too closely, the clinician stands the chance of missing vital information. Starfield and colleagues (1981) reported that, following 50% of visits, the patient and physician were found not to agree on the main presenting problem. Allowing for open-ended conversation and using fewer leading and canned questions were associated with more accurate diagnoses. Furthermore, patients are likely to disclose a greater amount of biomedical and psychosocial information to an interviewer who demonstrates a positive affect during an interview (Levinson & Roter, 1993). Allowing the patient to set the pace of the historical data collection session by providing a loosely formed structure that allows for random entry of information likely will result in a greater volume of information and increased patient confidence.

PATIENT INTERVIEW RECORD

Enter, in a narrative form, the conversation as it develops (Form 1–2). Enter the information for each numbered item according to the guidelines listed in the discussion.

❶ Chief Complaint

Some patients may pursue services independently or may come to the initial interview with an incomplete consultation or medical record. In these cases, a completely open-ended question that allows the patient great latitude in his or her response (such as, "What brings you here?") is most appropriate. This will provide the clinician with a context for the visit that would otherwise have to be constructed, at times less accurately, during the interview process.

If you are a member of a consulting service, paint the picture of the consult for the patient. Refer to the originator of the request for the examination by name, refer to his specialty or service, and tell the patient why you were consulted. Verbally review the patient's history as you see it in a few short sentences. This provides the patient with the context for an appropriate exchange of information and gives him the chance to correct any errors that may have occurred in the consulting process.

Example.

"Mr. Smith, I understand from your records that you were diagnosed with Parkinson's disease back in 1988. Your chart indicates that you have been losing some weight these

Form 1–2.
Patient Interview Record

❶ Chief Complaint: _____

_____

_____

❷ Patient's Perception of Problem: _____

_____

_____

❸ Character of Complaint: _____

_____

_____

❹ Course of Complaint: _____

_____

_____

❺ Activities of Daily Living: _____

_____

_____

❻ Previous Treatment: _____

_____

_____

_____

_____

_____

_____

_____

_____

_____

last 6 months. Dr. Wellman from neurology is concerned about your ability to swallow food and liquid and has asked us to provide you with an assessment of how well you swallow."

With the context established, it is likely a good idea to hand the exchange of information over to the patient. The clinician may wish to open with the question, "When was the last time you were fully healthy?" This question probably will provide the clinician with more information than is necessary, but it also provides a temporal placement of the appearance of symptoms in relation to disease onset or formal identification. The clinician also should be attuned to any co-occurring health problems even if their effect on the presentation of dysphagic symptoms appears unrelated.

❷ Patient's Perception of Problem

At the close of the patient's response to the initial question, the patient can be asked the following, "Why do you think you are having this problem with swallowing?" The patient's response to this question can provide valuable information regarding his or her perception of the illness and may uncover any phobias or misconceptions related to the primary disease process.

You may get a sense of the patient's fund of knowledge and his or her ability to learn new material. The patient's ability or inability to attend to the interview process will have an obvious effect on your subsequent interactions and can alter dramatically the scope of the assessment. The alert clinician should be looking beyond the assessment process to the eventual recommendations that may come out of it.

Much of the success of any therapeutic intervention administered by a clinician following the assessment will depend on the patient's acceptance of the program. The patient's responses during the interview may illuminate his or her belief system, revealing a patient who may be willing and capable of going to great lengths to follow instructions and carry out the sometimes difficult proscriptions of the clinician. Another patient may reveal himself or herself as a passive agent to an unstoppable force with little will to participate in a vigorous rehabilitation program. Yet another patient may deny the entire process and regard the clinician and assessment process

with contempt. The clinician should try to determine what his or her swallowing difficulty means to the client. Is the patient attending an appointment simply to comply with the referring professional's wishes or is he or she truly concerned about the symptoms and/or underlying disease? Determining the patient's attitude may greatly affect the scope of the assessment and eventual outcome of intervention. Regardless of the patient profile, allowing the patient to express his or her concerns gives the clinician a headstart in planning the patient education process that will follow the assessment.

Direct Questioning

During the initial phase of the interview you have allowed the patient to set the pace of the interaction and have estimated the patient's sense of physical well-being and attitude toward his or her dysphagic symptoms. When the patient appears to have reached an appropriate level of comfort, more direct questioning can begin.

Restate Chief Complaint

Make note of the symptom or symptoms that are of most concern to the patient. Be sure to have noted the severity and duration of the symptoms. Restate them to the patient to be sure that you have the captured the chief complaint accurately.

> "For the last 3 months you have been coughing and choking on your coffee. In the last two weeks it has gotten worse and now you don't even try to drink it anymore."

It is natural at this point to begin developing inferences about the nature of the dysphagia. It is important that these inferences are not reflected in your questioning. During direct questioning, the clinician should avoid leading questions (questions that suggest answers), such as, "So the only time you cough or choke is when you are drinking thin liquids, isn't that right?" This not only suggests that the answer is correct but also requires the patient to respond in a yes/no fashion. Using a direct question that does not lead the patient to a response will allow the patient to respond more openly: "What else brings on this coughing and choking?"

Once a chief complaint has been determined, the clinician should attempt to identify its specific components by examining the course of the complaint and its characteristics.

❸ Character of Complaint

A careful review of the distinctive traits of the swallowing complaint or complaints should follow. The most dramatic symptoms probably will have been addressed earlier in the interview process, particularly if they include events of coughing and choking. Other events such as food coming out of one's nose (nasal regurgitation), food falling out of the mouth, or food returning to the mouth in its original form hours or days after being consumed (pharyngeal pocket or Zenker's diverticulum) may be events that are identified as the primary complaint. Characterizing the complaint by looking at the specific components helps to create the framework by which the clinical picture is formed.

Litvan, Sastry, and Sonies (1997), suggested that combinations of complaints in patients with progressive neuromuscular disease were more predictive of abnormal swallowing on an instrumental examination than individual complaints. Coughing or choking on swallowing exclusively with thin liquids is a strong indicator of laryngeal penetration of swallowed material. By itself, this complaint may indicate a poor coordination of airway protection and bolus propulsion often associated with pharyngeal delay. When combined with complaints of excessive saliva or mucus, one can infer that there is a weakness in the propulsion of secretions during spontaneous nonbolus swallows. See Table 1–21.

Consistency of Food Associated with Event

Once a specific component is identified, the clinician should attempt to determine if it is associated with specific food consistencies. The identification of consistency should be very specific. Many clinicians tend to divide food types into several subtypes according to viscosity and/or cohesive qualities. Viscosity is a term used to describe the property of a fluid or semifluid to resist flow. High viscosity fluids flow slowly (e.g., honey), low viscosity fluids flow quickly (e.g., water). Cohesion describes the ability of material to stick together uniformly and typically is used to describe properties of solids (e.g., celery) or semisolids (e.g., noodles). Typically, patients will not cre-

Table 1–21. Complaints and possible physiologic causes for the complaint.

Complaint	Possible Physiologic Substrata
Coughing and choking	Laryngeal penetration or aspiration
Food coming out of nose	Poor velar closure during swallow
Food falling from mouth	Poor lip seal/oral containment
Food stuck in throat after swallow	Weakened pharyngeal stage
Something stuck in throat (not food)	Globus (reflux)
Throat burns on swallow	Reflux
Food returns to mouth in original condition	Pharyngeal pocket/Zenker's diverticulum
Food spread throughout mouth	Poor oral bolus formation/propulsion

ate a similar stratification of food types without some sort of prompting. Further, some food types defy classification or may undergo a change in properties during oral preparation. A mixture of fresh fruits in the form of a fruit cocktail will, for instance, change from a solid consistency to a mixture of solids and thin liquids during mastication. The patient typically will need to describe or name the food type that induces the problem in question (e.g., mushroom soup). The clinician then can provide annotation indicating the appropriate descriptors for viscosity and cohesion. Identifying food cohesion and viscosity properties will assist in planning for the materials needed in the clinical and instrumental examinations.

Frequency and Timing of Occurrence

The frequency of the symptom should be determined. The frequency should be characterized with respect to the number of times the symptom occurs during the meal. If the symptom does not occur during each meal, the number of times it occurs over the course of a day, week, or month should be determined.

Fatigue associated with physical activity or medication may occur at a specific time each day and time the symptoms associated with the dysphagia may also appear at the same time. Patients with myasthenia gravis, Parkinson's disease, or ALS may perform well at the beginning of a meal but demonstrate more difficulty at the close as the cumulative effort of feeding takes its toll.

Odynophagia

If there is a complaint of odynophagia (pain on swallowing) the pain should be characterized as burning, sharp, dull, aching, gnawing, or throbbing. The patient should provide an exact location by pointing to the area that hurts. An exact description of the onset of the pain also should be obtained. Patients who are status post head and neck surgery may complain of pain with swallowing during the acute recovery period as surgical wounds heal. Sudden onset of odynophagia could indicate the presence of infection or recurrence of cancer. Patients who recently have been trached or orally intubated often complain of pain on

swallowing that may subside a few days after decannulation or extubation. The management of the pain should be described and a description of the treatment measures should be noted.

Globus

"Globus" is the Latin word for "ball." The term is used commonly to describe a sensation of a "lump in the throat." Feelings of globus have been linked to hypertrophy of the lingual tonsils, sinusitis, spondylitis with cervical osteophytes, and gastoesophageal reflux. In the case of reflux, globus may be caused by local irritation of pharyngeal mucosa from stomach acid refluxed into the pharynx or by referred sensation due to irritation of vagal afferents in the distal esophagus. Patients with reflux-related globus might feel that there is a lessening of the symptoms when eating, as the food and liquid sooth the inflamed mucosa. The success of this strategy is such that these patients actually gain weight as the disease progresses. Common complaints of patients with globus are listed in Table 1–22.

The exact location of the feeling of food "getting stuck" should be determined. A determination of food consistency and body position at the time of globus also should be made. The frequency of occurrence during a meal, the number of times during the day or week, and the duration and character of the sensation should be noted. Does it get better, worse, or stay the same during the meal?

❹ Course of Complaint

During the interview, you should be able to make a determination as to whether the dysphagia was progressive or rapid in onset. An exact month or season likely will not be identi-

Table 1–22. Globus patients' most common complaints.

Feeling of something stuck in the throat

Discomfort/irritation in the throat

"Want to swallow all the time"

---

fied in a slowly progressing dysphagia. If an exact date is not available, attempt to determine when it was first noticed. The patient may identify the time of onset to be the moment he or she became alarmed enough to seek medical attention. The patient may be able to relate subclinical signs or symptoms if asked directly, or he or she may be able to relate when the problems became noticeable to others.

Onset times can vary widely depending on the disease process. Some disease processes are predictable in their progression, while others may wax and wane as the disease is exacerbated or controlled. It also should be determined if the symptom was constant or intermittent. Dates of onset of exacerbations and the duration of those episodes should be closely compared to changes in medication, surgeries, disease diagnoses, or acute lifestyle changes, such as the death of a spouse.

❺ Activities of Daily Living

The historical record should include information describing the patient's ability to perform activities related to feeding and oral hygiene. The interplay of disease progression and simultaneous reduction in ability to perform activities of daily living are typical of the patient with progressive neurological diseases. As a disease progresses and motor function becomes more impaired, the ability to feed one's self or perform oral hygiene tasks will decline simultaneously. Langmore et al. (1998) demonstrated that being reliant on another for feeding and oral hygiene puts the neurologically impaired patient at a significantly greater risk for developing pneumonia. If the patient is not performing these tasks independently, every effort should be made to determine the manner and frequency of assistance given by the caregiver.

❻ Previous Treatment

Some patients will struggle with their dysphagia for some time before seeking treatment. Many patients will take a variety of measures in an attempt to alleviate the symptoms of dysphagia on their own or take advice from friends or family. Measures tried can range from over the counter medications to self invented maneuvers. A patient may try following solid food boluses with liquids to relieve a sensation of globus, or applying a peppermint ointment to his or her chest after a bout of coughing that followed an event of aspiration. Record the success or failure of these remedies. Patients often are surprisingly intuitive in their approaches to self-healing.

THE GRAPHIC TIMELINE

When patients present with multiple medical problems and multiple symptoms, it sometimes is difficult to parse out the important contributing factors. Creating a graphic visualization of the different disease processes using a timeline may help enhance one's understanding of a patient's condition.

In Figure 1–2, a 5-year timeline graphically represents the progression of Parkinsonism with co-occurring COPD and the accompanying symptoms, and events experienced by a patient. The starting point of the timeline coincides with the onset of signs, symptoms, and events. The timeline for each subcategory is seen to thicken as conditions progress or are exacerbated. The ADL timeline grows thinner as the ability to maintain self-care diminishes. The spikes or "bumps" in the timeline for COPD are in tandem with hospitalizations and procedures. The weight loss is gradual until the progression of Parkinson's and the accompanying dysphagia occur. The placement of the feeding tube precedes a weight gain and stabilization.

While reviewing the timeline, it appears that, as the disease progresses, the consumption of adequate nutrition probably became laborious and fatiguing. Weight loss may occur more rapidly in single elderly persons who find themselves without the ability to perform simple daily tasks such as purchasing and preparing the foods they find easiest to consume. Even with attentive family members, the degeneration of function can be dramatic when the ability to perform simple ADLs is compromised. Compounding medical problems hasten the decline and interventions such as tracheostomy and feeding tube placement assist in stabilizing the patient for a period of time before eventual further decline and death.

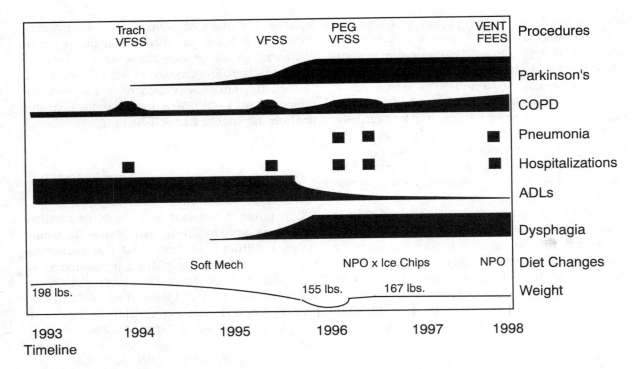

Figure 1–2. Graphic timeline.

SUMMARY

At this point we will review the goals of the history-taking session:

1. To determine if there is a swallowing problem and, if so, the nature and extent of the dysphagia.

2. To determine any causal factors that may contribute to the dysphagia.

3. To determine the patient's functional abilities and disabilities, with attention to adaptations and compensations that exist to make up for an impairment.

4. To provide a basis for determining the scope of the assessment.

A thorough medical record review and interview usually will yield enough information to achieve goals 1 through 3. Goal 4 sometimes is realized after the initial interview session. A patient may present with overwhelming signs and symptoms of dysphagia, or may have a well-developed history suggesting an instrumental examination. However, a clinical swallowing examination should always be performed, even in cases in which in-strumentation is obviously indicated. A properly performed clinical examination will allow for a more finely focused and efficient instrumental examination. The clinical examination protocol and guidelines follow in the next chapter.

REFERENCES

AbuRahma, A. F., & Lim, R. Y. (1996). Management of vagus nerve injury after carotid endarterectomy. *Surgery, 119,* 245–247.

Alberts, M. J., Bertels, C., & Dawson, D. V. (1990). An analysis of time of presentation after stroke. *Journal of the American Medical Association, 263,* 65–68.

Albrecht, J. T., & Canada, T. W. (1996). Cachexia and anorexia in malignancy. *Hematology/Oncology Clinics of North America, 10,* 791–800.

Aldoori, M. I., & Baird, R. N. (1988). Local neurological complication during carotid endarterectomy. *Journal of Cardiovascular Surgery (Torino), 29,* 432–436.

Barer, D. H. (1989). The natural history and functional consequences of dysphagia after themispheric stroke. *Journal of Neurology, Neurosurgery, and Psychiatry, 52,* 236–241.

Barer, D., Ebrahim, S., & Smith, C. (1984). Factors affecting day to day incidence of stroke in Nottingham. *British Medical Journal (Clin. Res. Ed.), 289,* 662.

Bassili, H. R., & Deitel, M. (1981). Effect of nutritional support on weaning patients off mechanical ventilators. *Journal of Parenteral and Enteral Nutrition, 5,* 161–163.

Bently, D. W., & Mylotte, J. M. (1991). Epidemiology of respiratory infections in the elderly. In M. S. Niederman (Ed.), *Respiratory infections in the elderly* (pp. 1–23). New York: Raven Press, Ltd.

Berger, G., Freeman, J. L., Briant, T. D., Berry, M., & Noyek, A. M. (1984). Late post radiation necrosis and fibrosis of the larynx. *Journal of Otolaryngology, 13,* 160–164.

Bertakis, K. D., Roter, D., & Putnam, S. M. (1991). The relationship of physician medical interview style to patient satisfaction. *Journal of Family Practice, 32,* 175–181.

Bird, M. R., Woodward, M. C., Gibson, E. M., Phyland, D. J., & Fonda, D. (1994) Asymptomatic swallowing disorders in elderly patients with Parkinson's disease: A description of findings on clinical examination and videofluoroscopy in sixteen patients. *Age and Ageing 23,* 251–254.

Blackburn, G. L., Bistrian, B. R., & Maini, B. S. (1977). Nutritional and metabolic assesssment of the hospitalized patient. *Journal of Parenteral and Enteral Nutrition, 1,* 11–22.

Bonanno, P. C. (1971). Swallowing dysfunction after tracheostomy. *Annals of Surgery, 174,* 29–33.

Born, L. J., Harned, R. H., Rikkers, L. F., Pfeiffer, R. F., & Quigley, E. M. (1996). Cricopharyngeal dysfunction in Parkinson's disease: Role in dysphagia and response to myotomy. *Movment Disorders, 11,* 53–58.

Boyer, G. S., Templin, D. W., Goring, W. P., Cornoni-Huntley, J. C., Everett, D. F., Lawrence, R. C., Heyse, S. P., & Bowler, A. (1995). Discrepancies between patient recall and the medical record: Potential impact on diagnosis and clinical assessment of chronic disease. *Archives of Internal Medicine, 155,* 1868–1872.

Branson, R. D., & Hurst, J. M. (1988). Nutrition and respiratory function: Food for thought [Editorial]. *Respiratory Care, 33,* 89.

Buchholz, D. W. (1994). Neurogenic dysphagia: What is the cause when the cause is not obvious? *Dysphagia, 9,* 245–255.

Buchholz, D. W. (1995). Oropharyngeal dysphagia due to iatrogenic neurological dysfunction. *Dysphagia, 10,* 248–254.

Burns, J. T., & Jensen, G. L. (1995). Malnutrition among geriatric patients admitted to medical and surgical services in a tertiary care hospital: Frequency, recognition, and associated disposition and reimbursement outcomes. *Nutrition, 11*(Suppl. 2), 245–249.

Buzzard, I. M., Faucett, C. L., Jeffery, R. W., McBane, L., McGovern, P., Baxter, J. S., Shapiro, A. C., Blackburn, G. L., Chlebowski, R. T., Elashoff, R. M., & Wynder, E. L. (1996). Monitoring dietary change in a low-fat diet intervention study: Advantages of using 24-hour dietary recalls vs. food records. *Journal of the American Dietetic Association, 96,* 574–579.

Cameron, J. L., Reynolds, J., & Zuidema, G. D. (1973). Aspiration in patients with tracheostomies. *Surgical Gynecology and Obstetrics, 136,* 68–70.

Chandler, J. R. (1979). Radiation fibrosis and necrosis of the larynx. *Annals of Otology, Rhinology, and Laryngology, 88,* 509–514.

Chernoff, R. (1995). Effects of age on nutrient requirements. *Clinics in Geriatric Medicine, 11*(4), 641–652.

Collen, M. F., Cutler, J. L., Siegelaub, A. B., et al. (1969). Reliability of a self-administered medical questionaire. *Archives of Internal Medicine, 123,* 664–681.

Daniels, S. K., Brailey, K., Priestly, D. H., Herrington, L. R., Weisberg, L. A., & Foundas, A. L. (1998). Aspiration in patients with acute stroke. *Archives of Physical Medicine and Rehabilitation, 79,* 14–19.

Daniels, S. K., & Foundas, A. L. (1997). The role of the insular cortex in dysphagia. *Dysphagia, 12,* 146–156.

Dary, I. J., Wilson, J. A., Harris, M. B., & Mac Dougall, G. (1995). Globus pharyngis: Development of a symptom assessment scale. *Journal of Psychosomatic Research, 39,* 203–213.

Davalos, A., Ricart, W., Gonzalez-Huix, F., Soler, S., Marrugat, J., Molins, A., Suner, R., & Genis, D. (1996). Effect of malnutrition after acute stroke on clinical outcome. *Stroke, 27*(6), 1028–1032.

de Larminat, V., Montravers, P., Dureuil, B., & Desmonts, J. M. (1995). Alteration in swallowing reflex after extubation in intensive care unit patients. *Critical Care in Medicine, 23,* 486–490.

Dettelbach, M. A., Gross, R. D., Mahlmann, J., & Eibling, D. E. (1995). Effect of the Passy-

Muir valve on aspiration in patients with tracheostomy. *Head and Neck, 17,* 297–300.

DeWys, W. D. (1977). Anorexia in cancer patients. *Cancer Research, 37*(7, Pt. 2), 2354–2358.

DeWys, W. D. (1979). Anorexia as a general effect of cancer. *Cancer, 43*(Suppl. 5), 2013–2019.

Doekel, R. C., Zwillich, C. W., Scoggin, C. H., et al. (1978). Clinical semi-starvation: Depression of the hypoxic ventilatory response. *New England Journal of Medicine, 295,* 358.

Driver, A. G., & Lebrun, M. (1980). Iatrogenic malnutrition in patients receiving ventilatory support. *Journal of the American Medical Association, 244,* 2195.

Eadie, M. J., & Tyrer, J. H. (1965). Alimentary disorders in Parkinsonism. *Australian Annals of Medicine, 165,* 13–22.

Edwards, L. L., Pfeiffer, R. F., Quigley, E. M., Hofman, R., & Balluff, M. (1991). Gastrointestinal symptoms in Parkinson's disease. *Movement Disorders, 6,* 151–156.

Evans, W. E., Mendelowitz, D. S., Liapis, C., Wolfe, V., & Florence, C. L. (1982). Motor speech deficit following carotid endarterectomy. *Annals of Surgery, 196,* 461–464.

Fagon, J. Y., Chastre, J., Trouillet, J-L, Domart, Y., Dombret, M. C., Bornet, M., & Gilbert, C. (1990). Characterization of distal bronchial microflora during acute exacerbations for chronic bronchitis. Use of protected specimen brush technique in 54 mechanically ventillated patients. *American Review of Respiratory Disease, 142,* 1004–1008.

Fainsinger, R., Miller, M. J., Bruera, E., Hanson, J., & Maceachern, T. (1991). Symptom control during the last week of life on a palliative care unit. *Journal of Palliative Care, 7,* 5–11.

Feldman, S. A., Deal, C. W., & Urquhart, W. (1966). Disturbance of swallowing after tracheostomy. *Lancet,* 954–955.

Ferrendelli, J. A. (1974). Cerebral utilizaton of non-glucose substrates and their effect in hypo-glycemia. In F. Plum (Ed.), *Brain dysfunction in metabolic disorders.* New York: Raven Press.

Finestone, H. M., Greene-Finestone, L. S., Wilson, E. S., & Teasell, R. W. (1995). Prolonged length of stay and reduced functional improvement rate in malnourished stroke rehabilitation patients. *Archives of Physical Medicine and Rehabilitation, 76,* 310–316.

Finestone, H. M., Greene-Finestone, L. S., Wilson, E. S., & Teasell, R. W. (1996). Length of stay and it's relation to malnutrition. *Archives of Physical Medicine and Rehabilitation, 77,* 340–345.

Finkelstein, M. S., Petkun, W. M., Greedman, M. L., & Antopol, S. C. (1983). Pneumococcal bacteremia in adults: Age-dependent differences in presentation and outcome. *Journal of American Geriatrics Society, 31,* 19–27.

Fitten, L. J., Morley, J. E., Gross, P. L., Petry, S. D., & Cole, K. D. (1989). Depression. *Journal of the American Geriatric Society, 37,* 459–472.

Frankel, R., & Beckman, H. (1989). Evaluating the patient's primary problem(s). In M. Steart & D. Roter (Eds.), *Communicating with medical patients* (pp. 86–98). Newbury Park, CA: Sage.

Giacosa, A., Frascia, F., Sukkar, S. G., & Roncella, S. (1996). Food intake and body composistion in cancer cachexia. *Nutrition, 12,* S20–S23.

Gordon, C., Hewer, R. L., & Wade, D. T. (1987). Dysphagia in acute stroke. *British Medical Journal (Clinical Research Edition), 295,* 411–414.

Green, G. M., Jakab, G. S., Low, R. B., & Davis, G. S. (1977). Defense mechanisms of the respiratory membrane. *American Review of Respiratory Disease, 115,* 479.

Grossman, J. H., Barnett, G. O., McGuire, M., & Swedlow, D. (1971). Evaluation of computer-aquired patient histories. *Journal of the American Medical Association, 215*(8).

Hambraeus, G. M., Ekberg, O., & Fletcher, R. (1987). Pharyngeal dysfunction after subtotal oesophagectomy. *Acta Radiologica, 28,* 409–413.

Hamdy, S., Aziz, Q., Rothwell, J. C., Singh, K. D., Barlow, J., Hughes, D. G., Tallis, R. C., & Thompson, D. G. (1996). The cortical topography of human swallowing musculature in health and disease. *Nature and Medicine, 2,* 1217–1224.

Heitmiller, R. F., & Jones, B. (1991). Transient diminished airway protection after transhiatal esophagectomy. *American Journal of Surgery, 162,* 442–446.

Herkowitz, H. N. (1988). A comparison of anterior cervical fusion, cervical laminectomy, and cervical laminoplasty for the surgical management of multiple level spondylotic radiculopathy. *Spine, 13*, 774–780.

Hughes, T. A., & Wiles, C. M. (1996). Palatal and pharyngeal reflexes in health and in motor neuron disease. *Journal of Neurology, Neurosurgery, and Psychiatry, 61*, 96–98.

Jeejeebhoy, K. N. (1994). Clinical and functional assessments. In R. S. Goodhart & N. M. M. E. Shils (Eds.), *Modern nutrition in health and disease* (6th ed., p. 805). Philadelphia: Lea & Febiger.

Kidd, D., Lawson, J., Nesbitt, R., & MacMahon, J. (1993). Aspiration in acute stroke: A clinical study with videofluoroscopy. *Quarterly Journal of Medicine, 86*, 825–829.

Kirkland, M. L. (1989). Enteral and parenteral access. In A. L. Skipper (Ed.), *Dietitian's handbook of enteral and parenteral nutrition* (pp. 263–277). Gaithersburg, MD: Aspen Publications.

Kirshner, H. S. (1989). Causes of neurogenic dysphagia. *Dysphagia, 3*, 184–188.

Kronenberger, M. B., & Meyers, A. D. (1994). Dysphagia following head and neck cancer surgery. *Dysphagia, 9*, 236–244.

Langmore, S. E., Terpenning, M. S., Schork, A., Chen, Y., Murray, J. T., Lopatin, D., & Loesche, W. J. (1998). Predictors of aspiration pneumonia: How important is dysphagia? *Dysphagia, 13*, 69–81.

Lavizzo-Mourney, R., Johnson, J., & Stolley, P. (1988). Risk factors for dehydration among elderly nursing home residents. *Journal of the American Geriatrics Society, 36*, 213–218.

Lazarus, C. L., Logemann, J. A., Pauloski, B. R., Colangelo, L. A., Kahrilas, P. J., Mittal, B. B., & Pierce, M. (1996). Swallowing disorders in head and neck cancer patients treated with radiotherapy and adjuvant chemotherapy. *Laryngoscope, 106*(9, Pt. 1), 1157–1166.

Lenssen, P. (1989). Monitoring and complications of patenteral nutrition. In A. L. Skipper (Ed.), *Dietitian's handbook of enteral and parenteral nutrition* (pp. 347–373). Aspen Publications.

Leopold, N. A., & Kagel, M. C. (1997). Laryngeal deglutition movement in Parkinson's disease. *Neurology, 48*, 373–376.

Levinson, W., & Roter, D. (1993). The effects of two continuing medical education programs on communication skills of practicing primary care physicians. *Journal of Internal General Medicine, 8*, 318–324.

Lichter, X. (1996). Nausea and vomiting in patients with cancer. *Hematology/ Oncology Clinics of North America, 10*, 207–220.

Litvan, I., Sastry, N., & Sonies, B. C. (1997). Characterizing swallowing abnormalities in progressive supranuclear palsy. *Neurology, 48*(6), 1654–1662.

Loesche, W. J., Bromberg, J., Terpenning, M. S., Bretz, W. A., Dominguez, B. L., Grossman, N. S., & Langmore, S. E. (1995). Xerostomia, xerogenic medications and food avoidances in selected geriatric groups. *Journal of the American Geriatrics Society, 43*, 401–407.

Magaziner, J., Bassett, S. S., Hebel, J. R., & Gruber-Baldini, A. (1996). Use of proxies to measure health and functional status in epidemiologic studies of community-dwelling women aged 65 years and older. *American Journal of Epidemiology, 143*, 283–292.

Mahowald, J. M., & Himmelstein, D. U. (1981). Infections in the nursing home. *Journal of the American Geriatrics Society, 35*, 796–805.

Maltoni, M., Fabbri, L., Nanni, O., Scarpi, E., Pezzi, L., Flamini, E., Riccobon, A., Derni, S., Pallotti, G., & Amadori, D. (1997). Serum levels of tumour necrosis factor alpha and other cytokines do not correlate with weight loss and anorexia in cancer patients. *Support Care Cancer, 5*, 130–135.

McConnel, F. M., Mendelsohn, M. S., & Logemann, J. A. (1986). Examination of swallowing after total laryngectomy using manofluorography. *Head and Neck Surgery, 9*, 3–12.

McConnel, F. M., Mendelsohn, M. S., & Logemann, J. A. (1987). Manofluorography of deglutition after supraglottic laryngectomy. *Head and Neck Surgery, 9*, 142–150.

McConnel, F. M., Pauloski, B. R., Logemann, J. A., Rademaker, A. W., Colangelo, L., Shedd, D., Carroll, W., Lewin, J., & Johnson, J. (1998). Functional results of primary closure vs. flaps in oropharyngeal reconstruction: A prospective study of speech and swallowing. *Archives of Otolaryngology— Head and Neck Surgery, 124*, 625–630.

McGuirt, W. F. (1997). Laryngeal radionecrosis versus recurrent cancer. *Otolaryngology Clinics of North America, 30*(2), 243–250.

Mercadante, S. (1996). Nutrition in cancer patients. *Support Care Cancer, 4*, 10–20.

Miller, D. K., Morley, J. E., Rubenstein, L. Z., & Pietruszka, F. M. (1991). Abnormal eating attitudes and body image in older undernourished individuals. *Journal of the American Geriatrics Society, 39,* 462–466.

Miller, P. D., Krebs, R. A., Neal, B. J. H., & McIntyre, D. O. (1982). Hypodipsia in geriatric patients. *American Journal of Medicine, 73,* 354–356.

Morley, J. E., & Silver, A. J. (1995). Nutritional issues in nursing home care. *Annals of Internal Medcine, 123,* 850–859.

Nash, M. (1988). Swallowing problems in the tracheostomized patient. *Otolaryngology Clinics of North America, 21,* 701–709.

Niederman, M. S., & Fein, A. M. (1991). *Community—Acquired pneumonia in the elderly: Respiratory infections in the elderly* (p. 45). New York: Raven Press.

Odderson, I. R., Keaton, J. C., & McKenna, B. S. (1995). Swallow management in patients on an acute stroke pathway: Quality is cost effective. *Archives of Physical Medicine and Rehabilitation, 76,* 1130–1133.

Pals, J. K., Weinberg, A. D., Beal, L. F., Levesque, P. G., Cunningham, T. J., & Minaker, K. L. (1995). Clinical triggers for detection of fever and dehydration, implications for long-term care nursing. *Journal of Gerontological Nursing, 21,* 13–19.

Panchal, J., Potterton, A. J., Scanlon, E., & McLean, N. R. (1996). An objective assessment of speech and swallowing following free flap reconstruction for oral cavity cancers. *British Journal of Plastic Surgery, 49,* 363–369.

Pauloski, B. R., Logemann, J. A., Rademaker, A. W., McConnel, F. M., Heiser, M. A., Cardinale, S., Shedd, D., Lewin, J., Baker, S. R., Graner, D., et al. (1993). Speech and swallowing function after anterior tongue and floor of mouth resection with distal flap reconstruction. *Journal of Speech and Hearing Research, 36,* 267–276.

Pauloski, B. R., Logemann, J. A., Rademaker, A. W., McConnel, F. M., Stein, D., Beery, Q., Johnson, J., Heiser, M. A., Cardinale, S., Shedd, D., et al. (1994). Speech and swallowing function after oral and oropharyngeal resections: One-year follow-up. *Head and Neck Surgery, 16,* 313–322.

Phillips, P. A., Roll, B. J., Ledingham, J. G., Forsling, M. L., Morton, J. J., Crowe, M. J., & Wollner, L. (1984). Reduced thirst after water deprivation in healthy elderly men. *New England Journal of Medicine, 311,* 753–759.

Robbins, J., & Levin, R. L. (1988). Swallowing after unilateral stroke of the cerebral cortex: Preliminary experience. *Dysphagia, 3,* 11–17.

Robbins, J., Levine, R. L., Maser, A., Rosenbek, J. C., & Kempster, G. B. (1993). Swallowing after unilateral stroke of the cerebral cortex. *Archives of Physical Medicine and Rehabilitation, 74,* 1295–1300.

Robbins, J. A., Logemann, J. A., & Kirshner, H. S. (1986). Swallowing and speech production in Parkinson's disease. *Annals of Neurology, 19,* 283–287.

Rocca, W. A., Fratiglioni, L., Bracco, L., Pedone, D., Groppi, C., & Schoenberg, B. S. (1986). The use of surrogate respondents to obtain questionnaire data in case-control studies of neurologic diseases. *Journal of Chronic Disease, 39,* 907–912.

Schoeller, D. A. (1989). Changes in total body water with age. *American Journal of Clinical Nutrition, 50,* 1176–1181.

Shapiro, J., Martin, S., DeGirolami, U., & Goyal, R. (1996). Inflammatory myopathy causing pharyngeal dysphagia: A new entity. *Annals of Otology, Rhinology and Laryngology, 105,* 331–335.

Shaw, D. W., Cook, I. J., Jamieson, G. G., Gabb, M., Simula, M. E., & Dent, J. (1996). Influence of surgery on deglutitive upper oesophageal sphincter mechanics in Zenker's diverticulum. *Gut, 38,* 806–811.

Smith, C. H. (1995). *Drug-food/food-drug interactions: Geriatric nutrition* (2nd ed.) New Yord: Raven Press, Ltd.

Smithard, D. G., O'Neill, P. A., Parks, C., & Morris, J. (1996). Complications and outcome after acute stroke. Does dysphagia matter? *Stroke, 27,* 1200–1204.

Starfield, B., Wray, C., Hess, K., Gross, R., Birk, P. S., & D'Lugoff, B. C. (1981). The influence of patient-practitioner agreement on ourcome of care. *American Journal of Public Health, 71,* 127–131.

Strand, E. A., Miller, R. M., Yorkston, K. M., & Hillel, A. D. (1996). Management of oral-pharyngeal dysphagia symptoms in amyotrophic lateral sclerosis. *Dysphagia, 11*(2), 129–139.

Teasell, R. W., Bach, D., & McRae, M. (1994). Prevalence and recovery of aspiration poststroke: A retrospective analysis. *Dysphagia, 9,* 35–39.

Theodotou, B., & Mahaley, M. S., Jr. (1985). Injury of the peripheral cranial nerves during carotid endarterectomy. *Stroke, 16,* 894–895.

Torun, B., & Chew, F. (1994). *Protein-energy malnutrition: Modern nutrition in health and disease* (Vol. 2, 8th ed., p. 951). Philadelphia: Lea & Febiger.

Venkatesan, P., Gladman, J., Mac Farlane, J. T., Bares, D., Berman, P., Kinnear, W., & Finch, R. G. (1990). A hospital study of community acquired pneumonia in the elderly. *Thorax, 45,* 254–258.

Watts, G. F., Morris, R. W., Khan, K., & Polak, A. (1988). Urinary albumin excretion in healthy adult subjects: Reference values and some factors affecting their interpretation. *Clin Chim Acta, 15(172),* 191–198.

Weber, P. C., Johnson, J. T., & Myers, E. N. (1993). Impact of bilateral neck dissection on recovery following supraglottic laryngectomy. *Archives of Otolaryngology—Head and Neck Surgery, 119,* 61–64.

Weissman, C., Askanazi, J., Rosenbaum, S., et al. (1983). Amino acids and respiration. *Annals of Internal Medicine, 98,* 41.

Williams, M. E., & Pannill III, F. C. (1982). Urinary incontinence in the elderly. *Annals of Internal Medicine, 97,* 895–907.

Yuhas, J. A., Bolland, J. E., & Bolland, T. W. (1989). The impact of training, food type, gender, and container size on the estimation of food portion sizes. *Journal of the American Dietetics Association, 89,* 1473–1477.

Ziegler, T. R., Szeszycki, E. E., Estivariz, C. F., Puckett, A. B., & Leader, L. M. (1996). Glutamine: From basic science to clinical applications. *Nutrition, 12(11–12 Suppl),* S68–S70.

Zwillich, C. W., Sahn, S. A., & Weil, J. V. (1977). Effects of hypermetabolism on ventilation and chemosensitivity. *Journal of Clinical Investigation, 60,* 900.

CHAPTER 2

The Clinical Swallowing Examination

"To blow and swallow at the same moment is not easy."

Plautus (254–184 B.C.)

The Clinical Swallowing Examination (CSE) allows a circumscribed exploration of a patient's muscle function, sensation, and airway protective functions. This direct inspection allows the clinician to develop a profile of health, disability, or probable risk for disability. Findings from the clinical examination are combined with information gathered during the historical data collection and interview session. At the close of the clinical swallowing examination, the clinician should be able to develop confidently a management program for the patient or determine the necessity of further instrumental assessment or sub-specialty referral.

Unlike the interview, the clinical examination should be executed in an orderly way so that a thorough examination is consistently performed. An ordered approach to the examination is proposed to the clinician in the form of the protocol presented in Form 2–1. This is a suggested progression that may be resequenced and either added to or subtracted from at the clinician's discretion and according to the needs of the patient population. The objective, administration/observation instructions, and scoring of each component of

the CSE protocol is described in detail in the first part of this chapter. The second part of this chapter provides expanded discussions of each component of the CSE.

THE CLINICAL SWALLOWING EXAMINATION PROTOCOL

The initial entries in the protocol will relate mental status, voice, and airway function. During the interview the attentive clinician will have had an opportunity to make a rudimentary determination of mental status, observe spontaneous speech patterns and judge phonatory quality. Following the assessment of the voice and airway comes the testing of motor and sensory systems and, finally, the presentation of food and liquid.

CSE 1. MENTAL STATUS

In this section the clinician observes the patient's behavior and applies the observed behaviors to a scale. Any number of scales can be used for the record. The notation should be

Form 2–1

Clinical Swallowing Evaluation Protocol Score Sheet

CSE 1. Mental Status:

Notes: _____

_____

_____

_____

CSE 2. Speech/Articulation

    A. Speech Intelligibility:

        100%   (Normal)   _____

        >50%   (Moderate)   _____

        35–50%   (Severe)   _____

        <35%   (Profound)   _____

    B. Rate:

        Accelerated   _____

        Normal   _____

        Slowed   _____

    C. Predominant Error: **Additional Notation:**

        Distortions   _____   _____

        Omissions   _____   _____

        Substitutions   _____   _____

CSE 3. Respiratory Function/Respiration

    A. Volitional Cough:

        1. Type of clearing maneuver:

            Cough   _____

            Forced expiration   _____

            Throat clearing   _____

            Hawking   _____

2. Production:

    Productive   _____

    Dry   _____

Additional notation: _____

3. Loudness:

Perception	Score
Normal	1
Weak/audible	2
Very weak/inaudible	3

Loudness Score: _____

B: Sustained Expiration While Counting:

Highest # Counted	Score
≥30:	1
20–29:	2
10–19:	3
≤9:	4

Counting Score: _____

C. Patient's Rating: *(Derived from interview)*

1. History of difficulty handling mucus/secretions

        no: 1

        yes: 2

2. Cough (patient rates as normal or weak/diminished in strength)

        normal: 1

        weak: 2

D. Index of Pulmonary Dysfunction*   **Summary Score:** _____

*Source: From Smeltzer, S. C., Skurnick, J. H., Troiano, R., Cook, S. D., Duran, W., & Lavietes, M. H. (1992). Respiratory function in multiple sclerosis. Utility of clinical assessment of respiratory muscle function. Chest: *Official Publication of the American College of Chest Physicians, 101,* 479–484.

(continued)

Form 2–1 *(continued).*

CSE 4. **Voice/Resonance**

    A. **Voice:**

        Normal   _____

        Hoarse   _____

        Hypophonic/breathy   _____

        Aphonic   _____

        Wet dysphonic   _____

      If yes to wet dysphonic:

        Spontaneously attempts to clear?   _____

        Clearing successful?   _____

    B. **Resonance:**

        Normal   _____

        Hypernasal   _____

CSE 5. **Positioning**

    A. **Habitual Body Position:**

        Sitting erect (normal)   _____

        Leaning with self support: Left   _____

                           Right   _____

        Supported by apparatus   _____

          Description: _____

                   _____

                   _____

        Reclined   _____

            If yes, degree reclined: _____

        Bedbound   _____

Alteration in positioning elicited?   Yes _____   No _____

    Describe _____

Independent positioning on instruction?   Yes _____   No _____

Ability to assist in positioning?   Yes _____   No _____

Describe: _____

_____

_____

B. Habitual Head Position:

Symmetrically supported (normal)   _____

Flexed (chin down)   _____

Extended (chin up)   _____

Lateralization   left _____   right _____

Rotation   left _____   right _____

Alteration in positioning elicited? (yes/no)

    Flexion   _____

    Extension   _____

    Lateralization   _____

    Rotation   _____

Independent positioning on instruction?   Yes _____   No _____

Ability to assist in positioning?   Yes _____   No _____

Describe: _____

CSE 6. Lip Sensation/Strength/Seal

A. Lip Sensation:

Upper right _____   left _____

Lower right _____   left _____

(continued)

Form 2–1 *(continued).*

    B. Lip Strength/Seal:

        Upper right _____   left _____

        Lower right _____   left _____

    C. Drooling:

        Upper right _____   left _____

        Lower right _____   left _____

    D. Habitual Oral Position

        Open _____

        Closed _____

    Awareness/notes: _____

CSE 7. Mouth Opening

    Normal _____

    Reduced _____

        Approximate size _____

        Draw shape of mouth and indicate dimensions.

CSE 8. Muscles of Mastication

    A. Masseter _____

        1. Palpation

        Normal _____

        Reduced: Left _____   Right _____

    B. Temporalis:

        1. Palpation

        Normal _____

        Reduced: Left _____   Right _____

2. Strength

      Normal   _____

      Reduced: Left   _____   Right _____

C. Pterygoids:

    1. Normal protrusion   _____

    2. Deviation on protrusion:

              Left   _____   Right _____

    3. Normal lateralization   _____

    4. Reduced lateralization:

              Left   _____   Right _____

D. Pain:

Notes: _____

_____

_____

CSE 9. Dentition/Periodontium

    A. Existing Dentition/Periodontium:

        None   _____

        Dentate   _____

        1. Maxillary arch
        (Figure 2–9)

Right quadrant   Left quadrant

        2. Mandibular arch
        (Figure 2–10)

Right quadrant   Left quadrant

Form 2–1 *(continued).*

Notes: _____

_____

_____

    B. Removable Prosthetics:

        1. Maxillary arch

            Complete denture _____

            Partial denture   _____

        2. Mandibular arch

            Complete denture _____

            Partial denture   _____

Notes: _____

_____

_____

CSE 10. Salivary Flow/Appearance of Oral Mucosa

    A. Salivary Flow:

        Normal   _____

        Hyposalivation   _____

    B. Appearance of Oral Mucousa:

Notes: _____

_____

CSE 11. Oral/Pharyngeal Sensation/Gag

    A. Oral/Pharyngeal Sensation

        1. Tongue

            Tip   Right _____   Left _____

            Blade   Right _____   Left _____

            Dorsum Right _____   Left _____

    2. Faucial pillar   Right _____   Left _____

    3. Posterior pharyngeal wall   Right _____   Left _____

B. Gag

    1. Lateral pharyngeal wall movement

        Bilateral/symmetrical   _____

        Unilateral   Right _____   Left _____

Notes: _____

_____

CSE 12. Tongue Movement/Strength

    A. Tongue observation

Notes: _____

_____

    B. Tongue maneuvers:

    1. Tongue protrusion:

        Normal   _____

        a. Atrophy   Right _____   Left _____

        b. Deviation   Right _____   Left _____

        c. Dyskinesia   _____

    2. Nasal respiration w/ puffed cheeks

        a. Normal _____   Altered   _____

Notes: _____

_____

    C. Tongue Strength:

    1. Superior/anterior

        Right   Normal _____   Weakened _____

        Left   Normal _____   Weakened _____

(continued)

Form 2–1 *(continued).*

    D. Tongue Range of Motion:

        1. Buccal sulcus

           a. Maxillary

                Normal   _____

                Altered   Right _____   Left_____

           b. Mandibular

                Normal   _____

                Altered   Right _____   Left_____

           c. Palate

                Normal   _____

                Altered   Right _____   Left_____

CSE 13. Velar Elevation

    Normal   _____

    Altered   Left _____   Right _____

Elicited Swallows

CSE 14. Volitional Swallows

    A. Laryngeal Elevation:

      Normal   _____

      Reduced   _____

      Absent   _____

Notes: _____

_____

CSE 15. Food and Liquid Swallows

Material					*Liquid*	
	Ice Chips	*Puree*	*Soft Solid*	*Solid*	*Thick*	*Thin*
A. Max Amount	_____	_____	_____	_____	_____	_____
B. Timing/Speed	_____	_____	_____	_____	_____	_____

Material	Ice Chips	Puree	Soft Solid	Solid	Liquid Thick	Liquid Thin
C. # of Swallows	_____	_____	_____	_____	_____	_____
D. Oral Sign	_____	_____	_____	_____	_____	_____
E. Airway Sign	_____	_____	_____	_____	_____	_____
F. Instrumentation	_____	_____	_____	_____	_____	_____
G. Intervention	_____	_____	_____	_____	_____	_____

Notes: _____

_____

_____

_____

entered as a short narrative with a reference to the scale used. A sample entry for mental status is found in Table 2–1.

Scoring Discussion: Mental Status

A functional swallow is certainly a minimum for the safe oral intake of food and liquid. There are, however, a number of skills that support and sustain oral hydration and nutrition. There is an interdependence between safe swallow function and cognitive and behavioral factors such as alertness, attention, memory, judgment, reasoning, orientation, and sequencing skill (Cherney & Halper, 1989; Logemann, 1990; Steele, Greenwood, Ens, Robertson, & Seidman-Carlson, 1997). In patients

Table 2–1. Scoring example for mental status.

CSE 1. Mental status:

Glasgow Coma Scale = 11. The patient is easily aroused and is responding to simple direct commands. The patient continues to self extract IV and feeding tube but is otherwise cooperative for short periods of time.

with head injuries, the frequency of swallowing disorders was found to decrease as patients' scores on the Level of Cognitive Function Scale (Hagen, Malkmus, & Durham, 1979) improved (Yorkston, Honsinger, Mitsuda, & Hammen, 1989).

When swallowing function is impaired, the implementation of compensatory strategies may be necessary to maintain self-feeding. The efficacy of teaching patients with reduced cognition to compensate for a swallowing impairment has not been determined. Clinicians have been found to bias treatment according to their perception of a patient's ability to respond to behavioral intervention. Bine, Frank, and McDade (1995) found that patients diagnosed as having Parkinson's disease with co-occurring dysphagia and dementia were more likely to receive tube feedings than non-demented dysphagic patients with Parkinson's. The clinician should attend to signs that reflect a patient's ability to sustain the activities necessary to independently maintain self-feeding or to learn new skills throughout the assessment process. The clinician's initial impression of the patient's mental status may change as the examination progresses. During the interview, dramatic improvements and/or visible languor with inattention may occur.

The clinician should note the patient's early performance and enter changes as the examination goes on. Any changes may mirror the patient's performance during mealtime or indicate the appropriate "rise time" for maximizing performance.

General Observations

During the interview, the clinician should be vigilant for indications of reduced mental function. Make note of indications in the solitary elderly that self-care might be compromised. Are the clothes clean or blotched with food particulate? Is there evidence of appropriate attention to cleanliness and hygiene? Although these signs could indicate the onset of a dementing process, they also could simply reflect the patient's personal "style." To avoid overzealous attention to subtle signs, it is good to look at the cumulative picture. Is the individual attending to the questions and answering appropriately or is there a "drift" during the session? Is the caretaker or spouse acting as a surrogate in the interview without invitation? This behavior may be a means of masking the patient's deficits or shielding the patient from the difficulties of the interview process. This behavior may be just a means for a knowing surrogate to expedite the interview process. Be sure to direct the interaction in a way that allows the patient to reveal deficits while maintaining personal dignity.

A continuum of consciousness is observed in the patient. This continuum is divided roughly by observations of the patients' spontaneous or elicited behavior in response to environmental stimuli. In the low end of the continuum is the comatose state. It may seem incongruent to list the various indicators for those patients in deep comas, as the profile does not intuitively indicate safe oral feeding. Many patients will wax and wane in coma states or require monitoring to determine readiness for assessment.

Many scales have been developed for measuring and monitoring mental status. The type of scale used may depend on the nature of the patient's impairment. The reader may use any scale that is found to be acceptable and reproducible. The Glasgow Coma Scale (Teasdale & Jennett, 1974) is a quickly administered standardized scale that measures observed and elicited behaviors in patients exhibiting various stages of consciousness. Scoring for the examination is made up of the cumulative marks recorded for three different behaviors: eye opening, verbal response, and motor response. The best response for each of these behaviors is recorded. The scores range from 3 (severe coma) to 15 (full awareness). The Ranchos Los Amigos Scale (Hagen et al., 1979) is used widely in many facilities for determining cognitive function in individuals with brain injury. This 8-level scale is administered quickly and can be used to monitor patients progress over time.

CSE 2. SPEECH/ARTICULATION

In this section, the clinician makes a gross determination of the precision of articulation, the rate of speech production, and the predominant errors observed in connected speech. The clinician will rely on the connected speech elicited from the individual during the interview for the speech sample. A scoring example is provided in Table 2–2.

Table 2–2. Example of scoring for speech and articulation.

Example 1. Patient with Parkinson's:

| **Distortion:** | ✕ | Patient with rapid burst of speech with diffuse multiple distortions. Imprecision at end of utterance greater than at beginning |

Example 2. Patient with glossectomy:

Distortion:	✕	Imprecise affricate production particularly /s/, /z /
Omission:	✕	/t/ /d/ in all positions
Substitution:	✕	/ŋ/ for /n/

Scoring Discussion

Speech Intelligibility

Audio recordings of the interview portion of the dysphagia evaluation are done rarely. For this reason, a thorough analysis of the individual's articulation via transcription and review is not only impossible but, in most settings, it also is completely impractical. A thorough assessment of a co-occurring speech problem likely will be indicated and pursued in those patients with poor intelligibility. This portion of the exam should be considered a screening of speech intelligibility for the purpose of uncovering signs of muscular weakness, imprecise motor movements, or possible structural insufficiency.

There is a longstanding recognition of the existence of co-occurring speech problems and dysphagia (Meader & Muyskens, 1950; Netsell, 1984; Shohara, 1932). Further, co-occurrence of dysarthria and dysphagia is common. In neurogenic dysphagic patients, Martin, Corlew, Celement, and Zablocki (1990) found a significant positive correlation between dysarthria and confirmed dysphagia as evidenced during videofluoroscopic examination.

Patients with resection of oral cancers also will demonstrate articulation problems. These articulation problems are due largely to reduced range of motion of the tongue due to surgical scarring or reduction in tissue mass of the tongue. The obvious effects of changes in oral morphology are reduced oral control during mastication and poor bolus positioning prior to the initiation of the pharyngeal phase of the swallow.

Rate

The clinician is again asked to make a rough estimation when judging speaking rate. Normal speaking rate and the slowed rates typical of hyperkinetic (spastic) dysarthrias will be easily identifiable. Spastic dysarthric patients will demonstrate longer mean syllable rates and longer inter- and intra-word pause times that are related to reduced neuromuscular efficiency (Linebaugh & Wolfe, 1984). This slowed rate is the result of slower and less precise movement of the articulators and contributes to reduced intelligibility.

Rate of speaking in hypokinetic dysarthric speakers may become increasingly fast during connected speech (festination), or there may be short rushes of speech separated by pauses (Ludlow & Bassich, 1984). These speech patterns are observed most typically in the patient with Parkinson's disease. Coates and Bakheit (1997) identified speech disturbances as the main predictors of dysphagia in patients with Parkinson's disease. The clinician should be cautious in identifying accelerated rates in patients with hypokinetic dysarthric speech. Several authors have shown that hypokinetic speakers often demonstrate overall speaking rates similar to or slower than normal controls. The listener may attend to the rapid short rushes of speech and not account for pauses in speech that are of greater length and/or placed at syntactically inappropriate locations in utterances (Hammen & Yorkston, 1996). The patient's speech often may be perceived as being rapid when intelligibility is poor.

Patients with amyotrophic lateral sclerosis (ALS) may have mixed flaccid/spastic dysarthria and may demonstrate a number of imprecisions in speech that contribute to reduced intelligibility. Turner, Tjaden, and Weismer (1995) found that lengthened vowel production in patients with ALS resulted in a slower rate of speech and was an important component of global estimate of speech intelligibility.

Predominant Error

Articulation errors generally are identified as substitutions, omissions or distortions. Dysarthric speakers are more likely to produce distortion errors during speech than substitutions or omissions. The dysarthric speaker will lose intelligibility due to impaired neuromuscular function that negatively affects the precision and speed of the movement of articulators. Likewise, the surgical patient will attempt to produce sounds as was done preoperatively but will be unable to accomplish the targeted physiological task due to reduced mobility or missing structures. This change results in predictable distortions and omissions (Panchal, Potterton, Scanlon, & McLean, 1996).

Additional notes as to what sounds likely are distorted or omitted may give the clinician some insight as to tongue function during mastication and bolus positioning tasks. For an expanded discussion of this component of the examination, see page 76.

CSE 3. RESPIRATORY FUNCTION/EXPIRATION

In this section, the respiratory system is assessed. The following items provide the clinician with an impression of the adequacy of the expiratory system. Some of the items will have been gleaned from the patient interview.

Volitional Cough

Instruction

Instruct the patient to put forth his best effort in producing a cough: "Take a breath and produce as great a cough as you possibly can."

Scoring

Characterize the cough or clearing maneuver according to the type of clearing maneuver that is performed and whether the maneuver is productive. An example scoring entry is found in Table 2–3.

Sustained Expiration While Counting

Instruction

"Inhale as deeply as possible and with a single breath count as high as you can."

Scoring

The score is derived from the number reached when the patient counts aloud on a single exhalation after maximum inspiratory effort.

Scoring Discussion

Volitional Cough

Type. There are a number of different behaviors that may be evoked when a subject is asked to cough. These behaviors all accomplish the mission of clearing material (sputum, oropharyngeal secretions, food particulate, etc.) out of the portions of the upper and lower airways where they are most effective (Figure 2–1).

Cough. Many patients will produce what is recognized as the familiar lung or tracheal/laryngeal cough. The features of this clearing maneuver include glottal closure with accompanying subglottic pressure rise and sudden glottal opening with audible pressure release.

Forced Expiration. Individuals with any form of paresis of the larynx that results in poor adduction of the vocal cords or patients with tracheostomy likely will produce a forced expiration. Some patients may be unable to coordinate glottic closure with expiration.

Throat Clearing. Patients with neuromuscular disease resulting in poor coordination of expiratory airflow may be able only to generate throat clearing. Patients with weakness and/or pain associated with thoracic or gut surgery also may substitute throat clearing for a full cough.

Hawking. Webster's *Third New International Dictionary* describes hawking as follows:

Hawk: To utter a harsh palatal or guttural sound in or as if in trying to clear the throat, an audible effort to force up phlegm from the throat.

In many parts of the United States, this behavior is referred to as "harking," a variation that likely is derived from "harkla," the Scandinavian term for the same behavior.

Production

A productive cough refers to the transport of material from the lower airways. Production also may indicate the effectiveness of the behavior (cough, throat clearing, etc.) in moving sputum, oropharyngeal secretions, or debris, if present, from the airway. If this material is expectorated or makes itself available for inspection via tracheostomy or suction device, take note of the volume, type, and appearance of the material produced. Does the material produced appear to be from the lungs or is it more likely oropharyngeal secretions? Is there food particulate in the material? Make notes in the area provided in this section. Auditory

Table 2–3. Example of scoring for volitional cough.

A. Volitional Cough

1. Type of clearing maneuver:

Cough   _____
Forced expiration   _×_
Throat clearing   _____
Hawking   _____

2. Production:

Productive   _×_
Dry   _____

Additional notation: The patient produces copious secretions via spontaneous forced expiration through the trach tube. Appears to be significantly fatigued after coughing.

3. Loudness:

Perception	Score
Normal	1
Weak/audible	2
Very weak/inaudible	3

Loudness Score: __2__

B. Sustained Expiration While Counting

Highest # counted	Score
≥=30:	1
20–29:	2
10–19:	3
≥=9:	4

Counting Score: __4__

C. Patient's Self-Rating: (Derived from interview)

1. History of difficulty handling mucus/secretions

no:	1
yes:	2

Secretion Self-rating: __2__

2. Cough (Patient rates as normal or weak/diminished in strength)

Normal:	1
Weak:	2

Cough Self-rating: __2__

D. Index of Pulmonary Dysfunction*

Summary Score: __10__

*Source: From Smeltzer, S. C., Skurnick, J. H., Troiano, R., Cook, S. D., Duran, W., & Lavietes, M. H. (1992). Respiratory function in multiple sclerosis. Utility of clinical assessment of respiratory muscle function. *Chest: Official Publication of the American College of Chest Physicians, 101,* 479–484.

cues may be present and should be noted. Is there a gurgle at the level of the larynx, indicative of oropharyngeal secretions? Do these sounds disappear after the clearing attempt? Make note of these auditory cues in the area provided.

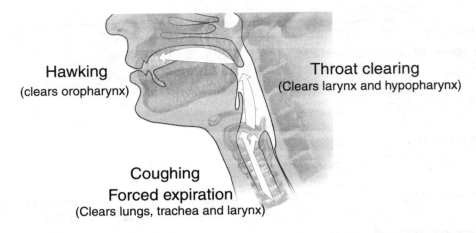

Figure 2–1. Different airway clearance behaviors will be effective in ejecting material from specific portions of the upper and lower airways.

Loudness

This auditory clue may give the clinician an idea of the expiratory force that is expended. Although loudness may not represent expiratory strength directly, it will provide the clinician with some perception of the power of the airstream produced during the behavior (Doherty, Wang, Donague, et al., 1997).

Sustained Expiration While Counting

There is much research relating to sustained speech task and respiration in dysarthric individuals (Clement & Twitchell, 1959; Hardy, 1964; Hixon, Putnam, & Sharp, 1983; Hixon & Hoit, 1984) and in normals (Netsell, Lotz, Peters, & Schulte, 1994). Poor performance on the task can be due to a number of factors other than weakened expiratory force. These factors could include poor initial inspiratory effort, poor laryngeal control during phonation, or reduced sustained attention, to name a few.

Index of Pulmonary Dysfunction

Smeltzer, Skurnick, Troiano, Cook, Duran, and Lavietes (1992) employed an index sensitive to pulmonary dysfunction (Medical Research Council, 1976) to predict poor maximal expiratory pressure, a key component in the production of an adequate cough. The index is comprised of clinical symptoms and signs that include "weakened cough" as rated by the examiner, the patient's ability to count on a single exhalation, and the patient's report of a weak cough and difficulty clearing pulmonary secretions. Smeltzer el al. (1992) demonstrated that observations regarding cough augmented with other clinical signs and symptoms provide an indicator for expiratory muscle strength. The possible range of scores is 4 (normal maximal expiratory pressure) to 11 (poor maximal expiratory pressure). No severity level was presented but, rather, the linear regression was very strong between the index score and the range of peak pressures measured. The Index has acceptable validity and reliability for use in clinical practice to identify those neurological patients with expiratory muscle weakness (Smeltzer, Lavietes, Troiano, & Cook, 1989).

For an expanded discussion of this component of the CSE protocol, see pages 76–77.

CSE 4. VOICE/RESONANCE

In this section, the clinician determines the presence or absence of dysphonia. If dysphonia is noted, a characterization of the dysphonia is recorded. The clinician will rely on the connected speech elicited from the individual during the interview as the voice sample. An example of scoring is found in Table 2–4.

Table 2–4. Example of scoring for voice and resonance.

A. Voice:

Normal	_____
Hoarse	_____
Hypophonic/Breathy	___×___
Aphonic	_____
Wet dysphonic	___×___

If yes to wet dysphonic:

Spontaneously attempts to clear?	No
Clearing successful?	Yes (when cued)

B. Resonance:

Normal	___×___
Hypernasal	_____

Scoring Discussion

Voice

Normal voice should display age- and gender-appropriate pitch, volume, and flexibility. The dysphonic voice shows an abnormality or combination of abnormalities in pitch, loudness, quality, or flexibility.

Hoarse. Voice is "hoarse" or harsh sounding. Loudness may be reduced. Pitch is low with little flexibility. This type of vocal quality is often referred to as "spastic dysphonia."

Wet Dysphonic. The voice sounds as if it is "percolating" through liquid. The percolating voice may be periodic, hoarse or hypophonic.

Hypophonic. Breathy quality. Intensity is low. Periodic vibration may vary from quiet voicing breaking to a whisper. This type of vocal qualities is often referred to as "flaccid dysphonia."

Aphonic. Consistent whisper-like voice.

Resonance

Hypernasality. The nasal cavity will resonate during vowel production. Oral plosives will be less distinct. Nasal emission of air may be audible during production of oral plosives and fricatives.

For an expanded discussion of this component of the CSE protocol, see pages 79–81.

CSE 5. POSITIONING

The clinician will observe the patient's habitual body and head position and examine the patient's adaptations or apparatus used to assist in support. The clinician then will attempt to elicit alterations in body and head positions. An example of scoring is found in Table 2–5.

Scoring Discussion

The scoring for the entries in this section is descriptive. Enter check marks for all of the items that apply in this section. Items that require more detailed notation are described below.

Body Positioning

Leaning with Self-Support. Patients with dense hemiplegia may lose support when attempting to feed themselves with the functional limb, resulting in a lean to the weakened side. These postures may not only directly increase the risk of aspiration but may make the process of self-feeding difficult and lead to fatigue before nourishment is achieved.

Supported by Apparatus. Note the device used for support. Is the patient belted into a wheelchair? Are cushions, wedges, or straps used to keep the patient upright? These devices may limit re-positioning during an instrumental examination and should be inspected closely for ease of manipulation should

Table 2–5. Example of scoring for positioning.

A. Habitual Body Position:

Sitting erect (normal)		_____
Leaning with self-support	Left	_____
	Right	___×___
Supported by apparatus		__yes__

Description: Chair with left lateral foam supports to keep patient from leaning to the left.

Reclined	_____
Degree	___90°___
Bedbound	_____

Alteration in positioning elicited?   Yes _____   No ___×___

If yes, describe: _____

Independent positioning on instruction?   Yes _____   No ___×___

Ability to assist in positioning?   Yes _____   No ___×___

Describe: Patient densely hemiplegic and with severe receptive aphasia

B. Habitual Head Position:

Symmetrically supported (normal)		_____		
Flexed (chin down)		___×___		
Extended (chin up)		_____		
Lateralization	left	___×___	right	_____
Rotation	left	_____	right	_____

Alteration in positioning elicited? (yes/no)

Flexion	_____
Extension	__no__
Lateralization	__no__
Rotation	__no__

Independent positioning on instruction?   Yes _____   No ___×___

Ability to assist in positioning?   Yes _____   No ___×___

Describe: *Severe left hemiplegia. Leans right to compensate. Head droops left. Dense receptive aphasia compromises ability to assist.*

the need arise. Care should be taken to ensure that the patient's safety and security are not compromised by changes in positioning.

Reclined. Patients may be placed in a wide variety of positions to accommodate the patient's needs by distributing weight to reduce pressure sores or to prevent contractures. Some positions, particularly reclined or semi-recumbent positions, at times will run counter to safe swallow recommendations. Determine the length of time the patient may be able to tolerate sitting upright. Is the window of time great enough to allow for con-

sumption of a full meal? Making these determinations during the clinical examination will allow the clinician to plan ahead for difficult position changes during the instrumental examination.

Head Positioning

Flexed. The individual habitually flexes the head downward. Note if there is a component of lateralization or rotation to the left or right.

Extension. The individual habitually extends the head upwards. Again note if there is a component of lateralization or rotation to the left or right.

Elicitation of Head Position Maneuvers

These maneuvers assume that the patient is starting from the habitual position. Request the patient to alter head position as necessary. Model the movement for those patients that require additional instruction. Make note of the patient's ability to perform these alterations. The patient may be able to perform some of the maneuvers fully while others may be problematic due to any number of conditions that may affect the range of motion of the cervical spine. Muscular weakness or fatigue also may play into the habitual position. Is the position sustained or of short duration? Examples of head positioning may be seen in Figures 2–2, 2–3, and 2–4. For an expanded discussion of this component of the CSE protocol, see pages 81–82.

CSE 6. LIP SENSATION/STRENGTH/ SEAL

The clinician will assess the sensation, strength, and range of motion of the lips. Equipment needed includes cotton tip applicators and a tongue blade. An example of scoring for this section is found in Table 2–6.

Scoring Discussion

Sensation

Use the cotton tipped applicator for this task. Ask the patient to close his or her eyes and respond either verbally or by raising a finger or hand in response to the stimulus. The stimulus consists of lightly touching the lip and lip margins with the cotton tip. The light touch should not be employed with enough pressure to dimple the surface of the skin but should, rather, be a very light, momentary brush over an area of 1–2 mm². As you move around the lips, randomly vary the rhythm of the stimulus. If no response to the initial stimulus is elicited, come back to the area and apply pressure great enough to dimple the skin. If there is no response to greater pressure, flip the cotton tipped applicator over and use the exposed wooden stick to apply the stimulus (see Figure 2–5).

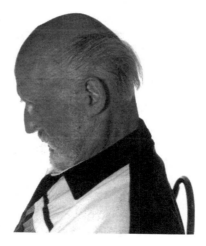

Figure 2–2. Head in flexing position.

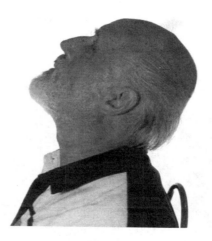

Figure 2–3. Head in extended position.

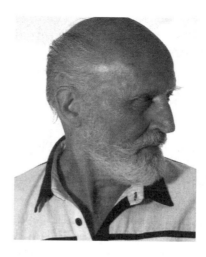

Figure 2–4. Head turned left.

Table 2–6. Example of scoring for lip sensation, strength, and seal.

A. Lip Sensation:

Upper   right ___1___   left ___3___

Lower   right ___1___   left ___3___

B. Lip Strength/Seal:

Upper   right ___1___   left ___2___

Lower   right ___1___   left ___2___

C. Drooling:

Left ___×___

Right _____

D. Habitual Oral Position:

Open ___×___

Closed _____

Awareness/notes: Patient with perpetual smile. Mouth rarely closed. Copious secretions stain clothes, appears completely unaware. Towel placed over left shoulder.

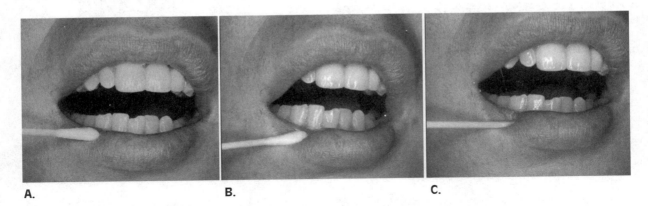

Figure 2–5. Lip sensation stimulus. **A.** Light brush. **B.** Light pressure with cotton tip **C.** Light pressure with stick.

Grade the patient's response by the area stimulated and the type of stimulus that elicited the response (Table 2–7). The vermillion of the middle of the lip may be more sensitive than the lateral vermillion (Rath & Essick, 1990; Wohlert & Smith, 1998). Attend to surgical sites affecting the lips and be sure to explore all areas thoroughly. Sensation may be impaired immediately postsurgery (Ono, Gunji, Tateshita, & Sanbe, 1997).

Lip Strength/Seal

Ask the patient to purse his or her lips with as much pressure as possible. Using the tongue blade, attempt to lift the upper lip up at several points along its entire length. Repeat with the lower lip, pushing down at several points. Patients often will place their lips between their teeth and use jaw-closing force to assist in the pursing pressure. To avoid this, have

Table 2–7. Scoring guide for sensation.

Stimulus	Score
Light brush with cotton tip	1
Light pressure with cotton tip	2
Light pressure with stick	3
No response	4

the patient smile first to insure that the teeth are placed together, then ask for them to purse their lips again. If this fails, have the patient pucker their lips, as if in preparation for delivery of a kiss. In this fashion, with the lips extended away from the teeth, continue with the assessment of strength.

If the lips are tender or a tongue blade is not readily available you may lift up on the skin above or below the margin of the lip and attempt to push the lip away from the opposing vermillion. If strength is in question, have the individual attempt to grasp the tongue blade between the lips on the left, right, and at midline with maximum effort. The patient with good lip seal should provide some resistance as the clinician attempts to pull the tongue blade away. If severe weakness or poor range of motion is present, the blade likely will droop from the lips or be easily extracted.

In a study using instrumentation, normal young individuals produced 17.6 kilo pascals (kPa) of pressure, with older individuals producing 12.6 kPa (Wohlert & Smith, 1998). Other research has described maximum lip pressure in newtons (Langmore & Lehmann, 1994) and in g/cm² (Chigira, Kazuhiko, Yoshiharu, & Yoshihiro, 1994). In the absence of pressure sensing instrumentation, such as strain gauge devices, an exact measurement of strength will not be possible. In an individual with normal strength it will be difficult to lift up or push down on the lip without the tongue blade bending under the strain. Table 2–8 provides a guide for scoring lip strength.

Do not attempt to lift or push too hard on the lip during this task. The objective of the task is to determine if enough strength is present to achieve a seal with the lips. The muscular effort used in achieving a lip seal is probably very much like the effort used during speech, in that it likely requires force levels well below maximum strength (Dworkin,

1980; Langmore & Lehman, 1994). Probing the lips with moderate pressure should give the clinician an idea as to where lip seal may break down (Figure 2–6).

Patients with a variety of neuromuscular diseases may present with unilateral or bilateral weakness of the obicularis oris complex of muscles that make up the oral sphincter. Patients with oral resections due to malignancy of the lip may have difficulty with range of motion of the reconstructed tissue. Radiation therapy also may cause fibrosis with reduced elasticity resulting in poor lip seal (Baker, 1983).

Drooling

Make note of any loss of control of saliva from the oral cavity. Note the site of release and the habitual oral position. Is the mouth open or closed? Does the patient appear aware of the drooling? Is there an attempt to clear the sputum away from the mouth or chin?

Drooling is associated with poor oral containment due to lip seal breakdown and a decrease in the frequency of swallowing which allows for the buildup of the oropharyngeal secretions (Sochaniwskyj, Koheil, Bablich, Milner, & Kenny, 1986). Drooling can be the cause of great social stigma. When poorly controlled, it can cause unpleasant odors and skin breakdown.

CSE 7. MOUTH OPENING

The clinician will assess the opening and closing of the mouth and associated physiologic movements that make up the components of mouth opening. Equipment needed includes tongue blades and gloves. An example of scoring for this section is found in Table 2–9.

Table 2–8. Lip strength scoring guide.

Response	Score
Normal strength (even resistance)	1
Weakness (lips separated with moderate pressure)	2
No apposition (lips do not touch when pursed)	3

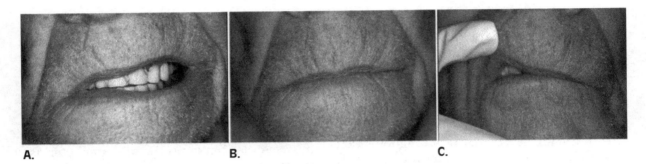

A.   B.   C.

Figure 2–6. A. Patient smiling, demonstrating right-sided weakness. **B.** Patient with lips pursed. **C.** Seal of lips is easily compromised with gentle lifting on right side.

Table 2–9. Example of scoring for mouth opening.

Normal	_____	
Reduced	✕	
Approximate size	1 cm	

Scoring Discussion

Mouth Opening

The patient is asked to open his mouth as widely as it will open. Note the symmetry and extent of opening. A normal adult should be able to achieve inter-incisal mouth opening distances of approximately 45–50 mm (Cox & Walker, 1997). Any reduction in size should be noted with attention to symmetry and shape of the opening. If the mouth is remarkably asymmetric, draw the basic shape of the open mouth on the illustration provided on the scoring sheet.

Mouth opening is the result of contraction of the lateral and medial pterygoid muscles, as well as the suprahyoid muscles (anterior belly of the digastric, mylohyoid and geniohyoid). All of the motor innervation for these muscles is supplied by the trigeminal nerve.

The clinician may want to palpate the commisure of the lips to assess the elasticity of the tissue in patients with resection of the lips or buccal tissue. Scar tissue or post-irradiation fibrosis can lead to reduced elasticity with resultant smaller opening of the mouth. Patients status post-mandibular surgery or surgery involving the suprahyoid muscles may present with reduced mouth opening.

Patients with small mouth openings may have great difficulty placing even small volumes of food in their mouths. The amount of time and effort needed to take in enough food to maintain nutrition may lead these patients to abandon oral solid foods in favor of liquid diets that are easily consumed by straw.

CSE 8. MUSCLES OF MASTICATION

The clinician will assess the muscles associated with mastication. Equipment needed includes tongue blades, gloves and gauss pads. A scoring example for this section is found in Table 2–10.

Scoring Discussion

Masseter and Temporalis

The masseter and temporalis act to move the mandible to a closing position (Figure 2–7). With the jaw muscles relaxed, ask the patient to clench down on a tongue blade placed along the length of the molars on the right or left side of the oral cavity. In edentulous patients, use a length of gauss pad to avoid lacerating the gums with the tongue blade. Palpate the muscle to determine tone and mass. A noticeable bulging and firmness should be present during the clench for both the temporalis and masseter. Pull on the blade to determine the strength of clench. The blade should not be easily removed from the patient's clenched jaws in normal strength. Ask the patient to relax the clench and repeat on the opposite side. The motor supply is innervated by the masseteric nerve, which emerges from the mandibular division of the trigeminal nerve.

Lateral and Medial Pterygoid

Protrusion. Place one hand behind the patient's head for stabilization. Place the base of the palm of your other hand against the chin. Apply pressure against the jaw as the patient protrudes the mandible. Patients with weakness will offer no effective protrusion against resistance. Remove your hands and observe the patient's ability to protrude the mandible without resistance.

Lateralization. Place one hand on the patient's temple and use the opposite hand to apply resistive pressure to the lateral mandible. A person with normal strength should be able to overcome the resistance and lateralize the mandible. In the absence of lateralization under pressure, remove your hands and observe the patient's lateral movement without resistance.

Table 2–10. Example of scoring for the muscles of mastication.

A. Masseter:
1. Palpation
   Normal _____
   Reduced   Left __×__   Right _____

B. Temporalis:
1. Palpation
   Normal _____
   Reduced   Left _×_   Right ___
2. Strength
   Normal _____
   Reduced   Left _×_   Right ___

C. Pterygoids:
1. Normal Protrusion _____
2. Deviation on Protrusion   Left___   Right _×_
3. Normal Lateralization _____
4. Reduced Lateralization   Left_×_   Right ___

D. Pain:

Notes: The patient complains of pain during chewing and talking. The pain is localized to the left TMJ area. Unable to fully open mouth greater than .5 cm. Due to sharp pain on left side. Currently eating only puree and liquid to avoid chewing.

Open   **Closed**

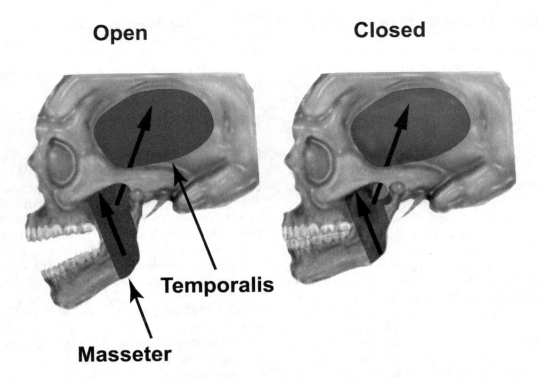

Temporalis

Masseter

Figure 2–7. Contraction of the temporalis and masseter act to move the mandible to a closed position.

The pterygoid is not as easily palpated as the masseter and temporalis muscles. The clinician must infer function from observable movements. The lateral pterygoid pulls the jaw laterally (Figure 2-8A). Contraction of the right lateral pterygoid pulls the jaw to the left side and vice versa. The medial and lateral pterygoids act together to move the mandible forward resulting in the protrusion of the jaw (Figure 2–8B). Motor innervation is supplied by the lateral pterygoid nerve and medial pterygoid nerve which emerge from the mandibular division of trigeminal nerve.

Protrusion and lateralization are essential movements for the grinding of food. These movements also are essential for contributing to changes in the shape of the oral cavity during manipulation of a bolus by the tongue. Weakness of these structures can impair chewing efficiency and lead to poor reduction of solid foods during oral preparation. This can in turn lead to fatigue during feeding and eventually food avoidance (Gilbert, Duncan, Heft, Dolan, & Vogel, 1997; Gilbert, Foerster, & Duncan, 1998; Hildebrandt, Dominguez, Schork, & Loesche, 1997; Locker, 1997).

Pain

Complaints of pain during any of these tasks could be an indicator of temporomandibular joint (TMJ) impairment. The TMJ is an unusual joint that articulates with both hinge-like and gliding motions. Probe the patient for information regarding the location and nature of the pain. Make note of whether the pain is unilateral or bilateral, localized to the TMJ or the muscles of mastication. When joint dysfunction occurs "popping" or "clicking" sounds may accompany jaw opening or closing. These sounds can be verified by using a stethoscope to auscultate the joint. The patient also should be asked about "grating" or "grinding" sounds in the joint as these could be signs of degenerative joint disease (Dierks, 1991). Previous trauma to the face or jaw and any previous treatment for the trauma should be recorded. The clinician also should be alert for any manifestations of oral habits that can be observed such as grating or grinding of the teeth (bruxism).

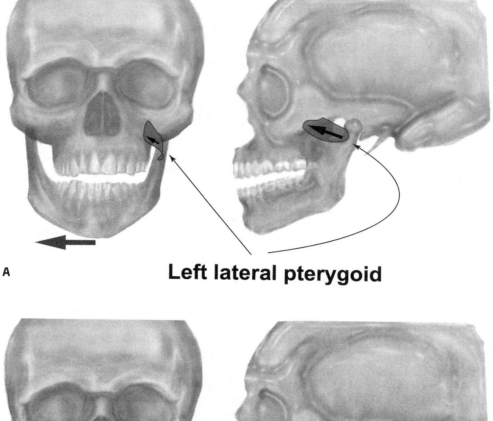

Left lateral pterygoid

A

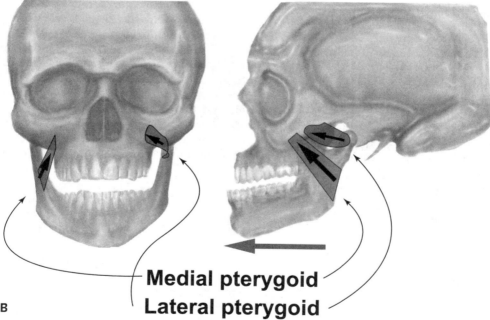

Medial pterygoid
Lateral pterygoid

B

Figure 2–8. A. Contraction of the left lateral pterygoid lateralizes the mandible to the right side. **B.** Contraction of the lateral and medial pterygoid muscles pull the mandible forward.

Pain from TMJ impairment can radiate to the head and muscles of mastication. This radiation of pain is representative of a syndrome known as myofascial pain-dysfunction syndrome or MPD (Laskin, 1969). Pain in the muscles of mastication has been shown to cause functional adaptations to the process of mastication. A reduction in the mean opening and closing velocities of the mandible have been found to be significantly reduced, and the distance of the jaw movement during chewing also is significantly smaller during pain (Svensson, Arndt-Nielsen, & Houe, 1996). This slowing and reduction in amplitude may have a negative effect on the efficiency of feeding, putting the patient at risk of fatigue and food avoidance. Symptoms of TMJ dysfunction are summarized in Table 2–11.

A complete workup of TMJ dysfunction should include consultation with an otolaryngologist and radiographic imaging studies of the temporomandibular joint and surrounding structures.

CSE 9. DENTITION/PERIODONTIUM

The clinician will assess the patient's dentition, prosthetic dentition, and gingiva. The equipment needed includes a pen light, gloves and a tongue depressor. A scoring example is provided in Table 2–12, which includes Figures 2–9 and 2–10.

Scoring Discussion

Existing Dentition

The tooth chart provided in the protocol is oriented to emulate the arrangement of the teeth while looking into the patient's open mouth. Using the pen light and tongue blade, inspect the oral cavity. Make note of the existing teeth and those that may be missing. Figure 2-11 shows normal teeth and periodontium.

Indicate missing dentition by placing an X over the appropriate tooth on the chart. Make note of the presence or absence of functional units (teeth or dentures on opposite arches that oppose one another and in tandem are employed in grinding food). Indicate the condition of the existing dentition by describing with notation and arrows any indication of decay or fractures. Telltale signs of decay are a greyish discoloration on the crown or root

surface of the tooth. Although discoloration may not always indicate decay, it may be an indicator for poor oral hygiene.

Additional attention should be directed to the buildup of plaque or calculus on the teeth and gums. Calculus is hardened plaque that has become mineralized. Calculus can adhere to tooth surfaces close to the gingiva and cause inflammation, which is a major contributor to the development of periodontal disease. Calculus is generally covered with plaque and can be located above or below the gingival margin.

The periodontium describes the structures that attach the tooth to the alveolar bone and is made up of the gingiva, periodontal ligaments, root cementum and alveolar bone. The gingival margin protects the subgingival area where the periodontal ligaments attach to the alveolar bone. The healthy gingival margin should form a band of tissue around the tooth. The interdental gingiva forms a papillae that fills the space between the roots of the teeth. Healthy gingiva should be pink and well vascularized.

The condition of the periodontium is reflected in the appearance of the gingiva and/or in the looseness or migration of the teeth. Patients who complain of loose teeth combined with an "itching" sensation or pain of the gums that is relieved by applying pressure, likely are experiencing a breakdown of the periodontium. Visual signs of poor health of the periodontium are erythema and/or bleeding of the gingival margin and gingival recession. The area likely to be first effected by the encroachment of plaque and calculus is the interdental gingiva. This may be the area of initial gingival recession and may be accompanied by inflammation. In the severely affected periodontium, the tissue of the gingiva may turn blue due to poor blood flow and the tissue may appear ulcerated and enlarged or be severely recessed to show the root of the tooth. Indicate the areas of concern

Table 2–11. Symptoms/signs relevant to TMJ dysfunction.

1. Pain during mastication
2. "Locking" or "sticking" of the jaw during opening or closing
3. "Clicking" or "popping" noises during mastication or jaw opening or closing
4. Pain of muscles of mastication radiating to head
5. Previous trauma to mandible or head
6. Report of or observation of bruxism
7. Wear of occlusal tooth surface related to bruxism

Table 2–12. Example of scoring for dentition and periodontium.

Existing Dentition/Periodontium

    None   _____
    Dentate _____

1. Maxillary Arch   2. Mandibular Arch

Notes: Patient with two molars on the left maxillary quadrant. One molar on the right maxillary with caries. The left mandibular quadrant is with two molars opposing the maxillary teeth. The right quadrant is with opposing molar to maxillary molar with caries. The attached gingiva of the maxillary molars is receding and reddened and bleeding. Evidence of plaque and calculus. Attached gingiva on mandibular molars ok.

Removable Prosthetics

1. Maxillary Arch
    Complete Denture _____
    Partial Denture   _____
2. Mandibular Arch
    Complete Denture _____
    Partial Denture   _____

Notes: Partial dentures for both mandible and maxilla. Somewhat loose due to recent weight loss. Appear to be in poor condition. Build up of plaque and food particulate throughout.

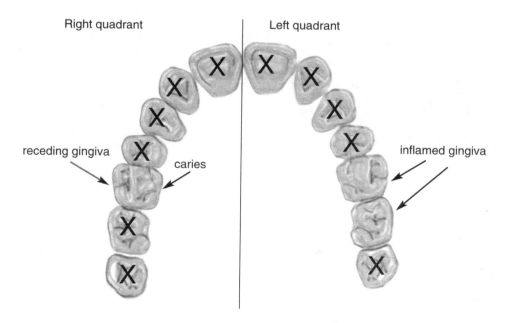

Figure 2–9. Maxillary teeth.

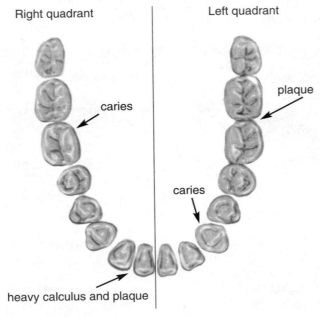

Figure 2–10. Mandibular teeth.

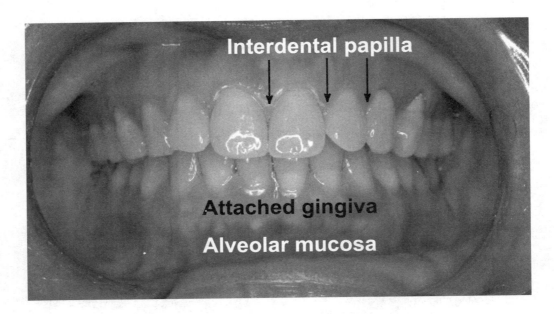

Figure 2–11. Normal dentition and periodontium.

on the diagram using arrows and narrative description. See Figure 2–12 for an example of severely affected periodontium and teeth.

Removable Prosthetics

While inspecting the mouth make note of removable partial or complete dentures. A partial denture replaces one or more teeth in one arch. A complete denture replaces most or all of the teeth in an arch. Indicate where the prostheses are in place and note their condition. With the patient's mouth wide open, grasp the denture and tug on it to determine the firmness of fit. Note the presence of food particulate or plaque on the surface of the denture. Inquire about the frequency of den-

Migrating teeth   **Receding gingiva**

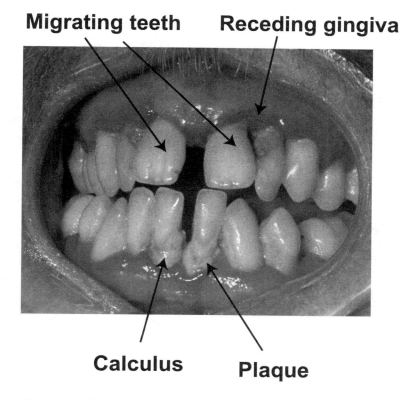

Calculus   **Plaque**

Figure 2–12. Poor dentition and periodontium. Migrating teeth, receding gingiva, plaque, and calculus are readily observable. (Courtesy of B. L. Dominguez, D.MD., M.S.)

ture cleaning and of oral hygiene if the dentures appear soiled.

Make note of the patient's report of existing dentures that are not worn or that may be unavailable temporarily due to emergent admission to the hospital. Probe the patient that reports the existence of dentures that are infrequently or never worn. Are the dentures not worn due to discomfort, malfunction, or poor fit? Make note of how long the patient has gone without the dentures and probe for any evidence of disability related to the missing teeth. Has weight loss accompanied the disuse of the denture? Are there food avoidance patterns present?

CSE 10. SALIVARY FLOW/ APPEARANCE OF ORAL MUCOSA

The clinician will judge the adequacy of salivary flow by inspecting the oral mucosa. The equipment needed includes a tongue blade, pen light, and gloves. A scoring example is found in Table 2–13.

Scoring Discussion

Salivary Flow/Hyposalivation

Quite simply, the oral cavity should appear wet. The mucosa of the tongue and palate should reflect light as the penlight illuminates the different structures. When hyposalivation occurs, the oral cavity will become dry. The tongue and palate will not demonstrate the same sheen observed in the mouth of an individual with normal salivary flow. Fissures or cracks may appear on the surface of the tongue. In severe cases of xerostomia (dryness of the mouth), the surface mucousa may flake. If there is some question as to whether the oral cavity appears dry, the patient should be queried as to the sensation of dry mouth. Record the responses in the notes section provided.

Appearance of Oral Mucosa

Make note of the color and surface texture of the gums and tongue if they appear outside of

Table 2–13. Example of scoring for salivary flow/appearance of oral mucosa.

A. Salivary Flow:

Normal _____

Hyposalivation __×__

B. Appearance of oral mucosa:

Notes: Surface of the tongue appears severely dry. Tongue with cracks and fissures.

---

the bounds of normal. Describe the location and characteristics of lesions or coatings of the tongue, gingiva , palate, or buccal tissue in the notes section provided.

For an expanded discussion of this component of the CSE protocol, see page xx.

CSE 11. ORAL/PHARYNGEAL SENSATION/GAG

The clinician will judge the adequacy of oral sensation and pharyngeal gag by stimulating the oral and pharyngeal mucosa. Equipment needed includes a tongue blade, cotton tipped applicator, pen light and gloves. A scoring example is found in Table 2–14.

Scoring Discussion

Oral/Pharyngeal Sensation

Have the patient open his or her mouth as you probe the surface of the tongue, faucial pillars, and posterior pharyngeal wall with a cotton tipped applicator. Probing of the faucial pillars and posterior pharyngeal wall may require the employment of the tongue blade to depress the tongue. Ask the patient to close his or her eyes and respond to each stimulus with a hand raise or a vocalization that does not require lingual movement (/ə/). The light touch should consist of a very light, momentary brush over an area of 1–2 mm². The initial stimulus should not dimple the tissue during the stimulation. As you move around the structures, randomly vary the rhythm of the stimulus. If no response to the initial stimulus is elicited, return to the area and apply enough pressure to dimple the tissue. If there is no response to greater pressure on the tongue, flip the cotton tipped applicator over and use the exposed wooden stick to apply the stimulus.

For each area stimulated, grade the patient's response and the type of stimulus that elicited the response. Remember to randomly time the application of the stimulus so as not to assist the patient in predicting the delivery and responding falsely. If the stimulus results in a gag response, indicate this next to the numeric score (Table 2–15).

The gag response may be elicited while probing any of the structures. Once observed, indicate the structure that was stimulated and record the pattern of pharyngeal wall movement. Make note of the symmetry of the movement. Variations in the amplitude of the response can be entered in the notes section as shown in Table 2–14.

For an expanded discussion of this component of the CSE protocol, see pages 88–89.

CSE 12. TONGUE MOVEMENT/ STRENGTH

The clinician will observe the tongue while the patient demonstrates strength and range of motion. Equipment needed includes a tongue blade, cotton tipped applicator, pen light and gloves. For an example of scoring for this section see Table 2–16.

Scoring Discussion

Tongue Observation

Request the patient to open his or her mouth and observe the tongue at rest. Make note of morphological changes due to surgery or irradiation. Note signs of atrophy. If dyskinesias are present, note whether these are rhythmic or random. Make additional note of the presence of fasciculations. A fasciculation is the twitching of a single muscle group served by a single motor nerve fiber or filament and is a sign of neurologic disease. This sign is well-vi-

Table 2–14. Scoring example for oral sensation.

Tongue

Tip	Right	1	Left	1
Blade	Right	1	Left	1
Dorsum	Right	1	Left	gag

Faucial Pillar

Right	1	Left	1

Posterior Pharyngeal wall

Right	gag	Left	gag

Gag

Lateral pharyngeal wall movement

Bilateral/symmetrical	×		
Unilateral	Right	_____	Left	_____

Notes: Strong gag response from posterior tongue and posterior pharyngeal wall.

Table 2–15. Stimulus scoring guide for gag.

Stimulus	Score
Light brush with cotton tip	1
Light pressure with cotton tip	2
Light pressure with stick (tongue only)	3
No response	4

---

sualized by shining a pen light across the surface of the tongue and monitoring the surface for the small random twitches.

Tongue maneuvers

Tongue protrusion. Ask the subject to protrude the tongue as far as possible. On protrusion, the tongue should be symmetrically supported and should not deviate to one side or the other. If the tongue is not protruded symmetrically, indicate whether the deviation is to the left or right of midline. Observe the position and stability of the tongue. Is this an easily organized task or is struggle involved? Do dyskinesias appear at the onset protrusion? Indicate the range of movement of the dyskinesia and duration of stability if observed.

Nasal Respiration During Cheek Puff.

Request the patient to puff his or her cheeks and breathe through the nose. Monitor breaths by observing thoracic movement. Is the patient capable of puffing the cheeks? A patient with normal strength and coordination should be able to breathe many cycles with the cheeks puffed. Push the cheeks in with both hands. The air should escape through the lips. If the cheeks are easily compressed without air leakage from the lips repeat the procedure and listen for nasal emission or "snoring" sounds of air leaking through the tongue and velar seal.

This task tests the posterior seal of the oral cavity. A patient with poor posterior tongue elevation or poor coordination of the tongue and velum will be unable to close the seal in the posterior oral cavity and the cheeks will not inflate. Poor lip seal will contribute to the inability to puff the cheeks. Make note of lip seal performance observed earlier in the clinical examination. Apraxic patients frequently also will have difficulty performing this task.

Tongue Strength

Superior/Anterior. Place the cotton tipped applicator along the blade of the tongue at the level of the gingival margin of the maxillary arch. Ask the patient push the swab against

Table 2–16. Example of scoring for tongue measures and observations.

Tongue Observation:

> **Notes:** Post surgical scarring on left lateral lingual surface. Erythmetous tissue along left lateral margin in area currently being irradiated. Some leukoplakia coating superior-anterior surface of tongue.

Tongue Maneuvers:

1. Tongue protrusion
   a. Normal _____
   b. Atrophy   Right _____   Left __×__
   c. Deviation Right _____   Left __×__
   d. Dyskinesia _____
2. Nasal respiration w/ puffed cheeks
   a. Normal _____   Altered __×__

Notes: Able to puff cheeks but loses pressure at the onset of nasal respiration. Likely unable to create lingual palatal seal.

E. Tongue Strength:

1. Superior/Anterior

Right	Normal	_____	Weakened	__×__
Left	Normal	_____	Weakened	__×__

F. Tongue Range of Motion:

1. Buccal Sulcus
   a. Maxillary
      Normal _____
      Altered   Right __×__   Left __×__

   b. Mandibular
      Normal _____
      Altered   Right __×__   Left __×__

   c. Palate
      Normal _____
      Altered   Right _____   Left __×__

his or her teeth and palate while you try to retract it. A patient with normal strength should be able to provide enough pressure so that the removal of the swab requires some moderate tugging. Repeat this procedure for the opposite side. The weakened patient will provide less resistance when removal of the swab is attempted.

As with many noninstrumental assessments of strength, this task requires a subjective judgement. In this case, we are attempting to judge the pressure exerted by the tongue. If you are unsure of your ability to decide, in a binary fashion, whether weakness exists, practice this task on friends or family to get a feel for what range of resistance is found in a normal subject. Keep in mind that the elderly will demonstrate less pressure on maximal exertion than young normals (Robbins, Levine, Wood, Roecker, & Luschei, 1995).

Tongue Range of Motion

Request the patient to move the tongue tip along the entire length of the maxillary and mandibular buccal sulci. Additionally, have the patient stroke the surface of the hard palate with the tip of the tongue. Demonstrate these maneuvers for the patient if necessary. To visualize the patient's tongue during this task, it may be necessary to open the buccal cavity by pulling the cheek to the side with a tongue depressor. Make note of reduced range of motion of the tongue.

This task does not assess full range of motion of the tongue. The range of motion of the tongue would include points well outside of the oral cavity. The task does give the examiner a chance to observe the patient's ability to clear the buccal pockets and the palate of material that may accumulate.

Some apraxic patients may struggle to volitionally coordinate this movement. This inability to complete the task should not be confused with reduced range of motion. If this occurs, assist them by tracing the desired path with a cotton tipped applicator. Request the patient to keep their tongue tip on the swab.

Patients with progressive neuromuscular disease such as Parkinson's disease may demonstrate bradykinesia (slow movement) or rigidity during this task. Make note of the presence of these findings.

For an expanded discussion of this component of the CSE protocol, see page xx.

CSE 13. VELAR ELEVATION

The clinician will assess velar elevation during phonation. Equipment needed includes a tongue blade, pen light, and gloves.

Scoring Discussion

Ask the patient to open his or her mouth and phonate /ə/. Observe the elevation of the velum from the onset of phonation. An unobstructed view of the velum may not be possible for some patients during phonation due to the position of the tongue. In this situation ask the patient to generate a yawn. The yawn depresses the tongue and elevates the palate, and usually provides adequate visualization.

Normal elevation of the velum should present as a superior arcing of the tissue of the soft palate. In unilateral weakness, the palate will droop on the affected side. Bilateral weakness will result in reduced symmetrical movement of palate.

For an expanded discussion of this component of the CSE protocol, see pages 92–93.

CSE 14. VOLITIONAL SWALLOWS/LARYNGEAL ELEVATION

The clinician will assess laryngeal elevation during dry and/or bolus swallows. Equipment needed includes spoon, cup, straw, ice chips, water and gloves. For an example of scoring for this section see Table 2–17.

Scoring Discussion

Laryngeal Elevation

Place the ring, middle, and index fingers along the anterior surface of the throat with the index finger in the superior position. Situate your fingers so that the thyroid notch is nestled between the ring and middle fingers (see Figure 2–13). When the fingers are located in this position, the index finger should be resting upon the suprahyoid muscles. Request the patient to swallow with the fingers lightly resting in this arrangement. There may be a moment of delay as the patient collects saliva within the oral cavity and prepares to swallow.

A number of patients may have difficulty performing this task. Patients with xerostomia may not have enough saliva available to initiate a dry (nonbolus) swallow. Individuals with apraxia may be unable to organize the motor coordination necessary to generate a swallow. Likewise, patients with poor auditory comprehension or those that are cognitively impaired may be unable to swallow on command. For all of these patients, the presentation of an ice chip, or very small water sip (1–2 cc) can be employed to initiate a pharyngeal swallow. Use the notation section to record the amount and type of bolus presented.

Once initiated, the swallow should occur briskly. The sublingual musculature should

---

Table 2–17. Example of scoring for laryngeal elevation.

A. Laryngeal Elevation:

Normal	___×___
Reduced	_____
Absent	_____

Notes: Unable to initiate a volitional dry swallow likely due to apraxia. Presented small sip of water (1–2 cc) from a cup and monitored elevation.

Laryngeal position at rest

Laryngeal position during elevation

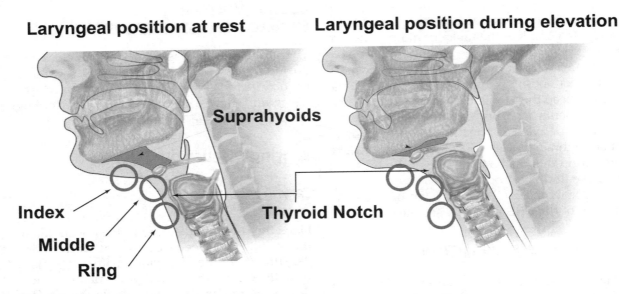

Figure 2–13. Guide for finger placement during laryngeal elevation.

pull away from the index finger slightly as the suprahyoid muscles contract. During elevation, the thyroid notch should move to a point above the middle finger and, at the apex of the swallow, may come in contact with the inferior margin of the index finger. A swallow following this pattern should be scored as "normal." Should the thyroid notch fail to elevate beyond the middle finger, elevation may be described as being reduced. If the clinician senses no evidence of movement of the structures, the attempt should be scored as absent.

This task may require several repetitions before a confident determination can be made. Normal subjects are not likely to repeatedly perform dry swallows more than three or four times in succession without requiring a bolus to assist in the initiation.

For an expanded discussion of this component of the CSE protocol, see pages 93–95.

CSE 15. FOOD AND LIQUID SWALLOWS

The clinician will elicit swallows by presenting food and liquid of varying volumes and consistencies to the patient. The clinician will observe and record signs and symptoms that are exposed during this session. Equipment needed includes spoons, cups, straws, applesauce, pudding, bread, solid foods, ice chips, water and gloves. Optional equipment consists of a stethoscope, pulse oximeter, suction device

and blue food dye. An example of scoring is provided in Table 2–18.

Scoring Discussion

Guidelines

Before proceeding with the presentation of food or liquid, the clinician must integrate thoroughly all of the historical information and findings that have been previously disclosed and/or revealed. The decision to initiate this portion of the exam or, once initiated, to move on to another, more challenging consistency or bolus volume, will depend on the existence of, or combination of, a great many factors.

As a basic guideline, the clinician should hold safety as the highest priority. At a minimum, before the presentation of food or liquid the clinician should be sure of the following parameters:

Medical Stability. If an event of aspiration has the potential to cause immediate and severe negative health effects, the decision to present food or liquid should be weighed carefully. The value of determining the safety of eating may be outweighed by the potential for respiratory distress. For close monitoring of

Table 2–18. Example entry for food and liquid swallows.

Material	Ice Chips	Puree	Soft Solid	Solid	Liquids Thick	Liquids Thin
A. Max Amount	1-chip	heaping teaspoon	heaping teaspoon	none	1/4 cup	teaspoon
B. Timing/Speed	2 s	5 s	5 s		5 s	2 s
C. # of swallows	2	6	8		3	2
D. Oral sign	none	L buccal	L buccal		none	none
E. Airway sign	none	none	hawk		cough	cough
F. Instrumentation	none	none	aus		aus	aus
G. Intervention	none	none	mend -		chin tuck +	Chin tuck -Ssglot-

Notes: Seated upright, alert for procedure. Edentulous, no solids presented. Laryngeal elevation was poor. Considerable effort to clear demonstrated with puree and soft solid. Multiple swallows and distress with larger boluses (>teaspoon). Patient unable to perform mendelsohn. Positive airway sounds on auscultation following initial swallow of thick and thin liquids. Clinical signs of aspiration (cough) and positive auscultation suggest aspiration of liquids. Chin tuck consistently effective in eliminating clinical signs with thick liquids thickened to a nectar-like consistency. Chin tuck ineffective with thins. Unable to perform super supraglottic maneuver.

Impression: Moderate pharyngeal dysphagia characterized by an inefficient and mistimed pharyngeal swallow. Poor laryngeal elevation coupled with multiple swallows per bolus would suggest poor propulsion of bolus through upper esophageal segment. Suspected aspiration of liquids is likely related to a delay in the transition between the oral and pharyngeal phases of the swallow.

Preliminary Plan/Recs

Interim diet change to puree with liquids thickened to a nectar consistency. Monitor intake via calorie count.
Perform videofluoroscopy to visualize biomechanics of pharynx/UES, identify impairment and verify aspiration.

the fragile patient, see the discussion regarding the use of pulse oximetry. The clinician may find that fragile patients in an intensive care unit already are being extensively monitored. Consult the attending physicians and nursing staff regarding specific precautions. Review the chart for indications of upcoming examinations that require NPO status before presenting food or liquids to the patient.

Alertness. The patient should be as fully alert as possible. An appropriate amount of time should be dedicated to orientation before introducing any food or liquid to a patient with reduced sensorium. See section CSE 1 for discussion regarding the assessment of mental status.

Cough. The clinician should be confident of his or her estimation of the patient's ability to volitionally reject material from the upper airways before introducing any material into the patient's mouth. This is not to say that the patient should be able to produce a strong cough on command before commencing with the clinical examination. However, if a strong cough is not present, the clinician should be prepared to provide upper airway clearance in the form of trans-oral, trans-nasal or transtracheal suctioning if severe aspiration is suspected. If the clinician is not trained, or able, to provide this service, the appropriate personnel should be alerted and agree to be on-call for its potential employment. Review the information regarding cough found in section CSE 3 of the clinical examination.

Order of Presentation

After determining the appropriateness of initiating the delivery of food and liquid, the clinician should present the materials in a manner that will reveal ability as well as impairment. The initial delivery should be of a volume and consistency that will be the easiest for the patient to consume. A catastrophic event of aspiration will cut the session short, preventing the clinician from testing the safety of various consistencies, bolus sizes, positions, and maneuvers. For example, a cognitively intact patient who complains confidently of coughing and choking with thin liquids should not be presented a full cup of water and ordered to drink. This approach may allow for the rapid

display of clinical signs of aspiration but does not allow for a full investigation of the patient's threshold of ability and disability. Further, a clinical sign (eg., wet gurgly dysphonia) may be sustained throughout the exam after the initial delivery of food or liquid. The sustained sign may obscure the successful employment of positioning maneuvers or manipulation of size or consistency later in the examination. Therefore, as a general rule, begin with small amounts of easily controlled materials that do not match the consistency, bolus size, or conditions that the patient has identified as being problematic.

Patients who display fragile health and demonstrate numerous clinical signs of dysphagia may be given benign testing materials, such as ice chips, to elicit swallows. Introducing ice chips as the first testing material provides a few advantages. First, the volume of the delivery is well controlled, as the ice chip size can be quite small (1cc or less) and is easily presented with a spoon or gloved hand. Second, the temperature of the ice may heighten the level of alertness in a patient with depressed sensorium who may need orientation before other test items are presented. Third, the cold ice chip may, theoretically, enhance the CNS afferent stimuli that triggers the pharyngeal swallow in the same way that tactile-thermal application does (Bisch, Logemann, Rademaker, Kahrilas, & Lazarus, 1994; Kaatzke-McDonald, Post, & Davis, 1996; Logemann, 1993; Logemann, 1996; Rosenbek, Robbins, Willford, et al., 1998; Rosenbek, Roecker, Wood, & Robbins, 1991; Rosenbek, Roecker, Wood, & Robbins, 1996).

Maximum Amount

Enter the maximum amount of food or liquid presented with that material. List the volume in whatever scale pleases you. Many clinicians find that using sizes familiar and meaningful to the patient or caretaker, such as a ¼ teaspoon, are more useful than employing unfamiliar measurement units, such as milliliters or cubic centimeters.

Many problems surface as the volume of the bolus increases. For this reason, start with smaller amounts than would normally be consumed in a meal. Move to larger boluses if no clinical signs are observed. After a few trials, the confident clinician may encourage the patient to demonstrate a "typical spoonful" or "typical drink" and allow the patient to self-feed. Enter the size of the bolus presented when clinical signs become clear and consistent. If unsure of the finding, repeat it.

The pharynx and larynx are configured to protect the lower airway from penetration of foreign objects. In a normally configured pharynx the protective structures are capable of holding a certain amount of material while preventing penetration of the laryngeal vestibule. The epiglottis acts much like a plow as it separates and divides an oncoming bolus. The bolus is guided into channels lateral to the laryngeal vestibule and falls, by means of gravity, to the pyriform sinuses. As long as the volume of the material presented does not exceed the capacity of these protective cavities, risk of penetration of the laryngeal airway is lessened. The configuration of the cavities, and their protective properties, can be altered due to poor positioning, edema, post surgical structural changes and the presence of large-bore nasogastric tubes.

When a swallow is weakened, the transit of the bolus through the pharynx will be incomplete and residual bolus will be found in the protective cavities of the pharynx. Low tongue driving force has been found to result in vallecular retention whereas diminished pharyngeal shortening results in pyriform sinus residue (Dejaeger et al., 1997). The capacity of these cavities to hold material will vary from patient to patient, but rarely safely exceeds 10 cc of material.

Scoring: Timing/Speed

While presenting food or liquid, the clinician can monitor laryngeal elevation in the manner described in section CSE 14. The timing of the onset often is dependent on the material presented (Hiiemae et al., 1995) with longer periods necessary as the "hardness" of the food increases. For material that is manipulated easily and/or requires no mastication (for example, liquids), the starting point can coincide with the entry of food into the mouth with the end point being the elevation of the larynx. For material that requires mastication, the clinician should monitor the suprahyoid muscles for the cessation of movement associated with chewing and begin to count the elapsed time until the initiation of laryngeal elevation.

Slowness of preparation prior to the initiation of the swallow can also be measured for all consistencies, if the clinician wishes. The elapsed time should begin as the food enters the mouth and end as the larynx elevates for the pharyngeal swallow.

Scoring: Number of Swallows

The clinician should count the number of swallows per bolus delivery by recording the number of elevations of the larynx. Because multiple boluses will be delivered to the patient during the examination, the clinician may wish to report the average number of swallows for the largest boluses presented. A normal subject will typically swallow only once or twice per teaspoon of food or liquid.

Scoring: Oral Signs

The clinician should look inside the patient's oral cavity following each food presentation in those patients who report oral stage difficulties. Be sure to attend to this task after the first few puree and solid food presentations regardless of patient complaint. Attention should be directed to inspecting all of the crevices and pockets where food could collect following the swallow. Pull the buccal cavity open with the tongue blade to determine if buccal pocketing is present. Inspect the palate and under the tongue for residue. Identify the specific areas where residue is present.

Patients with dyskinesias may demonstrate considerable trouble during food delivery to the mouth and with oral manipulation. Loss of control of the bolus and drooling should be noted.

Scoring: Airway Signs

Note the presence of adventitious sounds emanating from the airway after the presentation of food or liquid. The specific airway signs of interest are wet dysphonia and spontaneous cough. The clinician may wish to review the discussions regarding dysphonia and cough presented previously. See sections CSE 3 and CSE 4, respectively.

Does the individual continue to converse without attention to the wet dysphonia? Note attempts by the subject to clear his or her throat if dysphonia is present. Attention also should be directed to the timing and strength of the cough response. Coughs may occur before the initiation of laryngeal elevation in cases in which the duration of stage transition is extended. Compare this airway sign to the timing and speed findings.

Instrumentation

List the instrumentation used to monitor signs. See the expanded discussion for options.

Scoring: Intervention

Note the intervention techniques used for each consistency presented. Indicate success or failure by placing a "+" or "−" sign next to the notation. List modifications or additional information in the section reserved for notes.

For an expanded discussion of this component of the CSE protocol, see page 100.

DECISION POINT

The clinical examination, as presented to the reader in this text, is an extensive but not exhaustive review of a patient's swallowing function. The clinician, at this decision point, has reviewed the patient's medical history and inspected the structures of the oral cavity and throat involved in swallowing. The clinician has made fine and gross distinctions regarding muscle function as it relates to swallowing and protecting the airway and has presented food and liquid to the patient in an attempt to observe directly signs that are related to swallowing impairment. Finally, the clinician has attempted to make adjustments of bolus volume, consistency, viscosity, and rate of introduction, has implemented positioning and maneuvers where they are appropriate, and has observed the patient for subsequent resolution of clinical signs of dysphagia. All of the information gleaned from these tasks now must be integrated to establish an appropriate management program for the patient. Management objectives are presented in Table 2–19.

If the clinician can initiate confidently the execution of the first three management objectives at the close of the clinical examination, the assessment process can be considered complete. If, however, the findings are equivocal, the assessment process must continue.

There are a variety of instruments used to assess swallow function. The two most widely used instruments employ either fluoroscopy or flexible endoscopy. The choice of instrument often will depend on the nature of the query. Each instrument has strengths and weaknesses. A number of factors come into play during this decision-making process, including availability of the instrument, the area of interest to be studied, patient comfort, and personal preference. Chapters 3 and 4 will discuss the two instrumental examinations.

Table 2–19. Integration of patient management objectives.

1. Implement adjustments to a patient's diet to maximize nutrition, hydration, and safety

2. Implement changes in positioning and the use of maneuvers into a patient's behavioral repertoire to maximize safety and efficiency

3. Develop and carry out a treatment plan to address the physiological impairments that cause disability in the dysphagic patient

4. Determine the need for further instrumental assessment

5. Refer to another discipline as needed, to address diagnostic concerns revealed during the clinical exam that extend beyond the scope of practice of the clinician

EXPANDED DISCUSSIONS FOR CLINICAL SWALLOWING EXAMINATION

CSE 1. MENTAL STATUS

The following are special considerations that one may want to ponder when interacting with patients in their varying degrees of awareness.

No Response/Deep Coma

The nursing staff generally will have the clearest picture of the patient's responsiveness. If there is a question as to the status of the patient, the clinician may carefully squeeze the root of the fingernails or pectoralis muscle to elicit a response. Patients fitting into this category obviously are improbable candidates for oral feeding. The patient may be montiored daily or as often as necessary to determine readiness.

SemiComa

If the patient's status is in question, the clinician may carefully apply the stimuli listed above. More frequent monitoring of the patient to determine readiness for assessment may yield good results.

Confusion/Stupor

Engage the patient in conversation for more than a single sentence. Many patients require a few moments of "rise time" before their best responses are observed. Carrying food or liquid, or even a cup with water or ice may garner more attention than any series of questions. Use this to your advantage by placing the items in full view of the patient. Many patients fitting this profile are successful at achieving some type of oral intake with assistance. Special attention should be directed to the amount of time, and specific time during the day, that the patient is most alert. These may be the moments when testing is initiated or trial feeding attempted. This may vary greatly in a single patient and will vary greatly between patients.

Confused/Somnolent

This patient may be roused and perform well momentarily but return to a confused or sleepy state. This patient will need to be monitored for his or her best performance time.

Time of day and activity prior to interaction should be noted. Patients roused from sleep will not perform as well as those who are fully awake and seated upright. The nursing staff usually is aware of the patient's optimum time for performing tasks such as self-care or positioning that requires the patients cooperation.

Confused/Demented/Agitated

Patients with this profile generally will be capable of carrying out the tasks necessary for a complete assessment of swallowing function. Successful testing may require a highly orchestrated protocol with little time left for attention and cooperation to wane. Planning for patient comfort and ability to cooperate during instrumental procedures should be considered carefully. Many agitated patients will not allow a tongue depressor to enter the oral cavity much less keep barium impregnated paste in their mouth or have an endoscope placed transnasally.

Post-Stroke Rehabilitation Patients

The timing of testing may be particularly important for this patient. A patient with a full day of rehabilitation should not be tested right after physically demanding sessions in physical therapy. The same goes for those patients undergoing other physically challenging diagnostic tests or treatments.

Mild/Moderate Cognitive Impairment

This patient will present few problems during testing. Future planning regarding the effectiveness of complex therapeutic interventions for such a patient should be carefully weighed. A patient's insight into the nature of the swallowing problem often assists in implementing a successful therapy program. Planning for efficacious intervention should be considered during this initial meeting.

Mild Cognitive Impairment/Normal

This patient may cooperate fully during the examination, attend therapy sessions faithfully, thank the clinician profusely for his or her time and effort at the close of therapy, and then go home and disregard all previous instructions. Even fully capable and intelligent individuals will disregard instructions if they have not been afforded the appropriate patient education. The provision of therapy and the provision of patient education that leads to insight are too often mutually exclusive.

CSE 2. SPEECH/ARTICULATION

Motor speech function and swallowing function share many anatomic structures as well as efferent and afferent pathways to the central nervous system. Co-occurrence of pathological speech production and dysphagia should surprise no one. Early literature suggested that speech was an overlaid function that emerged from vegetative sucking, chewing, and swallowing (Meader & Muyskens, 1950; Netsell, 1984; Shohara, 1932). Most clinical bedside protocols call for some analysis of speech function based on the conventional wisdom that impairment in speech will correlate with dysphagia, and much of the literature supports this notion (Litvan, Sastry, & Sonies, 1997; Logemann, 1985; Martin, Corlew, Celement, & Zablocki, 1990).

The clinician should be cautioned that not every patient with a motor speech disorder will present with dysphagia (Kennedy, Pring, & Faucus, 1993; Martin et al., 1990). Litvan et al. (1997), in a study of patients with progressive supranuclear palsy, found that, although dysphagia is associated with dysarthria in this population, the two conditions are not always paired in the same patient. In stroke patients with co-occurring dysphagia and speech disorders, swallowing and speech may improve independently of each other (Netsell, 1984).

CSE 3. RESPIRATION FUNCTION

There are no hard and fast rules for ranking the efficiency of the different airway clearance behaviors. Poor volitional cough generally is considered to be a marker for poor airway clearance. By itself, it may be a sensitive marker for risk of aspiration in the dysphagic patient.

A number of investigators have included volitional cough as part of the data set in their clinical swallowing examinations without identifying specific attributes of the cough that should be considered (Daniels et al., 1998; Horner, Massey, & Brazer, 1990; Linden, Kuhlemeier, & Patterson, 1993; Linden & Siebens, 1983; Ott, David, Hodge, Pikna, Chen, & Gelfand, 1996). Many of the investigators presented a binary determination of adequacy of volitional cough (normal/abnormal). Daniels et al. (1998); Horner and Massey (1988); Horner et al. (1990, 1993) reported that abnormal volitional cough was an independent predictor of aspiration during videofluoroscopy. Linden et al. (1993) found that the identification abnormal cough was not associated significantly with aspiration during videofluoroscopy.

More importantly, the task does not relate the ability to clear material that may enter into the lower airways during feeding unless, by happenstance, material is expelled during the task itself. Even in this case, it is difficult to determine efficiency without direct visualization of the material as it is aspirated and the resulting effort to expel it.

Physiology of the Cough

The cough is one of the most important mechanisms for airway protection and maintainence. Developing an understanding of the physiology of airway clearance may assist the clinician in making critical distinctions while managing the dysphagic patient.

The cough begins with a quick inspiration of air. This inspiration is followed by the tight sphincteric closure of the laryngeal vestibule lasting approximately 200 msec (see Figure 4–17 in Chapter 4). The pharynx shortens and the lateral pharyngeal walls move medially to squeeze material out of the pyriform sinuses. While glottic closure is maintained abdominal and pleural pressure is raised. This rise in pressure is due to an expiratory effort from both the rib cage and diaphragm. The larynx reinforces the cough by storing and coordinating the release of pressure as the glottis is opened rapidly (Bucher, 1958). This rapid opening of the glottis releases an airstream that clears any material in its path to a place further up the airway.

The cough reflex develops over time. Less than half of newborns cough spontaneously or on direct laryngeal stimulation (Leith, 1985). Although newborns appear to be able to generate the inspiratory and expiratory pressures necessary for a cough, the lung structure lacks the recoil pressures and the reduced elasticity of the trachea curtail the peak flow rates necessary for cough. As the infant matures, lung structures become more elastic and are capable of generating the expiratory pressures that create high expiratory flow and a successful cough.

Exogenous debris and pulmonary secretions normally are removed by the beating of cilia that line the mucosal surface of the lungs. When this defense mechanism is impaired or overwhelmed by increased secretions, coughing and/or other clearing maneuvers become an important means of secretion removal. Clearing maneuvers fail when there is a reduction in compression of the airways to drive the stream of air, inadequate inspiration or structural failures (incompetent glottis, tracheostomy). The airflow to support coughing is diminished in chronic obstructive pulmonary diseases such as asthma, emphysema, and chronic bronchitis. When expiratory flows are very low, material is less likely to be forcefully directed out of the larger airways. When the clearing maneuvers fail, obstruction of airways occurs. Plugging of the airways with secretions leads to poor gas exchange, eventually leading to acute and chronic infection and ultimately, death.

Measuring volitional cough does not predict the ability of the patient to cough reflexively in the event of laryngeal penetration or aspiration. The reason for assessing volitional cough is primarily to prepare for the emergent clearance of the airway and, to a lesser degree, to predict respiratory strength.

The elicitation of volitional cough helps the clinician determine whether the patient is capable of organizing the motor movements necessary to clear the airway should an event of aspiration be suspected during the clinical exam or observed during the instrumental examination. Additionally, the clinician is able to determine whether maneuvers such as the supra-glottic maneuver or super-supra-glottic maneuver are viable options should they need to be employed during the assessment and/or treatment process.

Tracheostomy Tubes

The clinician should determine the type and configuration of the tracheostomy tube before the administration of the examination. Tracheostomy tubes can come in a variety of configurations to suit the specific needs of the patient. They generally are grouped into fenestrated, cuffed, and uncuffed varieties. Uncuffed tubes and fenestrated tracheostomy tubes allow for the passage of aspirated material around the trach tube body. This allows for the dyed-food particulate or secretions to be expelled from the trach tube during a cough, or to be suctioned from the lower airways via trans-tracheal suctioning.

The cuffed trach allows for the inflation of a small balloon that surrounds the distal body of the trach tube (Figure 2–14). Once inflated, the cuff forms a seal around the tube. This seal closes the lower airways off from the larynx and pharynx. The primary purpose of the cuffed tracheostomy tube is to provide a sealed airway for mechanical ventilation. With inflation, the positive pressures generated by the ventilator will be directed to the lower airways without diffusion into the pharynx.

CSE 4. VOICE/RESONANCE

CSE 4 A. Voice

If the individual was able to communicate verbally during the interview, the alert clinician will have had ample opportunity to assess voice and resonance. The presence of dysphonia has been shown repeatedly to be an independent indicator for risk of aspiration on an instrumental examination in patients with neurologic disorders (Daniels, Brailey, Priestly, Herrington, Weisberg, & Foundas, 1998; Horner et al., 1993; Linden & Seibens, 1983; Linden et al., 1993, Wilson, Pryde, White, Maher, & Maran, 1995).

The genesis of a dysphonia can be iatrogenic (as a result of treatment, e.g., surgical), physiologic (acid reflux), due to neurogenic disease or event (ALS, Parkinson's, stroke, etc.), or behavioral (conversion dysphonia). The dysphonic patterns of special interest to the dysphagia clinician are those that provide signs of swallowing difficulty or that suggest insufficient adduction of the vocal cords.

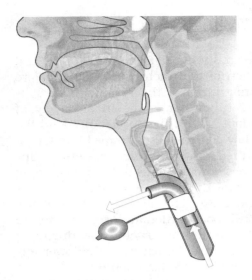

Cuff inflated

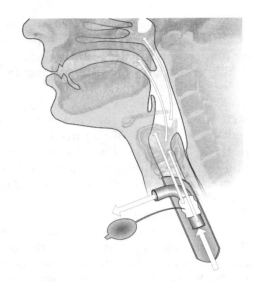

Cuff deflated

Figure 2–14. Cuffed tracheostomy tube. When inflated the cuffed tracheostomy tube seals the lower airway from the pharynx.

Wet Dysphonia

The "wet" dysphonic voice quality is one of the strongest indicators of a swallowing impairment. This vocal quality results from the accumulation of oropharyngeal secretions resting within the bounds of the laryngeal vestibule. The secretions fall by gravity to the level of the vocal cords, where, upon phonation, they interfere with the stream of air emitted from the vibrating glottis. As the phonatory air stream moves through the layer of secretions, a "gurgly" sound is heard.

Saliva and nasopharyngeal secretions are created and collect throughout the waking hours. The role of saliva in the masticatory process, as it lubricates the bolus in preparation for swallowing, is well known. Saliva also has antimicrobial and pH buffering properties that serve to control the propagation of oral bacteria and neutralize acid in the esophagus respectively (Helm, 1989; Terpenning et al., 1993). Resting saliva flow is approximately 0.4ml/min (Kapila, Dodds, Helm, & Hogan, 1984). This flow rate increases when the oral cavity is stimulated during speech or chewing. Saliva flow is reported to increase to approximately 2.8 ml/min during mastication (Navazesh & Christensen, 1982).

As salivary flow increases, so does the frequency of swallowing (Kapila et al., 1984). During sleep states, major salivary glands nearly cease production of saliva resulting in a drop-off of spontaneous swallowing. Lear et al. (1965) found the mean swallowing frequency of sleeping subjects to be 0.088 swallows/min whereas awake and alert normals registered 0.612 swallows/min. In short, normal subjects swallow as often as is needed in response to the accumulation of oropharyngeal secretions.

The passive flow pattern of material in a normally configured pharynx is illustrated in Figure 2–15. Oropharyngeal secretions either are stored in the vallecular space, or, because of the configuration of the epiglottis and aryepiglottic folds, are directed around the laryngeal vestibule to the pyriform sinuses, where they pool before being transported out of the pharynx during the pharyngeal swallow. If a clearing swallow does not occur before the capacity of these reservoirs is reached, they will overflow into the laryngeal vestibule. It is at this point that the conditions necessary for the creation of the wet dysphonic voice are fulfilled.

In normal subjects, any collection of material within the vestibule would be expelled

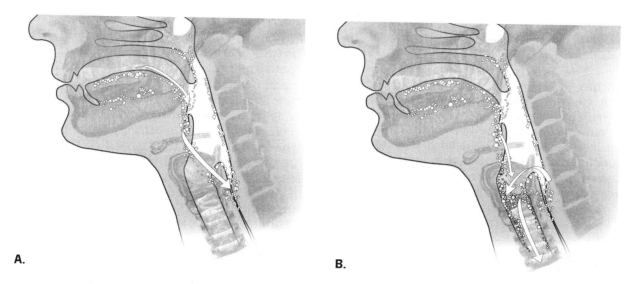

A.

B.

Figure 2–15. A. Path of secretions around the laryngeal vestibule. The secretions accumulate in the pyriform sinuses and vallecular space until swallowed or expectorated. **B.** If not swallowed or expectorated, secretions will flow into the airway.

with a combination of throat clearing and subsequent swallow. In dysphagic individuals, the material may not be cleared due to a reduced frequency of spontaneous swallowing, a weakened pharyngeal swallow, depressed sensorium, or a synergistic combination of all of these factors (Linden & Seibens 1993; Murray, Langmore, Ginsberg, & Dostie,1996).

Reduced sensation of the pharynx or larynx also may play a role in the accumulation of, and failure to clear, secretions. In severe cases of dysphagia the patient with intact pharyngeal and laryngeal sensation may clear his or her throat constantly and expectorate into a vessel such as a cup or emesis basin for relief. Patients with reduced awareness, reduced sensation, or the inability to expectorate due to weakness or incoordination will be observed to continue to converse with a wet dysphonic voice without attempts to clear.

Noting the patient's active attempts to clear oropharyngeal secretions may contribute to the clinician's overall impression of the individual's ability to sense and manage oropharyngeal secretions.

Hypophonic/Breathy Dysphonia

This vocal quality has been addressed specifically in many of the studies that have compared clinical and instrumental examinations for dysphagia (Daniels et al., 1998; Horner et al., 1993; Linden & Seibens, 1983; Linden et al., 1993). Hypophonic/breathy dysphonia was not identified in these studies as being associated independently with aspiration.

Horner et al. (1991), in a study of brainstem stroke patients, reported that the presence of vocal fold paralysis was significantly associated with aspiration. Vocal fold paralysis (paralysis of the vocalis and thyroarytenoid muscles) results in reduced tension and poor approximation of the vocal folds during phonation resulting in excessive emission of air through the folds with subsequent "breathy" voicing.

The term "vocal cord paralysis," or "vocal fold paralysis," often is used to describe a condition in which the arytenoid is in a fixed position, thereby preventing full adduction of the glottis. The term itself may be somewhat of a misnomer, in that the fixed position of the arytenoid is related to paralysis or paresis of the transverse and lateral cricoarytenoid muscles, the intrinsic musculature of the larynx employed in adduction of the vocal folds.

The inability to close the glottis puts an individual at much greater risk for entry of material into the lower airways. Fixed arytenoids often are the result of lower motor neuron damage to the recurrent laryngeal nerve (RLN), which supplies motor signals to the intrinsic musculature of the larynx. This damage can be the result of infection, disease process, and radiation treatments, or to trauma following surgery.

The RLN fibers of the vagus are found within the vagal trunk, which courses inferiorly from the inferior ganglion and passes the larynx before emerging from the trunk and ascending to the larynx bilaterally. The inferior course is asymmetrical with the right RLN looping under the subclavian artery and then ascending (see Figure 2–16). The left RLN travels slightly more inferiorly and loops under the aorta before ascending to the larynx. The close proximity of the left RLN to the aorta leads to complications due to heart disease and its treatment. Ortner's syndrome, first described in 1897, is a clinical entity with breathy dysphonia due to a left RLN palsy caused by cardiac disease. The typical course of the syndrome may include the development of a thoracic aneurysm that compresses the RLN nerve with resulting reduction in motor efferents and development of the clinical signs of breathy voice (Thirlwall, 1997).

Iatrogenic RLN often results from misadventures during carotid endarterectomy, cardiac surgery or other thoracic surgeries. Permanent damage can be caused by sharp dissection during surgery. Damage also can be caused by retractors, diathermy burns in the vicinity of the nerve, or inclusion of the nerve in arterial clamps. Ice or saline slush used for heart arrest in cardiac operations can cause hypothermic damage to the left recurrent laryngeal nerve. Left RLN damage of this type, in which actual resection of the nerve does not occur, is not usually permanent. A typical recovery period is 8 to 10 months before function returns (Curran et al., 1997).

Surgical procedures also can result in damage to other vagal nerves. Bilateral damage to the internal branch of the superior laryngeal nerve (SLN) usually produces loss of sensation of the mucosa in the laryngeal vestibule. The resulting loss of the afferent input that drives the cough reflex can put a patient at great risk of aspiration without spontaneous protective clearance. Patients with combined SLN and RLN damage will present a greater degree of dysphagia and aspiration. Vagal injuries also affect palatal and pharyngeal function and frequently are associated with other cranial nerve deficits.

Temporary hoarse/harsh dysphonia can be observed in patients recovering from any type of surgery or bouts of respiratory insufficiency that require oral intubation for anesthesia or ventilation. The hypopharynx and cervical esophagus are particularly vulnerable to intubation trauma (Tartell, Hoover, Friduss,

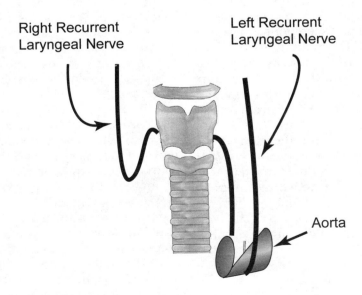

Figure 2–16. Assymetric pathway of the recurrent laryngeal nerves. The left recurrent laryngeal nerve courses below the aorta before ascending to the larynx.

& Zuckerbraun, 1990). Contributing factors include careless or rapid intubation by inexperienced personnel, malpositioning of the head during insertion, and the application of cricoid pressure. Forces on the arytenoid cartilage can be exerted by the distal part of the endotracheal tube may cause anterior and inferior displacement of the arytenoid cartilage (Rieger, Brunne, & Striebel, 1997; Shafei, el-Kholy, Azmy, al-Ebrahim, & al-Ebrahim, 1997). This type of trauma can lead to edema of the laryngeal vestibule, trachea, and surrounding pharyngeal structures, and in the patient with long-term intubation, may be a prognosticator for poor outcome and even death (Burns, Dayal, Scott, van Nostrand, & Bryce, 1979). The edema can lead to reduced range of motion of the structures of the pharynx and reduce the afferent input that is so important to triggering and organizing the pharyngeal stage of the swallow.

CSE 4 B. Resonance

The effect of an impairment of velopharyngeal closure on swallowing usually is fairly straightforward. At the time of the interview, the patient invariably will report events of nasal regurgitation (food or liquid entering the nasopharynx) during the swallow. The patient also may have difficulty in pulling liquid through a straw. Straw drinking requires closure of the nasal port to create negative interoral pressure that draws the material through the straw. The report of these symptoms invariably is accompanied by hypernasality during speech. The failure of the velum to close off the nasopharyngeal port during swallowing can be due to neurologic disease affecting the cranial nerves but it also can be due to surgical effects.

The velum rises and closes off the nasopharynx in a sphincter-like movement that is actualized by the contraction of the tensor veli palatini, levator palatini, and superior pharyngeal constrictor. During the height of the pharyngeal swallow, when pharyngeal pressures are being applied to the bolus, incomplete closure provides a path of least resistance for the moving bolus and it flows superiorly through the open sphincter. Patients who suffer from sleep apnea or demonstrate excessively troublesome snoring behaviors are treated surgically to make the nasopharynx more patent. The oropharynx is stripped of

the tonsils and the excessive mucosal folds of the nasopharynx are removed (Finkelstein, Talmi, Nachmani, Hauben, & Zohar, 1992). This procedure, known as uvulopalatopharyngoplasty, produces the beneficial effect of reduced apneic episodes during sleep and reduced snoring. It often has the negative result of velopharyngeal incompetence with subsequent nasal regurgitation (Katsantonis, Friedman, Krebs, & Walsh, 1987). A similar reduction in function of the velopharyngeal sphincter is seen in the surgical removal of tumors (Zohar, Buler, Shvilli, & Sabo, 1998).

CSE 5. POSITIONING

Eliciting changes in position during the clinical examination allows the examiner to probe for the patient's capacity to change position or posture later in the assessment process. Repositioning the head and trunk has been shown to cause changes in the biomechanics of the swallow and on bolus flow patterns (Chang, Rosendall, & Finlayson, 1996; DeToledo, Icovinno, & Haddad, 1993; Drake, O'Donoghue, Bartram, Lindsay, & Greenwood, 1996; Logemann, Rademaker, Pauloski, & Kahrilas, 1994; Ohmae, Karaho, Hanyu, Murase, Kitahara, & Inouye, 1997; Shaker, Junlong, Zafar, Achal, Jianmin, & Zhuei, 1994).

Head Positioning

Patients with glossectomy or other oral propulsive problems may benefit from the head extension position which allows gravity to act on the bolus causing to enter into the pharynx more readily (Logemann, 1995) (see Figure 2–2).

Some patients with a delayed pharyngeal stage or reduced oral containment of the bolus may benefit from the chin-down posture. In some patients, this position allows for better oral control as the bolus is held in a more anterior location in the oral cavity before the initiation of the pharyngeal stage of the swallow. It also changes the dimensions of the pharynx, positioning the tongue base closer in proximity to the posterior pharyngeal wall. However, this posture has not been shown to be uniform in its effect on changing the physical dimensions of the pharynx or on changing the physiology of the swallow (Shanahan, Logemann, Rademaker, Pauloski, & Kahrilas,

1993). This position may allow some patients with reduced posterior tongue base retraction to make tongue base contact with the posterior pharyngeal wall more easily increasing the effectiveness of the contraction (Logemann, 1995; Logemann, Kahrilas, Kobara, & Vakil, 1989). Head rotation toward the weakened side in patients with unilateral pharyngeal weakness has been found to guide the bolus away from the damaged side (Logemann et al., 1989).

Side-lying has been found to facilitate delivery of a more cohesive bolus resulting in the elicitation of a more coordinated oral and pharyngeal response in patients with pharyngeal delay due to lingual hypertonicity (Drake et al., 1997). The side-lying also allows pooled residue to rest along the lateral pharyngeal wall and prevents the residue from entering into the laryngeal inlet.

Patients that are capable of initiating purposeful position changes during the clinical examination likely will be able to perform them during an instrumental examination. Should the positioning yield a positive result, it can be assumed that the patient will begin to use it purposefully to reduce the effect of the swallowing impairment. Patients with substantial language or cognitive defects or restricted head movement will have more difficulty achieving beneficial results from postural and position changes (Rasley, Logemann, Kahrilas, Rademaker, Pauloski, & Dodds, 1993).

CSE 9. DENTITION/PERIODONTIUM

In the absence of trauma, tooth loss usually is preceded by poor oral hygiene. Decay eventu-ally leads to discomfort and the ultimate removal of offending teeth that do not fall out due to poor alveolar attachment associated with periodontal disease. Good oral health is thought to be largely dependent on the control of plaque. Plaque control requires a combination of natural defenses (adequate salivary flow) and proactive hygienic activities (toothbrushing). Saliva has both antibacterial and acid buffering qualities that, when combined with the physical properties of flow, wash away much of the plaque in the oral cavity. Some plaque will always remain behind and removal requires brushing of the teeth and gums. When either of these protective components is missing oral health is at risk of breaking down (see Figures 2–17 and 2–18). Colonization of the oral cavity with bacteria is exacerbated in patients with poor salivary flow and in patients that are dependent on another individual for the provision of oral care (Langmore, Terpenning, Schork, Chen, Murray, Lopatin, & Loesche, 1998).

Tooth decay begins with bacteria, found in plaque, contacting a tooth surface. Cariogenic bacteria strains, such as Streptococcus mutans, begin to produce acids that attack the tooth surface through a process of demineralization (McCabe, Adamkiewicz, & Pekovic, 1991).

The diagnosis of caries depends on the correct identification of demineralized enamel. This demineralization usually is identified as grayish blotches on the surface of crowns. They are more difficult to identify when positioned in the interproximal surfaces. It is important to remember that demineralization

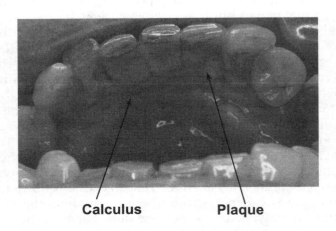

Calculus   Plaque

Figure 2–17. Severe plaque and calculus.

Broken teeth   Receding gingiva

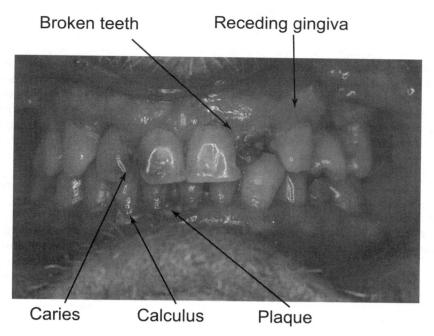

Caries   Calculus   Plaque

Figure 2–18. Poor dentition and periodontium. Receding gingiva, plaque, calculus, carious and broken teeth are evident.

precedes bacterial infection; therefore, dentine may be demineralized but remain uninfected. Visual evidence of carious lesions is not reliable and requires radiographic evidence to verify the extent of bacterial infection (Ricketts, Kidd, & Beighton, 1995).

When teeth are missing, or when malocclusion is present, the patient is at greater risk for the development of caries. This is because food particles and plaque are more likely to accumulate and remain where there is no occlusal contact with an opposing tooth (Ekstrand, Nielsen, Carvalho, & Thylstrup, 1993)

The number of residual teeth and chewing ability are closely related. As the number of missing teeth increases, chewing ability decreases (Oesterberg & Steen, 1982). Loss of posterior teeth without replacement leads to the greatest impairment in chewing (Van der Bilt, Olthoff, Bosman, & Oosterhaven, 1993). Replacing missing dentition with prostheses may improve the individual's chewing function but does not restore chewing function to that of an individual with full dentition (Agerberg & Carlsson, 1981)

Interestingly enough, a full denture wearer's self perception of chewing ability is thought to be too optimistic. In a study by Slagter, Olthoff, Bosman, and Steen (1992), full denture wearer's perception of masticatory ability was compared to actual performance in reducing a tough test food while chewing. There was a weak correlation between the objective score and the patient's own evaluation, with patients believing they performed better than they actually did.

As the number of functioning teeth and functional units decreases, patients adapt to their edentulousness (Liedberg, Spiechowicz, & Owall, 1995). Although some individuals may be able to adapt well and maintain nutrition without teeth, others see their impairment become a disability and, eventually, a handicap. A maladaptation includes food selection changes (Chauncey, Muench, Kapur, & Wayler, 1984; Wayler & Chauncy, 1983; Yurkstas & Emerson, 1964) that may yield less nutrients. Patients with dental functional impairments tend to consume soft, easily chewed foods that may be low in fiber and nutrient density (Hildebrandt et al., 1995). Further, fully edentulous individuals without dentures have long been observed to be deficient in serum levels of nutrients and in other nutrition markers compared with the dentate (Chen & Lowenstein, 1984; Makila, 1964).

Good medical health and good oral/dental health are linked. Edentulous individuals are known to be at a greater risk of mortality from any cause (De Stephano, Anda, Kahn, et al., 1993). A study of the dental/oral health of geriatric patients with diverse medical backgrounds was performed by Loesch, Abrams, Terpenning, and Bretz (1995). In this study it was found that only 6% of a group of patients with longevity (>80 years) and low reported medical disease were edentulous. In this healthy group those that were dentate had only 4.5 missing teeth on average. In the group of patients with poor health, it was found that they were younger (<70 years) and that 49% were edentulous. These patients with poor health had an average of 12 missing teeth and 5 decayed teeth.

The relationship between oral health and systemic health may be one of cause and effect, or the two may co-occur. Hildebrandt et al. (1995) indicated that there was a relationship between functional units and overall systemic health. It was theorized that the loss of functional occlusion in a patient occurs over a period of several years and that this slow development reflects the underlying philosophy or choice pattern of the individual in seeking medical and dental treatment. It was felt that the co-occurrence of poor oral health and poor systemic health was likely to be found in individuals who use dental and health professionals sporadically and place little value on preventive medicine. The institutionalized elderly in particular are more likely to have dental disease and less likely to seek dental services (Beck, 1992). Hildebrandt also found that patients with fewer functional units had increased gingival bleeding which can lead to the development of pathogenic microflora. It

has long been known that oropharyngeal colonization with gram-negative bacilli is associated with increasing severity of illness (Johanson, Blackstock, Pierce, et al., 1970; Valenti, Trudell, & Bentley, 1978). This development predisposes an individual to pneumonia (Bartlett 1979; Langmore et al., 1998; Limeback, 1988), acute myocardial infarction (Mattila, Nieminen, Baltonen, et al., 1989), and stroke (Syrjanen, Peltola, Baltonen, Iivanainen, Kastem, & Huttunen, 1989).

For the elderly dysphagic patient, maintenance of the health of the oral cavity is paramount. Patients with unilateral paresis affecting the dominant hand will not likely be able to coordinate toothbrushing in their premorbid fashion. If a patient is severely debilitated, dependence on another for oral care becomes a necessity. It has been reported that patients who need assistance with oral hygiene had more plaque and gingivitis than those who brushed their own teeth (Jette, Feldman, & Douglass, 1993; Vigild, 1988) (see Figure 2–19). It is important to remember that, during oral preparation, food and liquid come in contact with bacteria and that the bacteria will be transported with the food once propelled out of the oral cavity. In the dysphagic patient who demonstrates aspiration, this can be an important point. Langmore et al. (1998) found that several conditions were independent predictors of aspiration pneumonia. The predictors associated with oral health were the presence of decayed teeth, infrequent toothbrushing, and dependence on another for oral care. In the same publication, a model for the acquisition of aspiration pneumonia

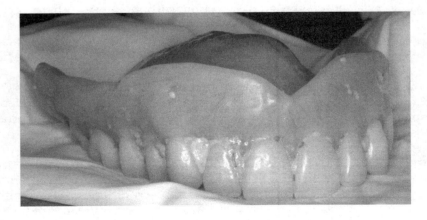

Figure 2–19. Poorly maintained dentures reflect poor oral hygiene. Oral hygiene is often ignored in elderly edentulous patients who are reliant on others for assistance.

was presented. The model lists the colonization of the oral cavity with altered oropharyngeal flora as a prerequisite.

CSE 10. SALIVARY FLOW/ APPEARANCE OF ORAL MUCOSA

Oral health is dependent on salivary flow for several essential protective duties. Salivary flow has antimicrobial properties. It keeps the oral mucosa moist, buffers destructive acids produced by bacteria, washes away plaques, lubricates the bolus during the oral stage of swallowing, and buffers gastric contents that find their way into the esophagus.

The flow of saliva originates from the major and minor salivary glands, which are distributed throughout the oral cavity (see Figure 2–20). Saliva is constantly being produced in a "resting" or unstimulated fashion. The parotid, submandibular, and sublingual glands make up the major salivary glands. During rest, the submandibular gland accounts for the bulk of salivary production, followed by the parotid and sublingual glands, respectively. During stimulation, however, the parotid gland accounts for two thirds of the saliva produced (Nachlas & Johns, 1991).

When salivary flow is compromised, oral health is compromised and the risk of systemic disease is elevated. The sequela to poor salivary flow is xerostomia, a "dry mouth" condition that is physically unpleasant for patients (see Figure 2–21). Rhodus and Brown (1990) found that the nearly one in five elderly patients who suffered from xerostomia avoided eating enough calories to maintain nutrition due to a decrease in taste sensation and inability to lubricate food adequately during mastication. In the same study, 100% of the seniors with xerostomia perceived the taste and quality of food to be "poor." None of the control subjects (without xerostomia) found the same food to be "poor," and 77% found it to be "good." During the course of the study, institutionalized elderly subjects with xerostomia demonstrated signs of compromised nutrition with albumin levels out of the normal range. Significantly fewer normals demonstrated the reduced albumin levels. This study illustrates the progressive diminution of function that may accompany impaired saliva production. A complaint of dry mouth may seem innocuous enough during the interview process but should be a red flag for the clinician to probe for associated signs of malnutrition.

Xerostomia has effects that go beyond the physical discomfort of a dry mouth and malnutrition. It is well-established that, when salivary flow is reduced, particularly from the parotid gland, the pH of the solution is lowered. Lowered pH in the oral cavity allows certain pathogenic organisms such as *Klebsiella pneumoniae* to adhere to buccal epithelial cells (Ayars, Altman, & Fretwell, 1982). The adherence of this and other pathogens puts the dysphagic patient with aspiration at greater risk of extended colonization and eventual pneumonia.

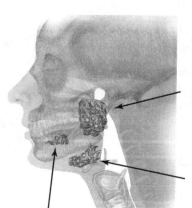

Parotid gland

Submandibular gland

Sublingual gland

Figure 2–20. Location of parotid and sublingual and submandibular glands.

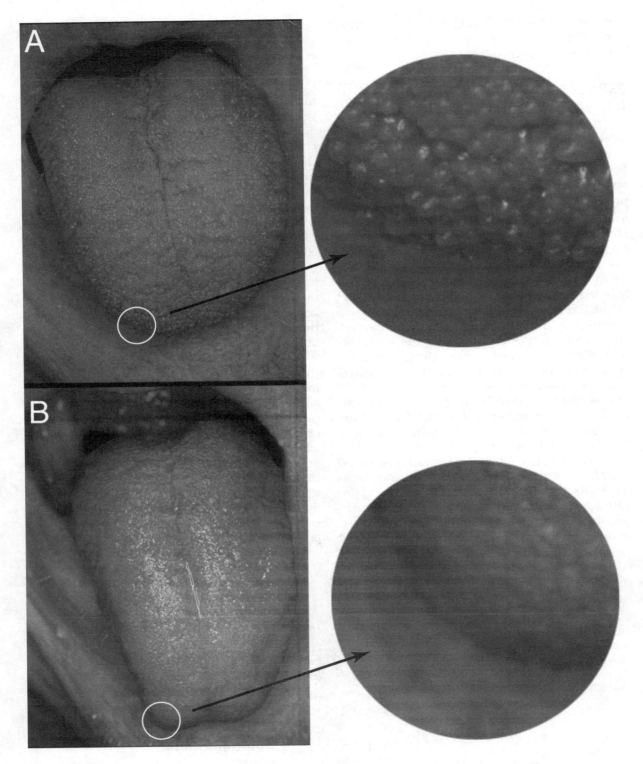

Figure 2–21. A. Severely dehydrated patient. **B.** Same patient after rehydration.

Hyposalivation with xerostomia can occur as a result of dehydration, iatrogenic origins related to the side effects of medication or irradiation, or as a symptom of systemic disease.

Dehydration

Although the association of dehydration and hyposalivation was perceived by many to be strong, objective evidence of this association was, until recently, lacking. Ship and Fischer (1997) found that dehydration was associated with decreased salivary gland flow rates. Unstimulated and stimulated parotid salivary flow rates were compared to lab values obtained from the blood that reflect hydration after a period of fasting. All subjects experienced a significant decrease in parotid gland salivary output and increased levels of hematocrit, hemoglobin, plasma protein, and creatinine during dehydration. Following the period of dehydration, patients were carefully rehydrated, but salivary flow did not return to baseline. This study makes evident the precarious balance of health and impairment in the fragile dysphagic senior, who may suffer sustained effects from an episode of dehydration.

Iatrogenic Hyposalivation

Irradiation

Hyposalivation occurs as the result of damage to salivary glands when they are included in the radiation field during treatment of head and and neck cancers. Taste loss and xerostomia were significantly correlated with the proportions of both tongue and parotid glands within the radiation treatment fields (Fernando, Patel, Billingham, et al., 1995).

Radiotherapy-induced hyposalivation encourages oral candidal colonization that often leads to oral/pharyngeal candidiasis. Candidiasiss is a designation for a group of mucosal conditions that originate from the colonization of the candida fungi. The organism usually presents as a whitish plaque and lives on the surface mucosa of different structures of the oral cavity. In a study of candidal colonization in patients undergoing irradiation, Ramirez, Amador, Silverman, Mayer, Tyler, and Quivey (1997) found that all patients complained of progressive xerostomia and that there was a significant increase in the prevalence of positive candidal cultures. At baseline, 43% of the patients had signs of colonization, at the completion of radiotherapy, 62%, and on follow-up, 75%.

Medication

Probably the most common cause of hyposalivation is the use of medication with a salivary secretion inhibitory side effect (Kaandorp, deBaat, & Michels, 1994). It has been shown that the longer an individual continues a xerostomic medication the lower the stimulated and unstimulated salivary output (Navazesh et al., 1996). Medication can affect salivation through a number of different mechanisms. A wide variety of drugs are capable of increasing or decreasing salivary flow by mimicking autonomic nervous system actions. Drugs also can indirectly affect salivation by altering fluid and electrolyte balance or by affecting blood flow to the glands (Schubert & Izutsu, 1987). Antihypertensives, sedatives, and female sex hormones have been found to be responsible for xerostomia (Hakeberg, Berggren, & Hagglin, 1997; Sullivan, 1997).

Tricyclic antidepressants such as clomipramine and anticholinergic medications are known to cause xerostomia (Lader, 1996; Leinonen, Lepola, Koponen, Mehtonen, & Rimon, 1997) by interfering with the perception of the stimuli of salivation (Ayars, Altman, & Fretwell, 1982).

Candida infection also often presents as a secondary infection produced by broadspectrum antibiotic use.

Oral Intubation

Oral intubation for ventilation support requires the oral cavity to be constantly open to accomodate the ventilation tube. Orally intubated patients are observed to display severe xerostomia, lesions of the lip, tongue, and buccal mucosa, and fungal colonizations (Treloar & Stechmiller, 1995).

The biomechanics of the pharyngeal swallow are clearly and severely compromised by the presence of the endotracheal tube. Aspiration of pathogenic oropharyngeal secretions likely contributes to the nosocomial pneumonias so often observed in the ventilated patient.

Systemic Disease

Sjögren's syndrome is the manifestation of an idiopathic autoimmune process. The disease is described classically as a grouping of three conditions: dry mouth, dry eyes, and the presence of an autoimmune disorder. Patients with Sjögren's syndrome are likely to be women with an average age of onset of 50 years. The xerostomia is associated with respiratory problems, specifically small airway disease (Constantopoulos, Papadimitrion, & Moutsopoulos, 1985), and autonomic neuropathies (Oobayashi & Miyawaki, 1995).

The patient with Sjögren's syndrome likely will experience chronic exacerbation and remission and are treated symptomatically with artificial saliva. The individual in the acute phase of the disease is advised to maintain a careful oral hygiene regimen to avoid oral infections. Table 2–20 summarizes the various etiologies of hyposalivation.

CSE 11. ORAL/PHARYNGEAL SENSATION/GAG

CSE 11 A 1. Tongue Sensation

The tongue is one of the most richly innervated structures in the human body. As food enters the mouth, there is a virtual bombardment of sensory input directed to the central nervous system. Almost one third of the cortical and thalamic sensory and receptive fields serve the face and mouth, with the tongue having a large individual share. There are a number of subconscious calculations made during the oral preparatory stage of the swallow that allow the individual to account for bolus size, consistency, temperature, and palatability.

For this task, we are assessing only the response to light touch. The anterior one third of the tongue is richly innervated with receptors that are very sensitive to light touch. The anterior tongue and upper lip are, for instance, much more sensitive to light touch than is the finger tip (Maeyama & Plattig, 1989). More posterior and lateral locations will be less senstive than anterior and midline locations (Ringel & Ewanowski, 1965). As aging occurs, sensation remains good, with some slight dimunition in sensation after age 80 years (Calhoun, Gibson, Hartley, Minton, & Hokanson, 1992).

The cranial nerves supplying sensory innervation to the tongue are: V (trigeminal), VII (facial), IX (glossopharyngeal), and (X) vagus. The anterior two thirds of the tongue are supplied by the lingual nerve from the mandibular branch of V (trigeminal nerve). The lingual branch of IX (glossopharyngeal nerve) breaks into two segments that provide sensation for the sulcus terminalis and postsulcal region, respectively. Proprioceptive nerve endings are innervated by the facial nerve (VII). The area of the tongue superior to the epiglottis is innervated by the vagus nerve (X).

There are a great number and variety of sensory end organs in the tongue. The sensory system includes receptors that respond to touch, pressure, vibration, position, pain, and temperature. At one time, it was believed that

Table 2–20. Etiology of hyposalivation and oral lesions.

Etiology	Clinical Presentation
Dehydration	Xerostomia
Systemic disease	
Sjögren's syndrome	Xerostomia, dry eyes, dry skin
Iatrogenic	
Medication	Xerostomia
Anticholinergics	Xerostomia
Tricyclics	Xerostomia
Antihypertensives	Xerostomia
Sedatives	Xerostomia
Female sex hormones	Xerostomia, burning mouth
Broad spectrum antibiotics	Xerostomia, candidiasis
Irradiation	Xerostomia, candidiasis
Oral intubation	Xerostomia, oral lesions, candidiasis
Behavioral	
Mouth breathing	Xerostomia, oral lesions, candidiasis

certain receptors only responded to specific stimuli; that is, thermal receptors only responded to changes in temperature, taste receptors to taste, and baroreceptors to pressure. Current thinking suggests that most receptors respond maximally to specific stimuli but also respond, to a lesser degree, to other stimuli. An individual's perception of a specific stimuli (e.g., bolus flow or temperature) is probably a sum of information sent from several types of peripheral receptors (Calhoun et al., 1992; Capra, 1995).

Sensation may become impaired after dental surgery or resection of the tongue or mandible. Irradiation also will diminish the effectiveness of the sensory end organs in the oral mucosa. Bolus formation and control will be diminished in these patients. Mapping of the oral cavity for sensation ability and disability will assist the clinician in planning treatment strategies for those patients with oral stage problems following surgery or irradiation.

CSE 11 A 2. Sensation: Faucial Pillars

The faucial pillars are formed by the palatoglossus muscle (anterior faucial pillar) and palatopharyngeus muscle (posterior faucial pillar). The anterior pillars form a vertical webbing that extends from the velum superiorly to the dorsum of the tongue inferiorly. The posterior pillars extend from velum superiorly, interdigitate with the the superior constrictor, and course inferiorly to insert in the lower lateral pharynx (Kennedy & Keuhn, 1989). Sensory innervation is provided by the glossopharyngeal nerve (IX) and the superior laryngeal nerve, a branch of the vagus (X). Some sensory nerves in the faucial pillars are touch/pressure specific and travel along the superior laryngeal nerve to the nucleus tractus solitarus in the brain stem (Rosenbek, Roecker, Wood, & Robbins, 1996).

Stimulation of the faucial pillars is thought to be an important component in the triggering of the pharyngeal stage of the swallow (Miller, 1982). Several authors have discussed the benefit of stimulating this region in hopes of eliciting a more timely onset of the pharyngeal stage of the swallow (Lazzara, Lazarus, & Longemann, 1986; Logemann & Kahrilis, 1990; Rosenbek et al., 1991, 1996; Selinger, Prescott, & Hoffman, 1994; Selinger, Prescott, & McKinley, 1990;). In these studies,

the stimulation is applied to the faucial pillars via a cold laryngeal mirror in the hopes of eliminating or reducing a delay in the initiation of the pharyngeal stage of the swallow. For a complete discussion of thermal tactile stimulation see the excellent review of this treatment in Huckabee and Pelletier (1998).

CSE 11 A 3./CSE 11 B. Posterior Pharyngeal Wall/Gag

The gag reflex is a sudden tonic reaction to noxious stimuli in the posterior oropharynx. It is thought to be a protective reflex that acts to expel material from the pharynx by means of shortening and narrowing the pharynx.

The elicitation of the gag requires the integration of sensory input (vomit, food particulate, reflux, or probing with the applicator) and a motor response (contraction of the pharynx, elevation of the velum, and depression of the tongue). The key visual sign that the gag has occurred is the motor response of velar elevation, narrowing of the oropharyngeal port, and depression of the tongue base. Davies, Kidd, Stone, and MacMahon (1995) found that interobserver reliability was quite good for determining pharyngeal sensation but less reliable when attempting to identify the gag reflex. When in doubt, it may be useful to ask those patients capable of responding whether they were gagging or just pulling away from aversive stimuli. The mucosa posterior to the facial pillars and along the posterior pharyngeal wall is thought to be the most likely location for the elicitation of a gag reflex and, in most patients, the gag will be elicited by stimulating the posterior pharyngeal wall (see Figure 2–22).

There will be a variety of responses to the probing of the oral cavity. Some patients will demonstrate a strong gag with the simple placement of a tongue blade in the oral cavity. Observing the posterior oropharynx may be difficult in these patients. The hyperactive gag reflex is well-recognized in the dental community and frequently hampers the treatment process (Ansari, 1994; Barsby, 1994; Daniel, 1982; Friedman & Weintraub, 1995; Robb & Crothers, 1996; Roberts, 1994). Patients with a hyperactive gag who require palatal prosthesis, obturators, or dentures often abandon the devices due to the constant stimulation and subsequent "gagging" reaction. When refer-

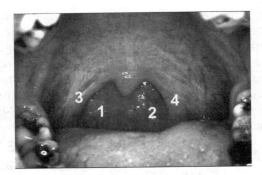

1– Right posterior pharyngeal wall
2– Left posterior pharyngeal wall
3– Right faucial pillar
4– Left faucial pillar

Figure 2–22. Location of stimulus points for eliciting the gag reflex.

ring a patient for the fitting of an oral prosthesis, it would be wise to characterize carefully the nature of the gag reflex to the prosthodontist. This information may assist in the planning for special fabrication of the device and may avoid costly return visits for fitting and refitting.

For a number of years, conventional wisdom has suggested that the absence of a "gag" reflex is associated with a swallowing impairment and increased risk of aspiration. This thinking is so pervasive that this single sign is often the catalyst that initiates the consultation for a swallowing assessment or, too often, initiates an order for a feeding tube. In fact, many normal individuals will perceive the sensation of posterior pharyngeal wall probing without demonstrating any sign of gagging. It is estimated that between 13% and 37% of normal subjects will demonstrate no gag response regardless of the pressure applied to the posterior wall (Bleach, 1993; Davies, Kidd, Stone, & MacMahon, 1995; DeVita, Spierer-Rundback, 1990; Leder, 1996, 1997; Smithard, 1996). The gag reflex is more likely to be absent in the elderly (Davies et al., 1995).

It is important to remember that the absence of the gag can be normal, but it also can be absent due to poor pharyngeal sensation, a weak or paretic motor response to sensory input or a poor conduction of sensory input and motor response through the brain stem. Linden and Siebens (1983) found that patients with pharyngeal dysphagia and absent gag

were more likely to penetrate the airway during a videofluoroscopic study of swallowing. Horner et al. (1990) studied aspiration in bilateral stroke patients and, through logistic regression, found that aspiration on videofluoroscopy could be best identified by the clinical signs of abnormal voluntary cough, abnormal gag reflex, or both. In a validation study (Horner et al., 1993), the presence of normal cough and gag identified patients at low risk for aspiration. When the presence of abnormal cough and abnormal gag co-occurred, patients were identified to be at high risk.

The presence of the gag reflex should not be considered a sign of safety. The same health professionals that entrust the absence of gag to signify risk likely will trust the presence of a gag to indicate safety. In a study of eight elderly men with myasthenia gravis, five experienced silent aspiration despite gag reflexes and the ability to cough on command (Kluin, Bromberg, Feldman, & Simmons, 1996). As always, it is best to integrate the findings from this section with the findings of the entire examination and interview before committing to an assessment or treatment paradigm.

CSE 12. TONGUE MOVEMENT/STRENGTH

Loss of motor control and/or strength of the tongue can have a great effect on the efficiency and safety of the swallow. During the clinical examination we are, unfortunately, only able to observe movements and make gross estimations of strength for the anterior two thirds of the tongue. Further, the tasks performed are surrogates for lingual movements that may be executed very differently during oral preparation, bolus containment, and bolus propulsion.

The tongue is divided into intrinsic and extrinsic muscle groups. The intrinsic muscles include the superior longitudinal , inferior longitudinal, transverse, and vertical muscles. The hypoglossal (VII) cranial nerve provides motor innervation to all of the intrinsic lingual muscles. The intrinsic muscles lift the tongue tip, depress the tongue tip, and flatten and narrow the blade of the tongue. The extrinsic muscles include the genioglossus, styloglossus, hyoglossus, and palatoglossus muscles. All of these muscles derive motor innervation from the hypoglossal (VII) cranial nerve, with the exception of the palatoglossus, which receives motor innervation from the spinal accessory nerve (IX). These muscles are attached to the soft palate, mandible, and hyoid bone, which provide a skeletal base from which these muscles act to protrude and retract the tongue.

Dyskinesia

Fasciculations, by themselves, will not affect the function of the swallow, but generally are a sign that neurologic dysfunction is present (Dworkin & Hartman, 1979; Jannetta & Robbins, 1980). Observation of this sign should trigger a referral to a neurologist for further workup (Talacko & Reade, 1990). Radiation therapy may damage the hypoglossal nerve and cause myokymia of the tongue which results in muscle twitches that appear similar to fasciculations (Poncelet, Auger, & Silber, 1996; Wang, Liao, Ju, Lin, Wang, Wu, & Chung, 1993).

Dyskinesias of the tongue are common in patients with tardive dyskinesia due to side effects from extended administration of neuroleptic drugs (Caliguri, Jeste, & Harris 1989; Fudge, Thailer, Alpert, Intrator, & Sison, 1991; Sachdev, 1992). These dyskinesias may appear to be of dramatic import during the clinical examination but there is very little research directly relating impaired swallow function and safety with lingual dyskinesia

(Hayashi, Nishikawa, Koga, Uchida, & Yamawaki, 1997; Yassa & Yal, 1986). Oral preparatory stage problems may predominate in these patients as delivery of food or liquid to the mouth and mastication may be problematic.

Intention tremor or action tremor may become obvious on protrusion. This is a tremor that does not become active until there is a purposeful movement of a limb or other structure. Tremor may play a part in the transition between oral and pharyngeal stages of the swallow. The tongue and, to a degree, the soft palate are employed to control the bolus prior to the initiation of the pharyngeal stage of the swallow. Early loss of control of the bolus results in premature leakage of material from the oral cavity and can result in penetration of the unprotected airway. An uncoordinated transition from oral stage to pharyngeal stage, also known as "pharyngeal delay," can result in the penetration of the unprotected airway. This occurs when the bolus is propelled out of the oral cavity without a timely, reflexive pharyngeal response to the oncoming bolus. Leopold and Kagel (1996, 1997) found that patients with progressive supranuclear palsy (PSP) and Parkinson's disease demonstrated a number of uncoordinated lingual movements. These movements included impaired posterior lingual displacement, noncohesive lingual transfer from the oral cavity to the pharynx, and excessive leakage of the oral bolus to the pharynx prior to active transfer.

It may be that patients with bradykinesia and tremor are incapable of overcoming the force of the rhythmic contractions during volitional acts. Slowness and multiple lingual pumping prior to the initiation of swallowing is frequently seen in patient's with Parkinson's disease. Hunker and Abbs (1984), in an excellent review of the physiology of Parkinsonian orofacial tremors, suggested that individuals with Parkinson's disease may demonstrate bradykinesia during volitional movements. The authors projected that the overall slowness of movement may be due to the fact that they are "unable to initiate a contraction until it coincides with the involuntary agonistic burst of a tremor oscillation. It is possible that this "forced" initiation of the contraction during bolus propulsion, will not be coordinated with subsequent airway protective movements that must be coordinated closely later in the pharyngeal swallow.

Protrusion

Unilateral weakness of the extrinsic and/or intrinsic muscles of the tongue will result in a deviation away from the weakened side. As the muscles move to extend the tongue outside of the oral cavity, the unilaterally weakened side will not provide an opposing force to the muscles of the stronger side. This results in the stronger side pushing the weaker side arcing over the midline point.

The patient may also suffer sensory loss on the weakened side. This finding should be compared to the data collected from the oral sensory section. Unilateral weakness and loss of sensation likely will impede the efficiency of mastication and bolus manipulation.

Strength

This task assesses anterior and superior pressure exerted by the tongue inside of the oral cavity. Although it cannot produce the precise measurement of pressures exacted by the tongue during the propulsion of a bolus from the oral cavity, it does allow the clinician to determine gross normality or weakness of the tongue, in a position at which tongue pressure is applied during the swallow.

Chi-Fishman and Stone (1996) used electropalatography to determine oral lingual movement patterns during swallowing. The authors found that the contact points of the elevating tongue and stationary palate are sequential, systematic, and stereotypical across patients. Movement from front to back and lateral to midline typified tongue contact during bolus propulsion.

Electropalatography allows the clinician to visualize placement of the tongue during the swallow but it does not measure pressure. Tongue blade pressures have been measured in normal young and elderly subjects using strain gauge devices during maximal pressure tasks and during swallowing (Robbins, Levine, Wood, Roecker, & Luschei, 1995). The maximal pressure task was a nonswallowing task and required the subject to push as hard as possible against several pressure sensing devices distributed across the tongue. Maximal isometric pressure tasks showed that young normals demonstrated significantly greater tongue blade pressure than during the swallowing task, a finding supported by the re-

search of Crow and Ship (1996). In the Robbins et al. (1995) study, the peak swallowing pressures were not significantly different for the young and elderly. This would indicate that the young have a reserve capacity of strength that is not used during swallowing and that the elderly have a decline in their reserve capacity. The authors suggested the following implications for this finding. Older people may be working harder to produce adequate swallowing pressures, and age-related illness may put geriatric patients at higher risk for dysphagia, thus further complicating recovery.

Miller and Watkin (1996) found that, in normal subjects, anterior lingual force varied with the viscosity of the material swallowed. A transducer array situated along the anterior margin of the tongue showed an increment of force that indicated greater force amplitude and force duration as viscosity increased. These findings are in agreement with a study of forceful and attenuated swallows (Ponderoux & Kahrilas, 1995). In this study, it was found that tongue propulsive force and clearing pressure during swallows showed substantial modulation for bolus viscosity. This increase in propulsive force was reproduced by volitional control during forcefully attenuated swallows (hard swallows). This suggests that, if a patient has the reserve strength capacity, a forceful swallow can overcome impairments seen during unattenuated swallows. According to Robbins et al. (1995), this may obviate the use of attenuated swallows for elderly subjects without reserve capacity. These finding would suggest that changes in the viscosity of materials can be tailored to a patient's ability. It would seem that thin liquids would require less effort to swallow for patients with lingual weakness. This solution may work for some patients with weakness and good oral control and coordination, but is problematic for patients with poor oral control.

CSE 13. VELAR ELEVATION

The clinician now will have had the opportunity to listen for signs of nasality during speech, assess movement of the palate during the elicitation of the gag, and assess movement during phonation.

The purpose of velar elevation is to isolate transiently the nasal port during speech, swallowing and expectoration. Although the velopharyngeal port is capable of many degrees of closure during speech, the closure during swallowing is complete.

The muscles of velar elevation are divided into intrinsic (musculus uvuli) and extrinsic muscles (tensor veli palatini, levator veli palatini, palatopharyngeus, and palatoglossus). The musculus uvuli's efferent signals are provided by the spinal accessory nerve (XI). When contracted, this muscle is thought to provide rigidity to the body of the velum, allowing more rapid excursion without distortion from forces applied by the extrinsic muscles during elevation. This muscle also provides midline bulk on the nasal aspect of the velum that contributes to the eminence of tissue contacting the posterior pharyngeal wall during the swallow (Huang, Lee, & Rajendran, 1997).

The tensor veli palatini muscle receives motor signals from the mandibular branch of the trigeminal nerve. This muscle is reported to function in a number of ways that include depressing and elevating the anterior velum (Kennedy & Kuehn, 1989).

The levator veli palatini, palatoglossus, and palatopharyngeus muscles all receive motor innervation from the the spinal accessory nerve (XI). The glossopharyngeal (IX) and vagus nerve (X) have also been identified as combining with the spinal accessory nerve in the motor suppy of the velopharynx by different authors (Kennedy & Kuehn, 1989). The levator veli palatini moves the velum superiorly and posteriorly. The body of the palatopharyngeus makes up the posterior faucial pillar and, when contracted, pulls the velum inferiorly. The palatoglossus muscle pulls the velum inferiorly and anteriorly. The body of the palatoglossus makes up the anterior faucial pillar. The muscles course through the velum and insert into the lateral aspect of the tongue (Kennedy & Kuehn, 1989). This muscle may assist in forming the posterior seal of the oral cavity by drawing the velum down to the dorsum of the tongue.

The velar elevation observed during the gag, yawn, and phonation is a surrogate for the velar elevation observed instrumentally during the swallow. Velopharyngeal closure patterns have been observed to vary with different tasks. Schneider (1997) observed different closure patterns via flexible transnasal endoscopy and found that the velum is moved independently during phonation, whereas additional lateral and posterior pharyngeal wall motion was observed during swallowing. The additional lateral movement during swallowing may be a function of the contraction of the palatopharyngeus and other longitudinal muscles of the pharynx acting to shorten the pharyngeal lumen during the swallow. The superior pharyngeal constrictor contributes additional posterior pharyngeal and lateral wall movement to close off the velopharynx during the swallow (Adachi, Kogo, Iida, Hamaguchi, & Matsuya, 1997).

CSE 14. VOLITIONAL SWALLOWS/ LARYNGEAL ELEVATION

Laryngeal elevation is one of the prime external indicators of a robust pharyngeal swallow. Among the functions of the elevating larynx is the anterior and superior movement away from the advancing bolus during the pharyngeal swallow. The principal function of laryngeal elevation is to open the upper esophageal sphincter (UES) by the application of traction to the anterior wall of the sphincter (see Figure 2–23). The UES is made up of the inferior pharyngeal constrictor, the cricopharyngeal muscle, and the circular muscle fibers of the upper esophagus. These muscles are surrounded by loose fatty tissue that allows the sphincter to travel as one unit with the larynx during laryngeal elevation (Nilsson, Isacsson, Isberg, & Schiratzki, 1989).

The larynx is elevated by the suprahyoid muscles: the mylohyoid, geniohyoid, anterior belly of the digastric, and the hyoglossus. The geniohyoid and hyoglossus receive motor innervation from the hypoglossal nerve (XII). Motor innervation for the mylohyoid and anterior digastric is supplied by the mylohyoid branch of the trigeminal nerve (V).

The event of laryngeal elevation, so often described in the literature, is in fact two distinct movements. The suspended hyoid bone moves separately from the thyroid and cricoid cartilages, which are fixed together by connective tissue. The initial contraction of the suprahyoid muscles apply traction to the hyoid bone from which the laryngeal cartilages are suspended. Once elevation of the hyoid is initiated, the thyrohyoid muscle contracts to pull the thyroid and cricoid cartilages superiorly along the same path as that of the elevating hyoid bone.

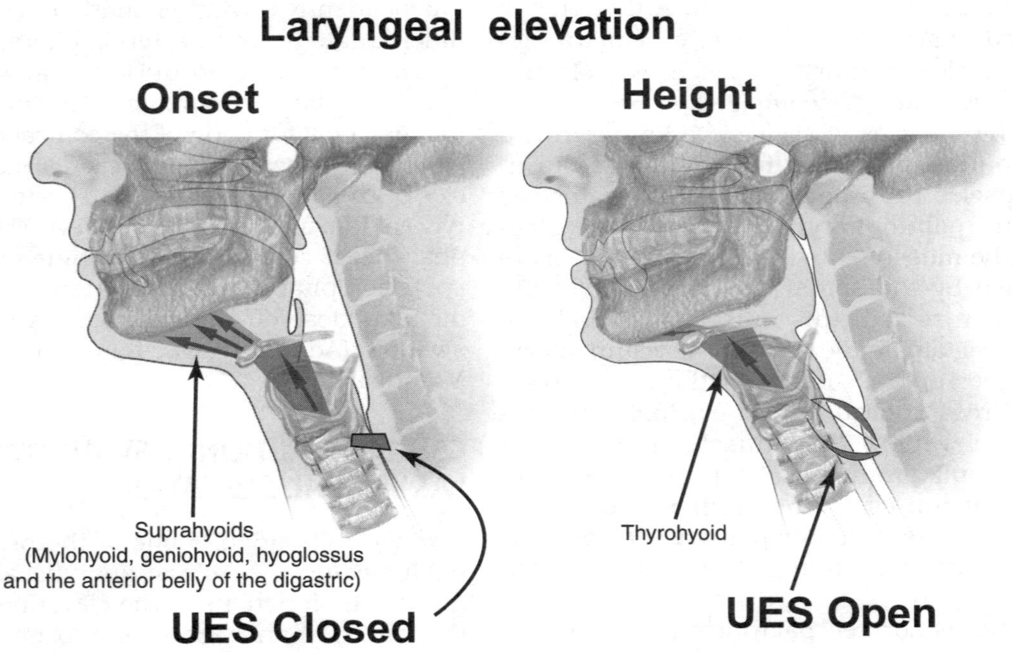

Laryngeal elevation

Onset

Height

Suprahyoids
(Mylohyoid, geniohyoid, hyoglossus
and the anterior belly of the digastric)

Thyrohyoid

UES Closed

UES Open

Figure 2–23. The supralaryngeal musculature contracts to elevate the larynx. The elevating larynx applies traction to open the relaxed UES.

The order of contraction of the suprahyoid muscles at the initiation of elevation varies in normal individuals. Spiro, Rendell, and Gay (1994) found that different individuals used all three muscles (geneohyoid, mylohyoid, and anterior belly of the digastric), whereas others used different combinations of the three muscles to raise the larynx.

Movement from rest to maximum elevation of the larynx occurs over a period of approximately one half-second and remains in the maximum position for approximately one-quarter to one third of a s (Doty & Bosma, 1956; Logemann, 1983; Spiro et al., 1994). A number of authors have investigated the range of motion of laryngeal elevation using fluoroscopy, ultrasound, and MRI (Cordaro & Sonies, 1993; Dantas, Kern, Bassey, Dodds, Kahrilas, Brasseur, Cook, & Lang, 1990; Dengel, Robbins, & Rosenbek, 1991; Furukawa, 1983; Hamlet, Ezzell, & Aref, 1993; Kahrilas, Lin, Chen, & Logemann, 1996; Lin, Chen, Hertz, & Kahrilas, 1996; Logemann et al., 1989; Nilsson et al., 1989; Sundgren, Maly, & Gullberg, 1993). The measurements of laryngeal elevation have included the tracking of vertical and horizontal movements of the hyoid, arytenoid, valleculae, and UES. In these studies, normal subjects

have been observed to move the larynx approximately 2–2.5 centimeters, from rest to maximum elevation.

All of the referenced studies have employed the use of digital plotters to determine objectively the extent of laryngeal elevation during the swallow during an instrumental examination. Even when experienced observers are employed, subjective visual estimation of adequacy of laryngeal elevation on fluoroscopic studies is highly variable, and has been shown to have poor interobserver reliability (Ekberg, Nylander, Fork, Sjoberg, Birch-Iensch, & Hillarp, 1988).

The clinician attempting to determine adequacy of elevation during the clinical examination using this method may have a difficult time judging the difference between normalcy and slight reductions in elevation. Given that the average diameter of a woman's ring finger is approximately 1.9 cm and average laryngeal elevation is over 2 cm, the failure of the thyroid notch to clear the span of the finger is a gross sign of reduced elevation.

When laryngeal elevation is impaired, it is expected that UES opening will be reduced. A reduction in UES opening prevents the unencumbered exit of food or liquid from the pharynx with resulting pharyngeal residue. Any aggregation of residue in the pharynx after the initial swallow increases the individual's risk of aspiration once respiration is resumed and the airway opens.

Laryngeal elevation can be impaired due to weakened suprahyoid musculature, as is observed in progressive neuromuscular diseases and/or in asthenia due to malnutrition. The larynx also can be prevented from elevating due to a "tethering" effect. "Tethering" can be the result of surgical scarring and/or fibrosis of the upper esophagus, as is often seen in patients that have undergone esophagectomy with irradiation of the tissues surrounding the site of anastomosis. A similar effect sometimes is observed in patients with tracheostomy tubes placed. In both scenarios, the suprahyoid and thyrohyoid muscles may contract with the same force as was observed premorbidly, but the traction forces are unable to overcome the tethering effect and a consequential reduction in UES opening occurs.

CSE 15-B. TIMING/SPEED

There is a large variation between and within normal subjects while preparing and swallowing foods of the same consistency (Hiiemae et al., 1995). The clinician seeking an objective measure will not find it here. The best that can be expected is an impression of slowness or delay. These numbers derived during this task also can be used as a baseline for later examinations.

In some subjects, a palpable struggle will occur before the initiation of the swallow. During this time, the bolus may be propelled volitionally from the oral cavity into the pharynx without initiation of the pharyngeal stage of the swallow. Alternately, the patient may hold the bolus in his mouth until the swallow is orchestrated and initiated. The clinician observing from the outside, without the ability to visually track the bolus through the pharynx, will, for the most part, be guessing as to when the bolus leaves the oral cavity and enters the pharynx. Another set of patients, typically with dementia or reduced sensorium, may take the bolus into their mouths and not attempt to manipulate the bolus for some time. In these cases, the clinician may request the patient to hold the material in their mouth until a command to swallow is issued. Elapsed time should start with the command and end

with laryngeal elevation. This will give the clinician a slightly better understanding of the coordination and speed of the onset of the reflexive swallow. In some patients, particularly those with cognitive deficits or apraxia, the clinician may observe considerable trouble organizing and executing the swallow on command. If this struggle is observed only when a command to swallow is issued, abandon this tact and accept the variability in timing to be a feature of the patient's swallow.

There are no hard and fast numbers that can be attached to this elapsed time as it is observed during the clinical examination. Inferring the presence of pharyngeal delay during the clinical exam is not easily accomplished. There are a number of studies that have identified pharyngeal delay times using fluoroscopy, but there have never been any published studies relating a noninstrumental means of accurately determining this measure.

The clinician can obtain a concrete measure of elapsed time, from the delivery of food or liquid until the completion of a swallow. This measure may serve the clinician by providing information about the appropriate rate of food delivery to a slow patient who relies on another for feeding assistance. Nathadwarawala, Nicklin, and Wiles (1992) reported that, during a timed test of swallowing capacity, neurological patients with a self-perceived dysphagia were more likely to swallow more slowly than those patients who did not perceive themselves to be dysphagic. The task involved the consumption of 150 ml^3 of water as quickly as the subject could comfortably consume it. A swallowing speed of less than 10 ml/sec was strongly associated with abnormal swallowing complaints with a sensitivity of 97%. Unfortunately, the existence or absence of dysphagia was not verified during an instrumental examination on these two groups of patients.

CSE 15-C. NUMBER OF SWALLOWS

The patient who swallows more than three times per bolus of food or liquid likely is perceiving the presence of residuals in the pharynx following the swallow. The clincian can consider one of a number of possible etiologies which are listed in Table 2–21.

When multiple swallows occur, the clinician should query the patient regarding the presence of "food sticking." If able, have the patient point to the perceived location of the

Table 2–21. Possible etiology for multiple swallows.

1. A biomechanical or structural impairment is present that has compromised pharyngeal and/or upper esophageal transit. The patient is sensitive to the resulting residue and is attempting volitionally to clear the residue.

2. An irritant unrelated to bolus propulsion or residuals, such as a tumor or other neoplastic structure, is present and the patient perceives its presence.

3. The sensation is referred from a more distal position along the vagal afferent tract. Esophageal stasis can be perceived to be residing in the pharynx.

4. Esophago-pharyngeal or gastroesophagopharyngeal reflux is taking place after the swallow.

residue. Make note of location in the section reserved for notation. An instrumental examination, preferably videofluoroscopy, is indicated in most cases. This examination will allow the clinician to screen fully the pharyngeal and esophageal stages of the swallow for a wide range of functional and pathological conditions.

CSE 15-D. ORAL SIGNS

Patients with poor tongue function and/or oral seal performance during earlier portions of the clinical examination may exhibit oral signs when presented with food or liquid. Patients with oral seal problems should be monitored for loss of control of the bolus and drooling. Observe whether these patients sense the loss of bolus or secretions from the mouth and record the compensations observed. Are the attempts to clear the drooled material successful? Because of the social stigma attached to this behavior, it is usually one very high on the prioritized list for remediation by both the dysphagic individual and family members.

Oral residue is common in patients with poor coordination, weakness, or structural changes to the tongue (see Figure 2–24). Baker, Fraser, and Baker (1991) compared oral surgery patient's perceptions of postoperative dysphagia to videofluoroscopic observations. Patients who perceived difficulty lifting the tongue and moving it from side to side and from front to back demonstrated adherence of food to the hard palate and difficulty lateralizing material during the fluoroscopic examination.

Make note of specific areas containing residue. Request the patient to move the tongue to the areas where the residue resides and attempt to clear it. In surgical resection patients, this may not be possible. In patients with neurological disease, attempt to determine if the patient senses the residue. Record the results of the clearing attempts.

CSE 15-E. AIRWAY SIGNS

During this task, the clinician is monitoring the patient for clinical signs of aspiration or penetration of food or liquid into the laryngeal inlet. Penetration is defined as the entry of material (oral, nasal, or pharyngeal secretions; food, liquid or gastric contents) into the protective vestibule of the larynx without passing below the level of the true vocal folds. Aspiration is defined as the entry of material into the laryngeal vestibule with further passage below the level of the true vocal folds into the trachea.

Dynamic visualization of the bolus and the laryngeal airway are not possible during the clinical examination. Although a laryngeal mirror may be employed to visualize the hypopharynx and larynx following the presentation of food and liquid, the vast majority of clinicians will rely on auditory cues to indicate an event of laryngeal airway penetration. The two classic auditory cues are wet dysphonia and cough.

Wet Dysphonia

The presence of wet dysphonia may be noted during the interview portion of the clinical exam and should be recorded in the appropriate section. Oropharyngeal secretions resting within the laryngeal vestibule typically cause the presence of wet dysphonia prior to the delivery of food or liquid.

Careful attention should be directed to the patient's voice quality prior to and after each delivery of food or liquid. Entry of test

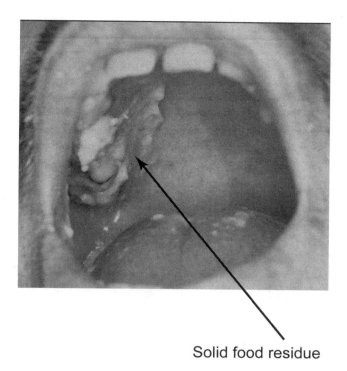

Solid food residue

Figure 2–24. Solid food residue on the hard palate in patient with reduced oral sensation.

material into the laryngeal vestibule before, during, or after the swallow can result in a wet dysphonia. The clinician should attend to the delay in time before the dysphonia makes itself evident. In cases of weakened oropharyngeal propulsion or UES dysfunction, residue may rest anywhere in the hypopharynx. This residue may be of a great enough volume so that it overflows the structural barriers that prevent material from entering into the laryngeal vestibule. Residue also could be distributed along the pharyngeal walls following the swallow and may be directed into the laryngeal vestibule by gravity or by the forces of a subsequent successive swallow. Residue also may build up following several presentations before accumulating to the point of overcoming the structural barriers.

Should a wet dysphonia be observed following the delivery of food or liquid the clinician should note the presence or absence of throat-clearing attempts by the patient. Patients who display no clearing attempts and continue to speak with a wet dysphonic voice may be insensitive to the presence of the material in the laryngeal vestibule.

Wet dyphonia observed on the clinical examination has been strongly linked to aspiration during an instrumental examination (Daniels et al., 1998; Horner et al., 1993; Linden & Seibens, 1983; Linden et al., 1993). The minimum requirement for the presence of a wet dysphonia is the collection of material on the true vocal folds (see Figure 2–25). Without direct visualization of the hypopharynx, it is impossible to differentiate laryngeal penetration from aspiration.

Coughing/Choking

Coughing after the presentation of any food or liquid is probably the single strongest indicator of penetration of the laryngeal inlet. The absence of this reflex in the presence of laryngeal airway penetration is commonly referred to as "silent aspiration." For additional discussion of the cough, see Chapter 4.

Careful attention should be directed to the timing of the onset of the cough. Does it occur before the swallow is initiated or can be completed? Does it occur immediately after the swallow or is there a delay (see Table 2–22)?

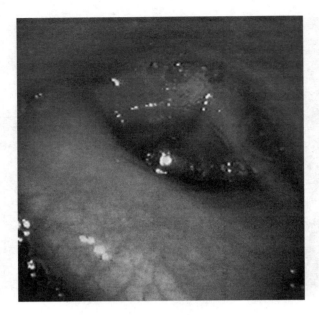

Figure 2–25. Endoscopic evidence of secretions within the laryngeal vestibule.

CSE 15-F. INSTRUMENTATION

Modified Blue Dye Test

A popular and fruitful means for determining the presence of aspiration in patients with tracheostomy is the "Evan's blue dye test." This test was introduced by Cameron, Reynolds, and Zuidema (1973) to determine the presence of aspiration in tracheostomized patients. This modification to the clinical examination requires the staining of test swallow materials with blue food dye or methyline blue dye. The dye is swallowed with the test material and, in the event of aspiration, is detected at the trach site after coughing or trans-tracheal suctioning. The method has gained great popularity due to its low cost and ease of administration. The minimum requirements for the examination are; the blue dye, test material for swallowing and a tracheostomy tube that is configured in a way that allows aspirated materials to flow out of the proximal opening after coughing or during suctioning.

Using the Modified Blue Dye Test

For the modified blue dye to be observed at the proximal opening of the tracheostomy tube, the cuff must be deflated. Many patients transitioning from mechanically supported ventilation to self-supported ventilation will have the cuff in various inflated and deflated positions. Before commencing with cuff deflation, be sure to review the planned procedure with the patient-care team and alert all related disciplines.

Conventional wisdom holds that the inflated cuff protects against aspiration of food, liquid, refluxed gastric contents, and oropharyngeal secretions. In fact, the seal provided by the cuff may prevent large amounts of aspirated materials from traveling to the distal airways, but likely does not provide a complete enough seal to prevent some small amounts of secretions and liquid to advance to the bronchi (Petring, Adelhoj, Jensen, Pedersen, & Lomholt, 1986) (see Figure 2–26). Further, when the cuff is deflated, all of the material previously resting above the cuff, will course down the trachea to the distal airways.

The clinician can be confident of positive findings from the modified blue dye test. The arrival of blue dye or food particulate at the trach site is a clear indicator of aspiration, and the chance of false positive readings are miniscule. False negative results are more problematic with this exam (Thompson-Henry & Braddock, 1995; Tippett & Siebens, 1996). In a study conducted by Thompson-Henry and Braddock (1995), five subjects known to

Table 2–22. Salient elements of cough during clinical examination.

Element	Possible Related Impairment/ Dysfunction	Possible Related Biomechanical Event
Timing		
Before	Impaired oral-palatal seal. Reduced CNS afferent input to cortex during oral stage	Premature spillage and/or pharyngeal delay, with entry of bolus into laryngeal vestibule before the swallow
During	Impaired glottic closure during pharyngeal propulsion of bolus. RLN damage	Entry of bolus into unprotected airway as the bolus is propelled through the pharynx
After	Weakend tongue base propulsion. Weakened pharyngeal peristalsis. Structural obstruction (tumor/cervical osteophytes)	Incomplete propulsion of the bolus through the pharynx with subsequent residue and overflow into the laryngeal vestibule
	Reduced laryngeal elevation. Hypertonic UES. Structural UES obstruction	Incomplete UES opening with resulting obstruction of the bolus passage and subsequent pharyngeal residue and overflow to the laryngeal vestibule
	Zenker's diverticulum	Collection of bolus material in the outpouching with subsequent escape and entry into the laryngeal vestibule
	Esophago pharyngeal reflux. Gastroesophageal reflux	Reverse flow of the bolus from the esophagus or stomach into the pharynx with overflow into the laryngeal vestibule
	Esophago-tracheal fistula	Flow through a fistular tract from the esophagus into the trachea
Delay	SLN impairment	Damage to the SLN reduces sensitivity to material resting in the pharynx. Material falls below the true vocal folds into the trachea whereupon a cough is produced
	RLN impairment	Material falls below the level of the true vocal folds and after a time reaches the bronchi whereupon a cough is produced
Strength	Reduced compression of the airways due to neurologic disease or COPD. Tracheostomy present (without plug or speaking valve)	Inadequate velocity of airstream through the pharynx prevents material from effectively being expelled from laryngeal airway

CNS = Central nervous system; UES = Upper esophageal sphincter; RLN = Recurrent laryngeal nerve; SLN = Superior laryngeal nerve; COPD = Chronic obstructive pulmonary disease.

aspirate were presented small volumes of food and liquid with blue dye added. Following the test swallows, the patients were suctioned without evidence of blue dye at the trach site. On subsequent instrumental swallowing examinations, all five were verified to have aspirated. This study was not without problems; the instrumental and modified blue dye tests were performed at an interval of 7–22 days apart. In this period of time, medically fragile ventilator-dependent patients could experience increments or decrements in swallow function. Further, aspiration on the instrumental examination was not described with the detailed precision necessary to understand fully the likelihood of positive or negative findings on the modified blue dye test. A dysphagic tracheostomized patient may aspirate material below the level of the true vocal folds and then expel the material from the trachea with a cough before it reaches the distal opening of the tracheostomy tube. If the authors had employed a precise penetration aspiration scale (Rosenbek, Roecker, Wood, &

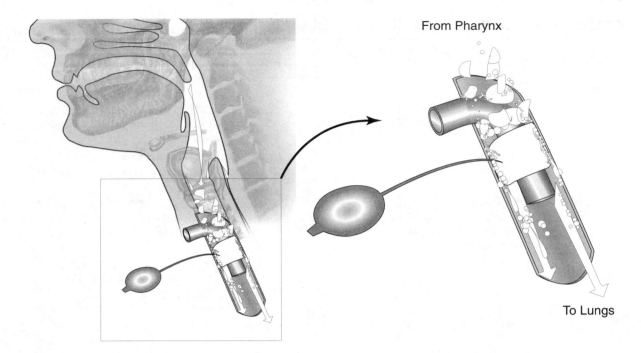

From Pharynx

To Lungs

Figure 2–26. Large particulate of food may remain above the inflated cuff but secretions and liquids may pass the cuff and travel to the distal airways.

Robbins, 1996), a better understanding of the false negative findings would have been realized. Even with the problems found in the design of this study, the authors described an intuitively well-founded wariness of negative findings on the modified blue dye test that has been expressed by others (Metheny & Clouse, 1997).

Blue dye also may be added to the enteral tube feedings of patients with tracheostomies that are suspected of aspirating refluxed gastric contents. Positive findings of blue dye at the trach site is a clear indicator of aspiration of refluxed material (Kocan & Hickisch, 1986; Treloar & Stechmiller, 1984).

CSE 15-G. INTERVENTION

In the course of the clinical examination the clinician will reveal or confirm clinical signs of dysphagia. The next step is to attempt to alleviate the sign with adjustments that may impact the physiology of the swallow in a positive way. Adjustments come in the form of :

- Manipulations of bolus volume
- Manipulation of bolus viscosity
- Manipulation of feeding rate

- Changes in means of delivery/use of device
- Application of postural changes
- Application of behavioral maneuvers

Manipulation of Bolus Volume

The alert clinician will note the increments in volume presented during the test swallows. Manipulate the volumes until a threshold for the sign is determined. I have encountered a great number of patients who are capable of safely consuming 2–3 cc of water but consistently aspirate slightly larger boluses. Determining threshold values for water sips can greatly augment the patient's sense of relief and comfort.

Manipulation of Bolus Viscosity

The clinician should attempt to provide a great variety of consistencies to the patient during the examination. Viscosity control has been enhanced greatly with the advent of prethickened products on the market today. However, maintaining viscosity stability in other foods that are not commercially prethickened remains a cursed task.

Manipulation of Feeding Rate

Some patients may require more time to consume a full meal. Push the patient that is at risk of fatigue during feeding to determine the threshold at which efficiency of chewing and swallowing begin to break down. These patients may benefit from smaller, more frequent meals. Other patients may consume foods more rapidly if they require less mastication.

If possible, make an effort to observe the consumption of a meal. Patients that are reliant on another person for feeding are at the mercy of the feeder to deliver the food and liquid in appropriate volumes and at a rate that is compatible with their ability.

Changes in Delivery/Use of Devices

Some patients may benefit from customized utensils. Anticipate the patient's needs prior to the administration of the exam. Patients with resections of the tongue often are unable to manipulate food in the anterior oral cavity and require the use of specially constructed spoons that allow delivery of a bolus in a position further back in the oral cavity where manipulation is more effective. Patients with weakened tongue and palatal function may be unable to generate enough negative pressure interorally to pull material through a straw. Be prepared to provide the patient with a variety of delivery options.

Application of Postural Changes

Employ head and body positioning to alleviate clinical signs. See the discussion in Chapter 1 regarding the elicitation of head and body positions.

Application of Behavioral Maneuvers

Behavioral maneuvers include the super glottic swallow, super supraglottic swallow, Mendelsohn maneuver, and Masako maneuver, to name a few. The maneuvers are discussed in the sections on instrumental examinations. After attempting behavioral maneuvers and determining their success, consider the patient's cognitive state and/or the likelihood of compliance.

ADDITIONAL INSTRUMENTATION

Pulse Oximetry

Some medically fragile patients will be at a higher risk for poor outcome following an episode of aspiration. In these patients, close monitoring of pulmonary and cardiac function may be desired. In such cases, the clinician may choose to employ pulse oximetry, an instrument that measures a patient's pulse and arterial-blood oxygen saturation. As the oxygen content of the blood increases, the blood color changes. Pulse oximetry exploits this property by utilizing small sensors that monitor the wavelengths of light emitted by a small light source. The light passes through tissue, usually the fingertip or earlobe.

The pulse oximeter measures the amount of light absorbed by the blood in the tissue and produces a number (saO_2) representing arterial oxygen saturation. The readings in modern pulse oximeters are considered to be accurate to ±2–3% for saO_2 readings between 50–100%. For normal subjects, saO_2 ranges between 97% and 99%. Some patients, such as chronic smokers, may have "normal" readings between 92% and 96%. Readings below 90% are considered low and usually indicate poor oxygenation. Some conditions can negatively affect the readings of the pulse oximeter. These can include cold extremities due to poor circulation, or hypervolemia.

Employing Pulse Oximetry for the Detection of Aspiration

Pulse oximetry can be employed during the clinical examination to monitor signs of distress in a patient who is at high risk of rapid decompensation. Other clinicians have employed pulse oximetry to detect events of aspiration during the clinical examination (Chapman & Rebuck, 1991; Collins & Bakheit, 1997; Lefton-Greif & Loughlin, 1996; Rogers, Arvedson, Msall, & Demerath, 1993; Rogers, Arvedson, Msall, & Shucard, 1993; Sellars, Dunnet, & Carter, 1998; Zaidi, Smith, King,

Park, & O'Neill, 1996). The premise of its employment is that aspiration results in a reflex bronchoconstriction that leads to a reduction in the oxygen saturation of arterial blood (Collins & Bakheit, 1997; Rodriguez-Roisin, Ferrer, Navajas, Agusti, Wagner, & Roca, 1991).

The employment of pulse oximetry during test swallows is relatively easy and safe. The device is simply attached to the finger-tip or earlobe and test swallows are elicited while the saO_2 levels are monitored. A typical, modern pulse oximeter measures light absorption and updates the estimated saO_2 every few seconds. However, the amount of time for an event of aspiration to affect saO_2 readings can vary. Collins and Bakheit (1997) performed simultaneous videofluoroscopy and pulse oximetry in 54 consecutive dysphagic stroke patients. Pulse oximetry readings were sampled at the time of the swallow and 2 and 10 min following the swallow. The authors found that more than half (55%) of those patients that aspirated showed a significant drop in saO_2 at the time of the aspiration event. When a two-min time delay in saO_2 reading was performed, the authors found that they were able to accurately predict aspiration, or lack of it, in 81.5% of the dysphagic stroke patients.

Using pulse oximetry to predict aspiration may result in false positive and false negative readings. Collins and Bakheit (1997) contended that false positive readings were observed in patients with chronic lung disease, smokers, and in the aged. The drop in saO_2 was also found to be more predictive of aspiration in younger male individuals who demonstrated high average baseline saO_2 readings. One-hundred percent of males under 65 years of age who aspirated on fluoroscopy also were identified as having siginificant drops in saO_2. However, older women (>65 years) who aspirated were less likely to show significant drops in saO_2 and, on average, returned to baseline saturation levels within 10 min of an aspiration event. It has been suggested that aspiration of water in most elderly subjects does not result in bronchoconstriction with subsequent hypoxemia (Teramoto, Fukuchi, & Ouchi, 1996).

Confidence of aspiration detection is enhanced considerably in those patients with reliable drops in saO_2 coupled with clinical signs of aspiration. In such patients, the clinician has the opportunity to alter the bolus size and consistency, incorporate positioning changes, or utilize maneuvers in a way that would lessen the hypoxemia and signs of aspiration (Rogers, Arvedson, Msall, & Demerath, 1993; Rogers, Arvedson, Msall, & Shucard, 1993). In this way, the clinician comes closer to identifying the safest means of oral intake without the use of instrumentation such as fluoroscopy or endoscopy.

Cervical Auscultation

Many clinicians employ cervical auscultation to amplify airway signs and/or the sounds emitted during the propulsion of the bolus through the pharynx and UES. A simple stethoscope can be used (see Figure 2–27) or, for improved fidelity and signal recording, stethoscopes fitted with accelerometers.

Swallow Sounds

As the bolus passes through the pharynx and the UES opens and closes around it, a number of sounds related to pressure change may be heard. The sound made as the bolus passes through the pharynx and UES has been described as a characteristic doubleclick (Hamlet, Penney, & Formolo, 1994; Selley, Ellis, Flack, Bayliss, Chir, & Pearce, 1994). The exact estimation of bolus position during the generation of these sounds has, however, been elusive (Hamlet, Nelson, & Patterson, 1990). There also is no data suggesting that the sounds of swallowing are different in a patient with dysphagia.

Takahashi, Groher, and Michi (1994a, 1994b) suggested placing the stethoscope along the lateral border of the trachea immediately inferior to the cricoid cartilage. This site was promoted over others because of the large magnitude and low variance of the signal. If the recognition and registration of this sound has any value, it is as a marker for the pharyngeal swallow. The clinician may wish to monitor the sounds of swallowing to determine the timing of swallow initiation, rather than monitoring for laryngeal elevation.

Airway Sounds

The stethoscope is capable of monitoring the breath sounds at the level of the larynx during the periods before and after the pharyngeal

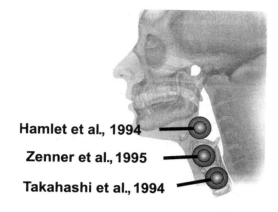

Hamlet et al., 1994

Zenner et al., 1995

Takahashi et al., 1994

Figure 2–27. Placement of stethoscope during the swallow.

swallow. One of the audible signals that clinicians look for is the start of adventitious airway sounds following a swallow. These are sounds that are produced as the inspiratory and expiratory airflow is effected by the presence of a foreign body in the laryngeal vestibule or trachea.

Zenner et al. (1994) performed clinical examinations using cervical auscultation prior to the administration of videofluoroscopic examinations on 50 residents of a long-term care facility. It was found that the clinician performing cervical auscultation during the clinical examination was able to distinguish subjects who aspirate from those who do not with a high level of agreement with videofluoroscopy. The authors went on to warn that successful employment of cervical auscultation requires proper training and clinical experience.

REFERENCES

Adachi, T., Kogo, M., Iida, S., Hamaguchi, M., & Matsuya, T. (1997). Measurement of velopharyngeal movements induced by isolated stimulation of levator veli palatini and pharyngeal constrictor muscles. *Journal of Dental Research, 76*, 1745–1750.

Agerberg, G., & Carlsson, G. E. (1981). Chewing ability in relation to dental and general health. *Acta Odontologica Scandinavica, 39*, 147–153.

Ansari, I. H. (1994). Management for maxillary removable partial denture patients who gag. *The Journal of Prosthetic Dentistry, 72*, 448.

Ayars, G. H., Altman, L. C., & Fretwell, M. D. (1982). Effect of decreased salivation and pH on the adherence of Klebsiella species to human buccal epithelial cells. *Infection and Immunity, 38*,179–182.

Baker, B. M., Fraser, A. M., & Baker, C. D. (1991). Long-term postoperative dysphagia in oral/pharyngeal surgery patients: Subjects' perceptions vs. videofluoroscopic observations. *Dysphagia, 6*, 11–16.

Baker, S. R. (1983). Management of osteoradionecrosis of the mandible with myocutaneous flaps. *Journal of Surgical Oncology, 24*, 282.

Barsby, M. J. (1994). The use of hypnosis in the management of 'gagging' and intolerance to dentures. *British Dental Journal, 176*, 97–102.

Bartlett, J. G. (1979). Anaerobic bacterial pneumonitis. *American Review of Respiratory Disease, 119*, 19–23.

Beck, J. D. (1992). Epidemiology of periodontal disease in older adults. In R. P. Ellen (Ed.), *Periodontal care for older adults* (pp. 9–35). Toronto: Canadian Scholars' Press, Inc.

Bine, J. E., Frank, E. M., & McDade, H. L. (1995). Dysphagia and dementia in subjects with Parkinson's Disease. *Dysphagia, 10*, 160–164.

Bisch, E. M., Logemann, J. A., Rademaker, A. W., Kahrilas, P. J., & Lazarua, C. L. (1994). Pharyngeal effects of bolus volume, viscosity, and temperature in patients with dysphagia resulting from neurologic impairment and in normal subjects. *Journal of Speech and Hearing Research, 37*, 1041–1059.

Bleach, N. R. (1993). The gag reflex and aspiration: A retrospective analysis of 120 patients assessed by videofluoroscopy. *Clinical Otolaryngology, 18*, 303–307.

Bucher, K. (1958). The physiology and pharmacology of cough. *Pharmacological Reviews. 10*, 43–58.

Burns, H. P., Dayal, V. S., Scott, A., van Nostrand, A.W., & Bryce, D. P. (1979). Laryngotracheal trauma: Observations on its pathogenesis and its prevention following prolonged orotracheal intubation in the adult. *Laryngoscope, 89*, 1316–1325.

Calhoun, K. H., Gibson, B., Hartley, L., Minton, J., & Hokanson, J. A. (1992). Age related changes in oral sensation. *Laryngoscope, 102*, 109–116.

Caligiuri, M. P., Jeste, D. V., & Harris, M. J. (1989). Instrumental assessment of lingual motor instability in tardive dyskinesia. *Neuropsychopharmacology, 2*, 309–312.

Cameron, J. L., Reynolds, J., & Zuidema, G. D. (1973). Aspiration in patients with tracheostomies. *Surgery, Gynecology, and Obstetrics, 136*, 68–70.

Capra, N. F. (1995). Mechanisms of oral sensation. *Dysphagia, 10*, 235–247.

Chang, M. W., Rosendall, B., & Finlayson, B A. (1998). Mathematical modeling of normal pharyngeal bolus transport: A preliminary study. *Journal of Rehabilitation Research and Development, 35*, 327–334.

Chapman, K. R., & Rebuck, A. S. (1991). Dysphagia as a manifestation of occult hypoxemia: The role of oximetry during meal times. *Chest, 99*, 1030–1032.

Chauncey, H. H., Muench, M. E., Kapur, K. K., & Wayler, A. H. (1984). The effect of the loss of teeth on diet and nutrition. *International Dental Journal, 34*, 98–104.

Cherney, L. R., & Halper, A. S. (1989). Recovery of oral nutrition after head injury in adults. *The Journal of Head Trauma Rehabilitation, 4*, 42–50.

Chi-Fishman, G. Stone, M. (1996). A new application for electropalatography: Swallowing. *Dysphagia, 11*, 239–247.

Chigira, A., Kazuhiko, O., Yoshiharu, M., & Yoshihiro, K. (1994). Lip closing pressure in disabled children: A comparison with normal children. *Dysphagia, 9*, 193–198.

Clement, M., & Twitchell, T. (1959). Dysarthria in cerebral palsy. *Journal of Speech and Hearing Disorders, 24*, 118–122.

Coates, C., & Bakheit, A. M. (1997). Dysphagia in Parkinson's disease. *European Neurology, 38*(1), 49–52.

Collins, M. J., & Bakheit, A. M. (1997). Does pulse oximetry reliably detect aspiration in dysphagic stroke patients? *Stroke, 28*, 1773–1775.

Constantopoulos, S. H., Papadimitrion, C. S., & Moutsopoulos, H. M. (1985). Respiratory manifestations in primary Sjogren's syndrome. *Chest, 88*, 226.

Cox, S. C., & Walker, D. M. (1997). Establishing a normal range for mouth opening: Its use in screening for oral submucous fibrosis. *British Journal of Oral Maxillofacial Surgery, 35*, 40–42.

Crow, H. C., & Ship, J. A. (1996). Tongue strength and endurance in different aged individuals. *Journals Of Gerontology. Series A, Biological Sciences And Medical Sciences, 51*, M247–M250.

Curran, A. J., Smyth, D., Sheehan, S. J., Joyce, W., Hayes, D. B., Walsh, M. A., & Coll, J. R. (1997). Recurrent laryngeal nerve dysfunction following carotid endarterectomy. *Surgery Edinborough, 42*, 168–170.

Daniel, B. (1982). A soft palate desensitization procedure for patients requiring palatal lift prostheses. *The Journal of Prosthetic Dentistry, 48*, 565–566.

Daniels, S. K., Brailey, K., Priestly, D. H., Herrington, L. R., Weisberg, L. A., & Foundas, A. L. (1998). Aspiration in patients with acute stroke. *Archives of Physical Medicine and Rehabilitation, 79*, 14–19.

Dantas, R. O., Kern, M. K., Bassey, B. T., Dodds, W. J., Kahrilas, P. J., Brasseur, J. G., Cook, I. J., & Lang, I. M. (1990). Effect of swallowed bolus variables on oral and pharyngeal phases of swallowing. *American Journal of Physiology, 258*, G675–G681.

Davies, A. E., Kidd, D., Stone, S. P., & MacMahon, J. (1995). Pharyngeal sensation and gag reflex in healthy subjects. *The Lancet, 345*, 487–488.

DeStephano, F., Anda, R. F., Kahn, H. S., et al. (1993). Dental disease and risk of coronary heart disease and mortality. *British Medical Journal, 306*, 688–691.

Detoledo, J., Icovinno, J., & Haddad, H. (1994). Swallowing difficulties and early CNS injuries: Correlation with the presence of axial skeletal deformaties. *Brain Injury, 8*, 607–611.

DeVita, M. A., & Spierer-Rundback, L. (1990). Swallowing disorders in patients with prolonged orotracheal intubation or tracheostomy tubes. *Critical Care Medicine, 18,* 1328–1330.

Dierks, E. J. (1991). Temporomandibular disorders and facial pain syndromes. In M. M. Paparella, D. A. Shumrick, J. L. Gluckman, & W. L. Meyerhoff (Eds.), *Otolaryngology* (Vol. 1, 3rd ed.). Philadelphia: W. B. Saunders Company.

Doherty, M. J., Wang, L. J., Donague, S., Pearson, M. G., Downs, P., Stoneman, S. A., & Earis, J. E. (1997). The acoustic properties of capsaicin-induced cough in healthy subjects. *The European Respiratory Journal, 10,* 202–207.

Doty, R. W., & Bosma, J. F. (1956). An electromyographic analysis of reflex deglutition. *Journal of Neurophysiology, 19,* 44–60.

Drake, W., O'Donoghue, Bartram, C., Lindsay, J., & Greenwood, R. (1997). Eating in side-lying facilitates rehabilitation in neurogenic dysphagia. *Brain Injury, 11,* 137–142.

Dworkin, J. P. (1980). Tongue strength measurement in patients with amyotrophic lateral sclerosis: Qualitative vs. quantitative procedures. *Archives of Physical Medicine and Rehabilitation, 61,* 422–424.

Dworkin, J. P., & Hartman, D. E. (1979). Progressive speech deterioration and dysphagia in amyotrophic lateral sclerosis: Case report. *Archives of Physical Medicine and Rehabilitation, 60*(9), 423–425.

Ekberg, O., Nylander, G., Fork, F. T., Sjoberg, S., Birch-Iensen, M., & Hillarp, B. (1988). Interobserver variability in cineradiographic assessment of pharyngeal function during swallow. *Dysphagia, 3,* 46–48.

Ekstrand, K. R., Nielsen, L. A., Carvalho, J. C., & Thylstrup, A. (1993). Dental plaque and caries on permanent first molar occlusal surfaces in relation to sagittal occlusion. *Scandinavian Journal of Dental Research, 101,* 9–15.

Fernando, I. N., Patel, T., Billingham, L., Hammond, C., Hallmark, S., Glaholm, J., & Henk, J. M. (1995). The effect of head and neck irradiation on taste dysfunction: A prospective study. *Clinical Oncology: A Journal of the Royal College of Radiology, 7,* 173–178.

Finkelstein, Y., Talmi, Y. P., Nachmani, A., Hauben, D. J., & Zohar, Y. (1992). On the variability of velopharyngeal valve anatomy and function: A combined perioral and nasoendoscopic study. *Plastic and Reconstructive Surgery, 89,* 631–639.

Friedman, M. H., & Weintraub, M. I. (1995). Temporary elimination of gag reflex for dental procedures. *The Journal of Prosthetic Dentistry, 73,* 319.

Fudge, R. C., Thailer, S. A., Alpert, M., Intrator, J., & Sison, C. E. (1991). The effects of electromyographic feedback training on suppression of the oral-lingual movements associated with tardive dyskinesia. *Biofeedback and Self Regulation, 16,* 117–129.

Furukawa, K. (1984). Cineradiographic analysis of laryngeal movement during deglutition. *Nippon Jibinkoka Gakkai Kaiho, 87,* 169–181.

Gilbert, G. H., Duncan, R. P., Heft, M. W., Dolan, T. A., & Vogel, W. B. (1997). Oral disadvantage among dentate adults. *Community Dentistry and Oral Epidemiology, 25,* 301–313.

Gilbert, G. H., Foerster, U., & Duncan, R. P. (1998). Satisfaction with chewing ability in a diverse sample of dentate adults. *Journal of Oral Rehabilitation, 25,*15–27.

Hagen, C., Malkmus, D., & Durham, P. (1979). Levels of cognitive functioning. In *Rehabilitation for the head injured adult: Comprehensive physical management* (pp. 39–44). Downey, CA: Professional Staff Association of Rancho Los Amigos Hospital, Inc.

Hakeberg, M., Berggren, U., Hagglin, C., & Ahlqwist, M. (1997). Reported burning mouth symptoms among middle-aged and elderly women. *European Journal of Oral Sciences, 105,* 539–543.

Hamlet, S., Ezzell, G., & Aref, A. (1993). Larynx motion associated with swallowing during radiation therapy. *International Journal of Radiation Oncology, Biology and Physics, 28,* 467–470.

Hamlet, S., Penney, D. G., & Formolo, J. (1994). Stethoscope acoustics and cervical auscultation of swallowing. *Dysphagia, 9,* 63–68.

Hamlet, S. L., Nelson, R. J., & Patterson, R. L. (1990). Interpreting the sounds of swallowing: Fluid flow through the cricpharyngeus. *Annals of Otology, Rhinology, and Laryngology, 99,* 749–752.

Hammen, V. L., & Yorkston, K. M. (1996). Speech and pause characteristics following speech rate reduction in hypokinetic dysarthria. *Journal of Communication Disorders, 29,* 429–444.

Hardy, J. C. (1964). Lung function of athetoid and spastic quadriplegic children. *Developmental Medicine and Child Neurology, 6,* 378–388.

Hayashi, T., Nishikawa, T., Koga, I., Uchida, Y., & Yamawaki, S. (1997). Life-threatening dysphagia following prolonged neuroleptic therapy. *Clinical Neuropharmacology, 20,* 77–81.

Hiiemae, K., Heath, M., Heath, G., Kazazoglu, E., Murray, J., Sapper, D., & Hamblett, K. (1996). Natural bites, food consistency and feeding behavior in man. *Archives of Oral Biology, 41,* 175–189.

Hildebrandt, G. H., Dominguez, B. L., Schork, M. A., & Loesche, W. J. (1997). Functional units, chewing, swallowing, and food avoidance among the elderly. *Journal of Prosthetic Dentistry, 77,* 588–595.

Hixon, T., & Hoit, X. (1984). Differential subsystem impairment, differential motor system impairment, and decomposition of respiratory movement in ataxic dysarthria: A spurious trilogy. *Journal of Speech and Hearing Disorders, 49,* 435–441.

Horner, J., Brazer, S., & Massey, E. (1993). Aspiration in bilateral stroke patients: A validation study. *Neurology, 43,* 430–433.

Horner, J., & Massey, E. (1988). Silent aspiration following stroke. *Neurology, 38,* 317.

Horner, J., Massey, E. W., & Brazer, S. R. (1990). Aspiration in bilateral stroke patients. *Neurology, 40,* 1686–1688.

Huang, M. H., Lee, S. T., & Rajendran, K. (1997). Structure of the musculus uvulae: Functional and surgical implications of an anatomic study. *Cleft Palate Craniofacial Journal, 34,* 466–474.

Isberg, A., Nilsson, M. E., & Schiratzki, H. (1985a). Movement of the upper esophageal sphincter and a manometric device during deglutition. *Acta Radiologica: Diagnosis, 26,* 381–388.

Isberg, A., Nilsson, M. E., & Schiratzki, H. (1985b). The upper esophageal sphincter during normal deglutition. *Acta Radiologica: Diagnosis, 26,* 563–568.

Jannetta, P. J., & Robbins, L. J. (1980). Trigeminal neuropathy—New observations. *Neurosurgery, 7,* 347–351.

Jette, A. M., Feldman, H. A., & Douglass, C. (1993). Oral disease and physical disability in community-dwelling older persons. *Journal of the American Geriatrics Society, 41,* 1102–1108.

Johanson, W. G., Blackstock, R., Pierce, A. K., et al. (1970). The role of bacterial antagonism in pneumococcal colonization of the human pharynx. *Journal of Laboratory and Clinical Medicine, 75,* 946–952.

Kaandorp, A. J., de Baat, C., & Michels, L. F. (1994). Xerostomia in the elderly: Causes, consequences, and treatment possibilities of dry mouth. *Tijdschrift Voor Gerontologie En Geriatrie, 25,* 145–149.

Kaatzke-McDonald, M. N., Post, E., & Davis, P. J. (1996). The effects of cold, touch, and chemical stimulation of the anterior faucial pillar on human swallowing. *Dysphagia, 11,* 198–206.

Kahrilas, P. J., Lin, S., Chen, J., & Logemann, J. A. (1996). Oropharyngeal accommodation to swallow volume. *Gastroenterology, 111,* 297–306.

Kapila, Y. V., Dodds, W. J., Helm, J. G., & Hogan, W. J. (1984). Relationship between swallow rate and salivary flow. *Digestive Diseases and Sciences, 29,* 528–533.

Katsantonis, G. P., Friedman, W. H., Krebs, F. J., & Walsh, J. K. (1987). Nasopharyngeal complications following uvulopalatopharyngoplasty. *Laryngoscope, 97,* 309–314.

Kennedy, G., Pring, T., & Fawcus, R. (1993). No place for motor speech acts in the assessment of dysphagia? Intelligibility and swallowing difficulties in stroke and Parkinson's disease patients. *European Journal of Disorders of Communication, 28,* 213–226.

Kennedy, J. G., & Kuehn, D. P. (1989). Neuroanatomy of Speech. In D. P. Kuehn, M. L. Lemme & J. M. Baumgartner (Eds.), *Neural bases of speech, hearing, and language* (pp. 134–156). Boston: College-Hill Press.

Kluin, K. J., Bromberg, M. B., Feldman, E. L., & Simmons, Z. (1996). Dysphagia in elderly men with myasthenia gravis. *Journal of Neurological Science, 138,* 49–52.

Kocan, M. J., & Hickisch, S. M. (1986). A comparison of continuous and intermittent enteral nutrition in NICU patients. *The Journal of Neuroscience Nursing, 18,* 333–337.

Lader, M. H. (1996). Tolerability and safety: Essentials in antidepressant pharmacotherapy. *Journal of Clinical Psychiatry, 57*(Suppl. 2), 39–44.

Langmore, S. E., & Lehman, M. E. (1994). Physiologic deficits in the orofacial system underlying dysarthria in amyotrophic lateral sclerosis. *Journal of Speech and Hearing Research, 37,* 28–37.

Langmore, S. E., Terpenning, M. S., Schork, A., Chen, Y., Murray, J. T., Lopatin, D., & Loesche, W. J. (1998). Predictors of aspiration pneumonia: How important is dysphagia? *Dysphagia, 13*, 69–81.

Laskin, D. M. (1969). Etiology of the pain-dysfunciton syndrome. *Journal of the American Dental Association, 79*, 147–153.

Lazzara, G. L., Lazarus, C., & Logemann, J. A. (1986). Impact of thermal stimulation on the triggering of the swallowing reflex. *Dysphagia, 1*, 73–77.

Lear, C. S. C., Flanagan, J. B., & Moores, C. F. A. (1965). The frequency of deglutition in man. *Archives of Oral Biology, 10*, 83–99.

Leder, S. B. (1996a). Comment on Thompson-Henry and Braddock: The modified Evan's blue dye procedure fails to detect aspiration in the tracheostomized patient: Five case reports. *Dysphagia, 11*, 80–81.

Leder, S. B. (1996b). Gag reflex and dysphagia. *Head Neck, 18*, 138–141.

Leder, S. B. (1997). Videofluoroscopic evaluation of aspiration with visual examination of the gag reflex and velar movement. *Dysphagia, 12*, 21–23.

Lefton-Greif, M. A., & Loughlin, G. M. (1996). Specialized studies in pediatric dysphagia. *Seminars in Speech and Language, 17*, 311–329.

Leinonen, E., Lepola, U., Koponen, H., Mehtonen, O. P., & Rimon, R. (1997). Long-term efficacy and safety of milnacipran compared to clomipramine in patients with major depression. *Acta Psychiatrica Scandinavica, 96*, 497–504.

Leith, D. E. (1985). The development of cough. *The American Review of Respiratory Disease, 131*(5), S39–S42.

Leopold, N. A., & Kagel, M. C. (1996). Prepharyngeal dysphagia in Parkinson's disease. *Dysphagia, 11*, 14–22.

Leopold, N. A., & Kagel, M. C. (1997a). Dysphagia in progressive supranuclear palsy: Radiologic features. *Dysphagia, 12*, 140–143.

Leopold, N. A., & Kagel, M. C. (1997b). Laryngeal deglutition movement in Parkinson's disease. *Neurology, 48*, 373–375.

Liedberg, B., Spiechowicz, E., & Owall, B., (1995). Mastication with and without removable partial dentures: An intraindividual study. *Dysphagia, 10*, 107–112.

Limeback, H. (1988). The relationship between oral health and systemic infections amoung elderly residents of chronic care facilities: A review. *Gerodontology, 7*, 131–137.

Linden, P., Kuhlemeier, K. V., & Patterson, C. (1983). The probability of correctly predicting subglottic penetration from clinical observations. *Dysphagia, 8*, 170–179.

Linden, P., & Siebens, A. (1983). Dysphagia: predicting laryngeal penetration. *Archives of Physical Medicine and Rehabilitation, 64*, 281–284.

Linder, S. H. (1993). Functional electrical stimulation to enhance cough in quadriplegia. *Chest, 103*, 166–169.

Linebaugh, C. W., & Wolfe, V. E. (1984). Relationships between articulation rate, intelligibility and naturalness in spastic and ataxic speakers. In M. R. McNeil, J. C. Rosenbek, & A. E. Aronson (Eds.), *The dysarthrias* (pp. 201–202). San Diego: College-Hill Press.

Litvan, I., Sastry, N., & Sonies, B. C. (1997). Characterizing swallowing abnormalities in progressive supranuclear palsy. *Neurology, 48*,1654–1662.

Locker, D. (1997). Clinical correlates of changes in self-perceived oral health in older adults. *Community Dentistry and Oral Epidemiology, 25*, 199–203.

Loesche, W. J., Abrams, J., Terpenning, M. S., Bretz, W. A., Dominguez, B. L., Grossman, N. S., Hildebrandt, G. H., Langmore, S. E., & Lopatin, D. E. (1995). Dental findings in geriatric populations with diverse medical backgrounds. *Oral Surgery, Oral Medicine, and Oral Pathology, 80*, 43–54.

Logemann, J. (1985). The relationship between speech and swallowing [preface]. In W. Perkins & J. Northern (Eds.), *Seminars in Speech and Language, 6*, 4.

Logemann, J. A. (1990). Factors affecting ability to resume oral nutrition in the oropharyngeal dysphagic individual. *Dysphagia, 4*, 202–208.

Logemann, J. A. (1993). The dysphagia diagnostic procedure as a treatment efficacy trial. *Clinics in Communication Disorders, 3*, 1–10.

Logemann, J. A. (1995). Dysphagia: Evaluation and treatment. *Folia Phoniatrica Logpaedics, 47*, 140–164.

Logemann, J. A., & Kahrilas, P. J. (1990). Relearning to swallow after stroke-application of maneuvers and indirect biofeedback: A case study. *Neurology, 40*, 1136–1138.

Logemann, J., Kahrilas, P., Kobara, M., & Vakil, N. (1989). The benefit of head rotation on pharyngoesophageal dysphagia.

Archives of Physical Medicine and Rehabilitation, 70, 767–771.

Logenann, J. A., Rademaker, A. W., Pauloski, B. R., & Kahrilas, P. J. (1994). Effects of postural change on aspiration in head and neck surgical patients. *Otolaryngology — Head and Neck Surgery, 110*, 222–227.

Ludlow, C. L., & Bassich, C. J. (1984). Relationships between perceptual ratings and acoustic measures of hypokinetic speech. In M. R. McNeil, J. C. Rosenbek, & A. E. Aronson (Eds.), *The dysarthrias* (pp. 193–204). San Diego: College-Hill Press.

Maeyama, T., & Plattig, K. H. (1989). Minimal two point discrimination in human tongue and palate. *American Journal of Otolaryngology, 10*, 342–344.

Martin, B. J., & Corlew, M. M. (1990). The incidence of communication disorders in dysphagic patients. *Journal of Speech and Hearing Disorders, 55*, 28–32.

Mattila, K. J., Nieminen, M. S., Baltonen, V. V., et al. (1989). Association between dental health and acute myocardial infarction. *British Medical Journal, 298*, 779–781.

McCabe, R. P., Adamkiewicz, V. W., & Pekovic, D. D. (1991). Invasion of bacteria in enamel carious lesions. *Journal of the Canadian Dental Association, 57*, 403–405.

Meader, C., & Muyskens, J. (1950). *Handbook of biolinguistics. Part 1: The structures and processes of expression.* Baltimore: Waverly Press.

Medical Research Council. (1976). *Index of pulmonary dysfunction: Aids to the examination of the peripheral nervous system* [Memorandum 45]. London: Pendragon House.

Miller, A. J. (1982). Deglutition. *Physiological Reviews, 62*, 129–184.

Miller, J. L., & Watkin, K. L. (1996). The influence of bolus volume and viscosity on anterior lingual force during the oral stage of swallowing. *Dysphagia, 11*, 117–124.

Murray, J., Langmore, S., Ginsberg, S., & Dostie, A. (1996). The significance of accumulated oropharyngeal secretions and swallowing frequency in predicting aspiration. *Dysphagia, 11*, 99–103.

Nachlas, N. E., & Johns, M. E. (1991). Physiology of the salivary glands. In M. E. Paparella, D. A. Shumrick, J. L. Gluckman, & W. L. Meyerhoff (Eds.), *Otolaryngology* (Vol. 1, (3rd ed., pp. 391–406). Philadelphia: W. B. Saunders Co.

Narhi, T. O. (1994). Prevalence of subjective feelings of dry mouth in the elderly. *Journal of Dental Research, 73*, 20–25.

Nathadwarawala, K. M., Nicklin, J., & Wiles, C. M. (1992). A timed test of swallowing capacity for neurological patients. *Journal of Neurology, Neurosurgery and Psychiatry, 55*, 822–825.

Navazesh, M., Brightman, V. J., & Pogoda, J. M. (1996). Relationship of medical status, medications, and salivary flow rates in adults of different ages. *Oral Surgery, Oral Medicine, Oral Pathology, and Oral Radiology Endodontics, 81*, 172–176.

Navazesh, M., & Christensen, C. M. (1982). A comparison of whole mouth resting and stimulated salivary measurement procedures. *Journal of Dental Research, 61*, 1158–1162.

Netsell, R. (1984). A Neurobiological view of the dysarthrias. In M. R. McNeil, J. C. Rosenbek, & A. E. Aronson (Eds.), *The dysarthrias.* San Diego: College-Hill Press.

Netsell, R., Lotz, W. K., Peters, J. E., & Schulte, L. (1994). Developmental patterns of laryngeal and respiratory function for speech production. *Journal of Voice, 8*, 123–131.

Nilsson, M. E., Isacsson, G., Isberg, A., & Schiratzki, H. (1989). Mobility of the upper esophageal sphincter in relation to the cervical spine: A morphologic study. *Dysphagia 3*, 161–165.

Oesterberg, T., & Steen, B. (1982). Relationship between dental state and dietary intake in 70-year-old males and females in Goteborg, Sweden: A population study. *Journal of Oral Rehabilitation, 9*, 509–552.

Ohmae, Y., Karaho, T., Hanyu, Y., Murase, Y., Kitahara, S., & Inouye, T. (1997). Effect of posture strategies on preventing aspiration. *Nippon Jibiinkoka Gakkai Kaiho, 100*(2), 220–226.

Ono, I., Gunji, H., Tateshita, T., & Sanbe, N. (1997). Reconstruction of defects of the entire vermilin with a buccal musculomucosal flap following resection of malignant tumors of the lower lip. *Plastic and Reconstructive Surgery, 100*, 422–430.

Oobayashi, Y., & Miyawaki, S. (1995). Ataxic sensory and autonomic neuropathies associated with primary Sjögren's syndrome: A case report. *Ryumachi, 35*, 107–111.

Ott, David, J., Hodge, R. G., Pikna, L. A., Chen, M. Y., & Gelfand, D. W. (1996). Modified Barium swallow: Clinical and adiographic correlation and relation to feeding recommendations. *Dysphagia 11*, 187–190.

Panchal, J., Potterton, A. J., Scanlon, E., & McLean, N. R. (1996). An objective assessment of speech and swallowing following free flap reconstruction for oral cavity cancers. *British Journal of Plastic Surgery, 49*, 363–369.

Petring, O. U., Adelhoj, B., Jensen, B. N., Pedersen, N. O., Lomholt, P. (1986). Prevention of silent aspiration due to leaks around cuffs of endotracheal tubes. *Anesthesia and Analgesia, 65*, 777–780.

Poncelet, A. N., Auger, R. G., & Silber, M. H. (1996). Myokymic discharges of the tongue after radiation to the head and neck. *Neurology, 46*, 259–260.

Pouderoux, P., & Kahrilas, P. J. (1995). Deglutitive tongue force modulation by volition, volume, and viscosity in humans. *Gastroenterology, 108*, 1418–1426.

Ramirez-Amador, V., Silverman, S., Jr., Mayer, P., Tyler, M., & Quivey, J. (1997). Candidal colonization and oral candidiasis in patients undergoing oral and pharyngeal radiation therapy. *Oral Surgery, Oral Medicine, Oral Pathology, and Oral Radiology Endodontics, 84*, 149–153.

Rasley, A., Logemann, J. A., Kahrilas, P. J., Rademaker, A. W., Pauloski, B. R., & Dodds, W. J. (1993). Prevention of barium aspiration during videofluoroscopic swallowing studies: Value of change in posture. *American Journal of Roentgenology, 160*, 1005–1009.

Rath, E. M., & Essick, G. K. (1990). Perioral somesthetic sensibility: Do the skin of the lower face and the midface exhibit comparable sensitivity? *Journal of Oral and Maxillofacial Surgery, 48*, 1181–1190.

Rhodus, N. L., & Brown, J. (1990). The association of xerostomia and inadequate intake in older adults. *Journal of the American Dietetic Association, 90*, 1688–1692.

Ricketts, D. N., Kidd, E. A., & Beighton, D. (1995). Operative and microbiological validation of visual, radiographic and electronic diagnosis of occlusal caries in non-cavitated teeth judged to be in need of operative care. *British Dental Journal, 179*, 214–220.

Rieger, A., Brunne, B., & Striebel, H. W. (1997). Intracuff pressures do not predict laryngopharyngeal discomfort after use of the laryngeal mask airway. *Anesthesiology 87*, 63–67.

Rieger, A., Hass, I., Gross, M., Gramm, H. J., & Eyrich, K. (1996). Intubation trauma of the larynx—A literature review with special reference to arytenoid cartilage dislocation *Anasthesiologie, Intensivmedizin, Notfallmedizin, Schmerztherapie, 31*, 281–287.

Ringel, R. L., & Ewanowski, S. J. (1965). Oral perception: Two-point discrimination. *Journal of Speech and Hearing Research, 8*, 389–398.

Robb, N. D., & Crothers, A. J. (1996). Sedation in dentistry: Part 2. Management of the gagging patient. *Dental Update, 23*, 182–186.

Robbins, J., Levine, R., Wood, J., Roecker, E. B., & Luschei, E. J. (1995). Age effects on lingual pressure generation as a risk factor for dysphagia. *Journals of Gerontology. Series A, Biological Sciences and Medical Sciences, 50*, M257–M262.

Roberts, E. W. (1994). The failed dental appointment case report: The phobic gagger. *Texas Dental Journal, 111*, 19–20.

Rodriguez-Roisin, R., Ferrer, A., Navajas, D., Agusti, A. G., Wagner, P. D., & Roca, J. (1991). Ventilation-perfusion mismatch anfter methacholine challenge in patients with mild bronchial asthma. *American Review of Respiratory Disease, 144*, 88–94.

Rogers, B. T., Arvedson, J., Msall, & M., Demerath, R. R. (1993). Hypoxemia during oral feeding of children with severe cerebral palsy. *Developmental Medicine Child Neurology, 35*, 3–10.

Rogers, B., Msall, M., & Shucard, D. (1993). Hypoxemia during oral feedings in adults with dysphagia and severe neurological disabilities. *Dysphagia, 8*, 43–48.

Rosenbek, J. C., Robbins, J., Fishback, B., & Levine, R. L. (1991). Effects of thermal application on dysphagia after stroke. *Journal of Speech and Hearing Research, 34*, 1257–1268.

Rosenbek, J. C., Robbins, J., Willford, W. O., Kirk, G., Schiltz, A., Sowell, T. W., Deutsch, S. E., Milanti, F. J., Ashford, J., Gramigna, G. D., Fogarty, A., Dong, K., Rau, M. T., Prescott, T. E., Lloyd, A. M., Sterkel, M. T., & Hansen, J. E. (1998). Comparing treatment intensities of tactile-thermal application. *Dysphagia, 13*, 1–9.

Rosenbek, J. C., Roecker, E. B., Wood, J. L., & Robbins, J. (1996). Thermal application reduces the duration of stage transition in dysphagia after stroke. *Dysphagia, 11*, 225–233.

Sachdev, P. (1992). Drug-induced movement disorders in institutionalised adults with mental retardation: Clinical characteristics and risk factors. *Australian New Zealand Journal of Psychiatry, 26,* 242–248.

Schneider, H. J. (1997). Gross dysarthric movement disorders of the velopharynx *HNO, 45,* 460–465.

Schubert, M. M., & Izutsu, K. T. (1987). Iatrogenic causes of salivary gland dysfunction. *Journal of Dental Research, 66,* 680–688.

Seidel, H. M., Ball, J. W., Dains, J. E, & Benedict, G. W. (1996). Chest and lungs, examination and findings. In *Mosby's Guide to Physical Examination* (2nd ed., pp. 290–293). St. Louis: C. V. Mosby.

Selinger, M., Prescott, T. E., & Hoffman, I. (1994). Temperature acceleration in cold oral stimulation. *Dysphagia, 9,* 83–87.

Selinger, M., Presott, T., & McKinley, R. (1990). The efficacy of thermal stimulation: A case study. *Rocky Mountain Journal of Communication Disorders, 8,* 21–23.

Sellars, C., Dunnet, C., & Carter, R. (1998). A preliminary comparison of videofluoroscopy of swallow and pulse oximetry in the identification of aspiration in dysphagic patients. *Dysphagia, 13,* 82–86.

Selley, W., Ellis, M., Flack, F., Bayliss, C., Chir, B., & Pearce, M. (1994). The synchronization of respiration and swallow sounds with videofluoroscopy during swallowing. *Dysphagia, 9,* 162–167.

Shafei, H., el-Kholy, A., Azmy, S., Ebrahim, M., & al-Ebrahim, K. (1997). Vocal cord dysfunction after cardiac surgery: An overlooked complication. *European Journal of Cardiothoracic Surgery, 11,* 564–566.

Shaker, R., Junlong, R., Zafar, Z., Achal, S., Jianmin, L., & Zhuei, S. (1994). Effect of ageing, position and temperature on the threshold volume triggering pharyngeal swallows. *Gastroenterology, 107,* 396–402.

Shanahan, T. K., Logemann, J. A., Rademaker, A. W., Pauloski, B. R., & Kahrilas, P. J. (1993). Chin-down posture effect on aspiration in dysphagic patients. *Archives of Physical Medicine and Rehabilitation, 74,* 736–739.

Ship, J. A., & Fischer, D. J. (1997). The relationship between dehydration and parotid salivary gland function in young and older healthy adults. *Journals of Gerontology. Series A, Biological Sciences and Medical Sciences, 52,* M310–M319.

Shohara, H. (1932). *Genesis of articulatory movements in speech* [Unpublished doctoral dissertation], University of Michigan, Ann Arbor.

Slagter, A. P., Olthoff, L. W., Bosman, F., & Steen, W. H. (1992). Masticatory ability, denture quality and oral conditions in edentulous subjects. *The Journal of Prosthetic Dentistry, 68,* 299–307.

Smeltzer, S. C., Lavietes, M. H., Troiano, R., & Cook, S. D. (1989). Testing of an index in pulmonary dysfunction in multiple sclerosis. *Nursing Research, 38,* 370–374.

Smeltzer, S. C., Skurnick, J. H., Troiano, R., Cook, S. D., Duran, W., & Lavietes, M. H. (1992). Respiratory function in multiple sclerosis. Utility of clinical assessment of respiratory muscle function. *Chest: Official Publication of the American College of Chest Physicians, 101,* 479–484.

Smithard, D. G. (1996). Percutaneous endoscopic gastrostomy feeding after acute dysphagic stroke. Gag reflex has no role in ability to swallow. *British Medical Journal, 312,* 972.

Sochaniwskyj, A. E., Koheil, R. M., Bablich, K., Milner, M., & Kenny, D. J. (1986). Oral motor functioning, frequency of swallowing and drooling in normal children and in children with cerebral palsy. *Archives of Physical Medicine and Rehabilitation, 67,* 866–874.

Spiro, J., Rendell, J. K., & Gay, T. (1994). Activation and coordination patterns of the suprahyoid muscles during swallowing. *Laryngoscope, 104,* 1376–1382.

Steele, C. M., Greenwood, C., Ens, I., Robertson, C., & Seidman-Carlson, R. (1997). Mealtime difficulties in a home for the aged: Not just dysphagia. *Dysphagia, 12,* 43–50.

Sundgren, P., Maly, P., & Gullberg, B. (1993). Elevation of the larynx on normal and abnormal cineradiogram. *The British Journal of Radiology, 66,* 768–772.

Sversson, P., Arendt-Nielsen, L., Houe, L. (1996). Sensory-motor interactions of human experimental unilateral jaw muscle pain: A quantitive analysis. *Pain, 64,* 241–249.

Syrjanen, J., Peltola, J., Baltonen, V., Iivanainen, M., Kaste, M., & Huttunen, J. K. (1989). Dental infections in association with cerebral infacrion in young and middle-aged men. *Journal of Internal Medicine, 225,* 179–184.

Takahashi, K., Groher, M. E., & Michi, K. (1994a). Methodology for detecting swallowing sounds. *Dysphagia, 9,* 54–62.

Takahashi, K., Groher, M. E., & Michi, K. (1994b). Symmetry and reproducibility of swallowing sounds. *Dysphagia, 9,* 168–173.

Talacko, A. A., & Reade, P. C. (1990). Progressive bulbar palsy: A case report of a type of motor neuron disease presenting with oral symptoms. *Oral Surgery, Oral Medicine, and Oral Pathology, 69,* 182–184.

Tartell, P. B., Hoover, L. A., Friduss, M. E., & Zuckerbraun, L. (1990). Pharyngoesophageal intubation injuries: Three case reports. *American Journal of Otolaryngology, 11,* 256–260.

Teasdale, G., & Jennett, B. (1974). Assessment of coma and impaired consiousness. A practical scale. *Lancet, 2,* 81–84.

Teramoto, S., Fukuchi, Y., & Ouchi, Y. (1996). Oxygen desaturation on swallowing in patients with stroke: What does it mean? [Editorial]. *Age and Ageing, 25,* 333.

Terpenning, M., Bretz, W., Lopatin, D., Langmore, S., Dominguez, B., & Loesche, W. (1993). Bacterial colonization of saliva and plaque in the elderly. *Clinical Infectious Disease, 16*(Suppl. 4), S314–S316.

Tewari, P., & Aggarwal, S. K. (1996). Combined left-sided recurrent laryngeal and phrenic nerve palsy after coronary artery operation. *Annals of Thoracic Surgery, 61,* 1721–1722.

Thirlwall, A. S. (1997). Ortner's syndrome: A centenary review of unilateral recurrent laryngeal nervepalsy secondary to cardiothoracic disease. *The Journal of Laryngology and Otology, 111,* 869–871.

Thompson-Henry, S., & Braddock, B. (1995). The modified Evan's blue dye procedure fails to detect aspiration in the tracheostomized patient: Five case reports. *Dysphagia, 10,* 172–174.

Tippett, D. C., & Siebens, A. A. (1996). Reconsidering the value of the modified Evan's blue dye test: A comment on Thompson-Henry and Braddock (1995). *Dysphagia, 11,* 78–79.

Treloar, D. M., & Stechmiller, J. (1984). Pulmonary aspiration in tube-fed patients with artificial airways. *Heart & Lung, 13,* 667–671.

Treloar, D. M., & Stechmiller, J. K. (1995). Use of a clinical assessment tool for orally intubated patients. *American Journal of Critical Care, 4,* 355–360.

Turner, G. S., Tjaden, K., & Weismer, G. (1995). The influence of speaking on vowel space and speech intelligibility for individuals with amyotrophic lateral sclerosis. *Journal of Speech and Hearing Research, 38,* 1001–1013.

Valenti, W. M., Trudell, R. G., & Bentley, D. W. (1978). Factors predisposing to oropharyngeal colonization with gram-negative bacilli in the aged. *New England Journal of Medicine, 298,* 1108–1111.

Van der Bilt, A., Olthoff, L. W., Bosman, F., & Oosterhaven, S. P. (1993). The effect of missing postcanine teeth on chewing performance in man. *Archives of Oral Biology, 38,* 423–429.

Vigild, M. (1988). Oral hygiene and periodontal conditions among 201 dentate institutionalized elderly. *Gerodontics, 4,* 140–145.

Wang, V., Liao, K. K., Ju, T. H., Lin, K. P., Wang, S. J., Wu, Z. A., & Chung Hua, I. (1993). Myokymia and neuromyotonia of the tongue: A case report of complication of irradiation. *Hsueh Tsa Chih, 52,* 413–415.

Wayler, A. H., & Chauncey, H. H. (1983). Impact of complete dentures and impaired natural dentition on masticatory performance and food choice in healthy aging men. *The Journal of Prosthetic Dentistry, 49,* 427–433.

Wilson, J. A., Pryde, A., White, A., Maher, L., & Maron, A. G. (1995). Swallowing performance in patients with vocal fold motion impairment. *Dysphagia, 10,* 149–154.

Wohlert, A. B., & Smith, A. (1998). Spatiotemporal stability of lip movements in older adult speakers. *Journal of Speech, Language, and Hearing Research, 41,* 41–50.

Yassa, R., & Lal, S. (1986). Respiratory irregularity and tardive dyskinesia. A prevalence study. *Acta Psychiatrica Scandinavica, 73,* 506–510.

Yorkston, K. M., Honsinger, M. J., Mitsuda, P. M., & Hammen, V. (1989). The relationship between speech and swallowing disorders in head injury patients. *The Journal of Head Trauma Rehabilitation, 4,* 1–16.

Yurkstas, A. A., & Emerson, W. H. (1964). Dietary selections of persons with natural and artificial teeth. *The Journal of Prosthetic Dentistry, 14,* 696–697.

Zaidi, N. H., Smith, H. A., King, S. C., Park, C., O'Neill, P. A., & Connolly, M. J. (1995). Oxygen desaturation on swallowing as a potential marker of aspiration in acute stroke. *Age and Ageing, 24,* 267–270.

Zenner, P. M., Losinski, D. S., & Mills, R. H. (1995). Using cervical auscultation in the clinical dysphagia examination in long-term care. *Dysphagia, 10,* 27–31.

Zohar, Y., Buler, N., Shvilli, Y., & Sabo, R. (1998). Reconstruction of the soft palate by uvulopalatal flap. *Laryngoscope, 108*(1, Pt. 1), 47–50.

CHAPTER 3

Videofluoroscopic Examination

"Even a single hair casts its shadow."
Publius Syrus (Circa. 42 B.C.)

INTRODUCTION

The first dynamic fluoroscopic image was observed by Wilhelm Roentgen in Wurzburg, Germany in 1895. While experimenting in his crowded laboratory with an early version of a cathode ray tube, a nearby plate coated with bariumplatinocyanide began to fluoresce. When various objects made of wood and metal were moved between the tube and the plate, it was observed that shadows, in the form of the manipulated material, were cast upon the plate.

In the early days of fluoroscopy, the clinician turned all of the room lights off and pulled a dark tent over the fluoroscope so that direct viewing of the fluorescent screen was possible. This, as we realize today, led to the early demise of many of the turn-of-the-century radiologists. Although viewing the image today is considerably safer than it was at the turn of the century, the acquisition of the image remains almost exactly the same. X-rays emanating from a diode tube are cast upon a fluorescent screen, on which an image is formed, allowing for the viewing of shadows cast by the differing densities of tissue and

bone. The only dramatic difference between today's imaging and that in Roentgen's time is in our ability to record the dynamic image on videotape.

The dynamic imaging of swallow function (see Figure 3–1) is enhanced by the visualization of the bolus during the swallow. Adding a contrast material dense enough to absorb the X rays, such as barium sulfate ($BaSO_4$), allows for visualization of the bolus as it travels through the alimentary tract.

VIDEOFLUOROSCOPIC IMAGING OF OROPHARYNGEAL SWALLOWING

To make a confident determination of safety and efficiency, the clinician must strive to integrate all of the elements that contribute to a viable oropharyngeal swallow. The components of the fluoroscopic assessment are listed in Table 3–1.

By integrating all of these components, the clinician hopes to estimate efficiency and ensure safety. Further, the clinician now will be armed with detailed information, which often will allow for the realization of the biomechanical basis of impairment. It is from this foundation that appropriate treatment goals are formulated.

VIDEOFLUOROSCOPIC PROTOCOL

The clinician will elicit swallows by presenting food and liquid with barium contrast of varying volumes and consistencies to the patient. Equipment required is listed in Table 3–2.

Food Presentation Guidelines

Food and liquid are presented in the same manner as they were in the clinical swallowing examination. The objective of the examination is to show ability as well as disability. The initial careful presentation of measured

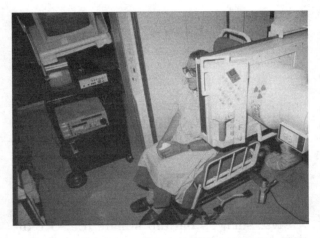

Figure 3-1. Patient seated in special fluoroscopy chair and positioned for lateral projection.

amounts will pay off later in the examination. The microphone will provide a soundtrack for the examination. The clinician should announce the amount and manner of presentation for each bolus. When reviewing the tape afterwards, even a few months or years later, this will serve to remind you what or how much was presented. More important, the soundtrack will provide verification of whether a patient's cough was spontaneous or cued. This is an important distinction when considering recommendations later in the management process.

Carefully conducted examinations with judicious presentations of food and liquid are not likely to yield catastrophic events of aspiration. The examination should not be aborted when a small amount of aspiration occurs. Aborting the examination prevents the implementation of the various adjustments that may alleviate the event of aspiration.

Scoring

Swallowing traditionally has been divided into stages that roughly describe the anatomic boundaries along the path of the advancing bolus. The traditional boundaries have been identified as the oral, pharyngeal and upper esophageal stages or phases of the swallow. Popular terms for the videofluoroscopic evaluation of swallowing (three-phase swallow test, or triple-phase swallow test) reflect this construct. An additional stage, the oral preparatory stage, has been recognized widely as being separate from the oral propulsive stage of the swallow. These stages do not adequately describe the continuum of movement or the

---

Table 3-1. Components of the fluoroscopic assessment.

Identification of:

    Normal and abnormal anatomy

    Discrete structural movements

    Temporal coordination of anatomic movements relative to bolus advancement

    Trajectory of the bolus through the aero-digestive pathway

Evaluation of the efficacy of:

    Adjustments to the bolus volume, consistency, and rate of delivery

    Adjustments in positioning

    Implementation of maneuvers

Table 3–2. Equipment needed for videofluoroscopic examination.

Equipment Needed	Optional Equipment
Spoons/cups/straws	Time/date character generator
Puree/solids with $BaSO_4$	Surface electromyography
Premixed $BaSO_4$ liquids of varying viscosity	Pharyngeal manometry
$BaSO_4$ tablet or capsule	Ball bearing/coin
Videotape recorder	
Microphone	
Lead-shielded protective apparel	

interplay of structural forces that are transferred from one of these arbitrary stages to another. For this reason, the swallow will be evaluated according to the components outlined on the scoring sheet (Form 3–1). A completed videofluoroscopic examination form is included as a model (see Form 3–2).

Observation/Projection

Anatomy

The initial task, once the patient is seated and the fluoroscope is positioned appropriately is to determine deviations in anatomic structures. If the clinician is aware of surgical or developmental structural deviations, care should be taken to scan the areas in question. In the absence of known structural deviations, scanning should include a gross census and inspection of these anatomic structures that can not be visualized during the clinical examination.

Some structures may not be well-visualized without some amount of contrast coating the surface mucosa. The clinician may present a small amount of contrast (1–2 cc) to the patient to highlight these structures, if necessary. Presenting this small amount also very likely will generate a pharyngeal swallow and the first impression of function will be formed.

Projection

The patient may be positioned between the tube and screen in several ways. The most frequent positions are lateral, anterior-posterior (AP), and oblique.

Lateral Projection. The lateral view provides the clinician with an unobstructed visualization of the aerodigestive path (see Figure 3–2). Of particular value is the clear demarcation of the lower pharynx, laryngeal inlet, and upper esophagus provided in this projection. This view allows the clinician to carefully track the trajectory of the bolus during its proper advancement through the pharynx and into the upper esophagus or, during an event of aspiration/penetration, its entry into the laryngeal inlet.

In the lateral projection, movements of the tongue, velum, epiglottis, and arytenoids can be observed. Because of the properties of fluoroscopy, structures that lie underneath surface mucosa are well-visualized. These structures include the hyoid bone, the thyroid and cricoid cartilages, and the upper esophageal sphincter (UES). Normal configuration of the cervical spine also is well-appreciated in this projection, as are abnormal configurations of the anterior cervical spine, such as cervical osteophytes (Figure 3–3).

Other spaces of the pharynx serve a protective function. These spaces, the valleculae and pyriform sinuses, collect and channel material away from the laryngeal inlet before and after a swallow.

The lateral projection compounds bilaterally represented anatomical structures. For this reason, it is very difficult to discern the left arytenoid or left pyriform sinus from the right.

Anterior-Posterior Projection. For this projection, the patient is positioned facing the fluorescent screen. The anterior-posterior projection allows for better visualization of the bilaterally represented structures that were compounded and visually obscured using the

Form 3–1
Videofluoroscopic Examination

VFE-1. Anatomic Notes:

_____

_____

VFE-2
Biomechanical Notation:

a-Tongue   _____

b-Velum   _____

c-Epiglottis   _____

d-Laryngeal Ele.   _____

e-P. Ph. Wall*   _____

f-UES*   _____

g-Esophagus   _____

h-Airway Closure   _____

Material	Puree	Soft Solid	Solid	Liquids	
				THIN	THICK
VFE-3 **Max Amount:**	_____	_____	_____	_____	_____
VFE-4 **Duration:** a-DST*	_____	_____	_____	_____	_____
b-OTD*	_____	_____	_____	_____	_____
c-PTD*	_____	_____	_____	_____	_____
d-OPSE*	_____	_____	_____	_____	_____
VFE-5 **Asp/Pen:**	_____	_____	_____	_____	_____
VFE-6 **Intervention:**	_____	_____	_____	_____	_____

VFE-7
Narrative: _____

OTD*	= oral transit duration
PTD*	= pharyngeal transit duration
DST*	= duration of stage transition
OPSE*	= oral pharyngeal swallow efficiency
P. Ph. Wall*	= posterior pharyngeal wall
UES*	= upper esophageal sphincter

Form 3–2

Videofluoroscopic Examination (Completed Form)

VFE-1. Anatomic Notes:

Small cervical osteophytes noted at the level of c3-4 and c6-7. Anatomy is grossly normal otherwise.

VFE-2
Biomechanical Notation:

a-Tongue	Good lingual velar seal and control of bolus. Contact along tongue base to posterior wall incomplete at level of c-3.
b-Velum	Velar elevation unremarkable.
c-Epiglottis	Epiglottal retroflexion incomplete. Noted to move to horizontal position when well visualized.
d-Laryngeal Ele.	Reduced hyoid excursion. Laryngeal cartilages noted to elevate to meet hyoid.
e-P. Ph. Wall*	Posterior pharyngeal wall anterior movement indiscernable. No contact with tongue base beyond the level of c-2-3.
f-UES*	Bolus that was propelled into the UES was cleared into the esophagus without obstruction. Majority of the bolus remained in pyriforms or rested atop post cricoid area.
g-Esophagus	Esophageal transit slow but complete and grossly normal.
h-Airway Closure	Arytenoid contact with base of epiglottis appeared to occur late during elevation as evidenced by airspace between arytenoid and epiglottic base at height of elevation.

Material	Puree	Soft Solid	Solid	Liquids THIN	Liquids THICK
VFE-3					
Max Amount:	15 cc	15 cc	20 cc	5 cc	25 cc
VFE-4 **Duration:**					
a-DST*	2 s	4 s	7 s	2 s	4 s
b-OTD*	1.2	3	3	1	1
c-PTD*	1.8	3.8	3.6	1.5	1.7
d-OPSE*	30	12	10	38	34
VFE-5 **Asp/Pen:**	1	1	1	7	4

(continued)

VFE-6

Intervention:	none	none	none	chin tuck −	chin tuck −

VFE-7

Narrative:

Patient strapped securely in procedure chair. Somnolent prior to exam. Fully alert prior to presentations of food. Slow oral manipulation. Labored mastication. Swallow typically initiated when bolus at the level of valleculae for puree and solids and at pyriforms for liquids. Thin liquids noted to flow into pyriforms and overflow into laryngeal vestibule and deeply into tracheal airway prior to swallow initiation. Appeared sensitive to aspirate as severe coughing ensued. Coughing marginally successful at clearing aspirate with some evident in right middle bronchus. Unable to follow instructions to perform chin tuck. Nectar thins aspirated in similar manner. Liquids thickened to honey consistently safely swallowed in all volumes up to 25 cc. Poor tongue base retraction and posterior wall apposition. Laryngeal elevation reduced, epiglottal retroflexion incomplete.

Impression:

Moderate pharyngeal dysphagia characterized by mistimed airway protection and bolus propulsion resulting in aspiration of quickly flowing liquids. Reduced amplitude of pharyngeal stage results in residue remaining after the initial swallow attempt that is easily cleared with successive spontaneous swallows. Patient unable to follow commands, poor candidate for behavioral intervention.

Plan:

Make diet recommendation in report to upgrade to soft solids with liquids thickened to a honey consistency. Perform calorie count to determine adequacy of intake. Monitor closely and re-examine in 2 days to determine change.

OTD* = oral transit duration
PTD* = pharyngeal transit duration
DST* = duration of stage transition
OPSE* = oral pharyngeal swallow efficiency
P. Ph. Wall* = posterior pharyngeal wall
UES* = upper esophageal sphincter

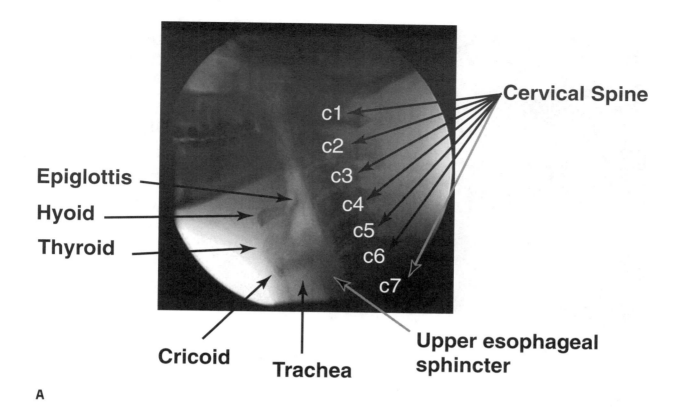

Cervical Spine

c1
c2
c3
c4
c5
c6
c7

Epiglottis
Hyoid
Thyroid

Cricoid

Trachea

Upper esophageal sphincter

A

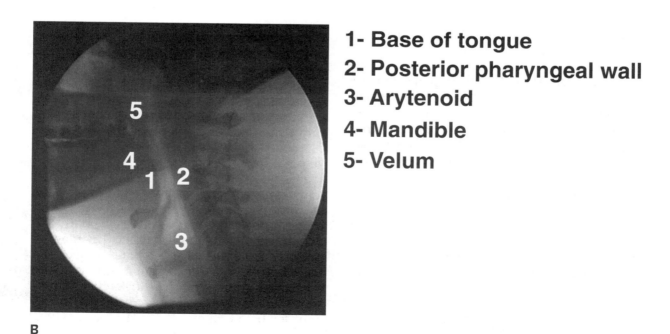

5

4

1 2

3

1- Base of tongue
2- Posterior pharyngeal wall
3- Arytenoid
4- Mandible
5- Velum

B

Figure 3-2. Lateral fluoroscopic projection of the oral, pharyngeal and upper esophageal regions.

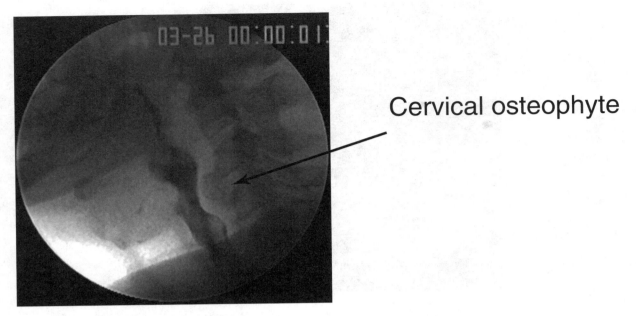

Figure 3-3. Cervical osteophyte emanating in the area of c3-4.

lateral projection (Figure 3–4). This view also allows for a view of the true and false vocal folds. As the projection continues inferiorly, the upper esophagus is seen to form an arch as it traverses around the aorta before continuing inferiorly to the lower esophageal sphincter and stomach. In this projection, much of the detail of the air space of the pharynx is obscured because of the density and centered position of the cervical spine.

Oblique Projection. In this projection, the subject is positioned at a 45° angle to the fluorescent screen. This projection allows for better visualization of the anterior midline structures that would be obscured by the density of the spine in the AP projection (Figure 3–5).

Corpulent patients that do not fit comfortably between the diode tube and the fluorescent screen frequently are positioned for an oblique projection.

The following sections provide descriptions of each of the components of the videofluoroscopic examination (VFE) listed on Form 3–1.

VFE-1. SCORING: ANATOMIC MOVEMENTS

Presenting food and liquid to a patient under fluoroscopy allows the clinician to observe the discrete movements of oral, pharyngeal, and upper-esophageal structures. Some anatomical structures move independently during the advancement of the bolus from the oral cavity to the stomach whereas additional structures impart traction on, and displace, other structures. The movements will be discussed in terms of the projection that provides the best visualization.

VFE-2. SCORING: BIOMECHANICAL MOVEMENT

Enter, in narrative form, information regarding impaired movement in the Biomechanical Notation section of the score sheet.

VFE-2A. SCORING: TONGUE

Tongue movement is well-observed in both the lateral and AP projections. The body of the tongue largely is observed to move with the jaw during mastication (Palmer, Hiiemae, & Liu, 1997). The tip of the tongue pushes the bolus from side to side as the food particulate is reduced gradually to a consistency appropriate for swallowing. Lateral tongue movement for bolus manipulation during mastication is best viewed in the AP projection.

Bolus control and propulsive movements are well-visualized in the lateral projection. The bolus typically is cradled in the oral cavity prior to the initiation of the swallow. During

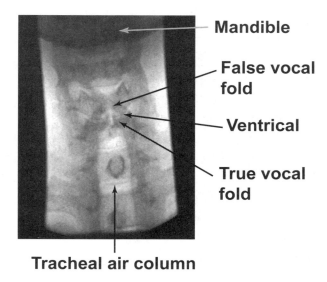

Figure 3-4. Anterior-posterior projection or the head and neck.

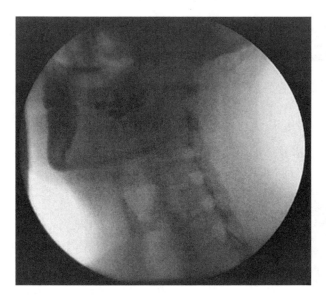

Figure 3-5. Oblique projection of the head and neck.

this time, the lateral margins of the tongue will stay in contact with the alveolar mucosa while a central groove is formed in the tongue to accommodate the bolus. The dorsum of the tongue and soft palate contact posteriorly to form a seal. In some subjects, the bolus may be cradled below the tip of the tongue and, at initiation of the oral stage, the tongue will dip down to collect the bolus (Dodds et al., 1989). The authors attached the moniker of "dipper" to this pattern of bolus storage and retrieval often seen in subjects over the age of 60.

At the onset of the swallow, the tongue has formed a propulsive chamber that expels the bolus from the oral cavity by applying pressure in a progressive, arcing, peristaltic motion, starting anteriorly and progressing posteriorly against the hard palate and elevated soft palate (Shaker, Cook, Dodds, & Hogan, 1988). While the tongue continues to thrust the bolus toward the oropharynx in a "piston-like motion" (Dodds et al., 1989), the base of the tongue flattens and moves anteriorly to provide space for the oncoming bolus. As the bolus enters the oropharynx, the base of the tongue continues the peristaltic arc by progressively contacting the posterior pharyngeal wall at the tail of the bolus until it is squeezed inferiorly to the border of the valleculae.

Abnormal Tongue Movement

A number of postoperative and/or postirradiation changes can be observed in patients with oral cavity cancers. These changes can result from loss of tissue, changes in the elasticity of the tissue, reduced strength, and reduced sensation. For problems involving the anterior tongue tip and blade, information from the clinical examination should be carefully integrated. Specifically, the clinician should integrate the clinical findings related to strength, sensation, and ROM of the tongue and compare that information with the radiographic findings (Table 3–3).

The effect of structural changes can be wide-ranging and highly variable between patients with identical surgeries and irradiation schedules. Patients with anterior lesions may demonstrate residue throughout the oral cavity but, more frequently it is seen to be lateralized to the site of the surgery (Panchal, Potterton, Scanlon, & McLean, 1996).

Posterior tongue resection compromises posterior tongue retraction, one of the main components of safe and efficient bolus advancement through the pharynx. Stachler et al. (1994) found that head and neck cancer patients with anterior resections had better postoperative outcomes than did patients with posterior resections of the tongue. However, in a study by Colangelo, Logemann, Pauloski, Pelzer, and Rademaker (1996), it was found that patients with anterior resection and posterior resections have similar functional outcomes.

Table 3-3. Abnormalities in the preparatory and oral phases of swallowing.

Radiological Findings	Type of Impairment
Cannot hold barium in mouth anteriorly	Reduced lip closure
Cannot form bolus	Reduced range or coordination of tongue movement
Cannot chew	Reduced tongue lateralization
Hesitancy initiating swallow	Impaired cognitive function, neural function, or oral sensation
Stasis in buccal sulci	Reduced labial or buccal tension
Stasis in floor of mouth	Reduced tongue shaping
Stasis in midtongue depression	Tongue scarring
Abnormal lingual peristalsis	Impaired tongue motion
Poor tongue to palate contact	Reduced tongue elevation
Repetitive tongue rolling	Parkinson's disease
Premature spillage of bolus	Reduced tongue or palatal control
Slow oral transit time	Impaired tongue movement

Source: From Dodds, W., Stewart, E., & Logemann, J. (1990). Physiology and radiology of the normal oral and pharyngeal phases of swallowing. *American Journal of Roentgenology, 154*, p. 966. Reprinted with permission.

The posterior tongue also contributes to the lingual-palatal seal of liquids prior to the intiation of the swallow. Loss of control of the bolus will result in premature spillage into the lower pharynx with the possible consequence of penetration of the laryngeal inlet.

Patients with dyskinesia often demonstrate tongue-pumping behaviors prior to the final initiation of the oral stage of the swallow. The amount of time necessary to initiate the swallow might be extended, but the swallow, once initiated, can be performed with adequate amplitude and safety. The main consideration in these patients is the loss of oral control of the bolus prior to the initiation of the swallow with subsequent premature leakage of material into the laryngeal inlet.

Patients with diffuse weakness may demonstrate residue along the surface of the tongue from the tip to the vallecular space. Low tongue driving force has been found to result in vallecular retention (Dejaeger, Pelemans, Ponette, & Joosten, 1997). In these patients, the amplitude of tongue pressure on the bolus as it is squeezed along the hard and soft palates and posterior pharyngeal wall is reduced. In patients with intact sensation of this residue, puree and solid food stasis often is seen to fall to the vallecular space where multiple swallows are implemented for clearance. Liquid stasis will fill the vallecular space and, if of a volume great enough to overflow the vallecular space, will travel, by gravity, alongside the laryngeal vestibule to the pyriform sinuses.

VFE-2B. SCORING: VELUM

The velum contributes to the posterior closure of the oral cavity prior to the onset of the swallow. The palatoglossus muscle contracts and bends the body of the soft palate against the elevated dorsum of the tongue which, together, form a glossopalatal sphincter (Rubesin, Jones, & Donner, 1987). This seal prevents the premature leakage of material into the pharynx, reducing the chance of bolus entry into the laryngeal inlet prior to the commencement of airway protection. For further discussion regarding the glossopalatal seal, refer to pages 55–57 of the clinical exam.

The velum also elevates, during the onset of the pharyngeal stage of the swallow, to close off the nasopharynx, thus preventing the entry of food or liquid into the nasal cavity. The arrival of the bolus head into the pharynx occurs approximately 0.200 seconds after the complete closure of the nasopharynx (Dua, Shaker, Ren, Arndorfer, & Hofmann, 1995). The closure is augmented by the palatopharyngeus muscle and the superior constrictor muscles (Schneider, 1997) to form a tight seal during the swallow.

Abnormal Velar Elevation

A unilateral or bilateral weakening of the palatoglossus will result in a poor glossopalatal seal. When palatoglossus muscle depression or tongue dorsum elevation is not adequate, boluses may be released into the pharynx prior to volitional propulsion, resulting in "premature spillage." If the spillage reaches an unprotected laryngeal inlet, aspiration is possible. Causes of velopharyngeal insufficiency are listed in Table 3–4.

When velar elevation is insufficient, food or liquid may enter into the nose through the compromised nasopharyngeal seal resulting in nasoregurgitation. This occurs due to the increasing pressure that is exerted by the bolus on the pharyngeal tissue as the tongue and pharyngeal constrictors close around it. The pressurized bolus will flow along the path of least resistance, and, if an opening occurs anywhere in the propulsive chamber, as is the case with a compromised nasopharyngeal seal, the path of least resistance will be the nasopharyngeal port.

VFE-2C. SCORING: EPIGLOTTIS

The epiglottis provides protection to the laryngeal inlet in a manner that is both active and static. It is primarily a static structural barrier to the lower airway. The epiglottis rises above the base of the tongue and forms a plow-shaped shield, that directs the advancing bolus laterally to channels that terminate at the

Table 3–4. Causes of velopharyngeal insufficiency.

Cleft palate

Congenital palatal incompetence

Deep pharynx

Submucous cleft palate

Anomalies of cervical spine

Palatal neuromuscular dysfunction

Traumatic or surgical defects

---

pyriform sinuses. At the lingual base of the epiglottis is the vallecular space, a space that is a temporary reservoir for the early arrival of portions of a bolus prior to a swallow.

Even in its role as an active protective mechanism, the epiglottis moves passively, and is affected by traction forces from the tongue, hyoid, and laryngeal cartilages. During the height of the pharyngeal swallow, the epiglottis is observed to invert over the laryngeal inlet as it provides another, redundant, layer of protection to the already closed airway.

Epiglottal inversion is composed of three distinct components, all of which occur as a result of the application and release of traction forces from elevating and descending laryngeal structures and tongue forces. The three movement components are (1) onset of descent to a horizontal position, (2) movement below horizontal, and (3) return to rest (Logemann et al., 1992).

The anterior movement of the elevating hyoid bone applies traction to the hyoepiglottic ligament. This traction pulls the base of the epiglottis anteriorly, resulting in a tilting of the epiglottis to a horizontal position. As the elevating thyroid and cricoid cartilages ascend to the elevated hyoid bone, the epiglottis downfolds (Perlman, Van Daele, & Ottervacher, 1995; Van Daele, Perlman, & Cassell, 1995). The retraction of the base of tongue and bolus pressure forces also are said to contribute to the downfolding from horizontal (Logemann et al., 1992). Although tongue base retraction could promote downfolding, the contribution of the bolus to inversion may be in question, as complete epiglottal inversion is seen commonly during nonbolus, "dry" swallows. The epiglottis returns to rest when the larynx begins to descend and the longitudinal muscles of the pharynx relax to allow for pharyngeal lengthening and return to a baseline configuraton.

Abnormal Epiglottic Function

The epiglottis functions by standing passively and deflecting an advancing bolus around the airway prior to the initiation of the pharyngeal swallow. Structural defects in the formation of the cartilage or mucosa surrounding the cartilage, which compromise the deflecting and channeling properties of the epiglottis may, in turn, compromise airway protection by allowing food, liquid, or secretions to enter the airway. This can occur as a result of congenital defect, surgical resection, or edema. An edematous epiglottis may rest along the surface of the base of the tongue, eliminating its barrier effect by obliterating the vallecular space. In this configuration, prematurely spilled material is guided into the open airway (Figure 3–6).

Function may be compromised during the swallow as well, usually as a result of poor hyoid bone and laryngeal cartilage elevation. When hyoid elevation is reduced, traction on the hyoepiglottic ligament is, in turn, reduced, as is laryngeal cartilage elevation. The cumulative effect of this poor initial movement is incomplete downfolding of the epiglottis during the pharyngeal swallow.

Cervical osteophytes that extend anteriorly into the hypopharynx may render a structural impediment for inversion during the swallow. Large bore nasogastric tubes may have a similar effect.

In a study by Perlman, Grayhack, and Booth (1992), patients with vallecular residue were more likely to have deviant epiglottic function, characterized by an absence of epiglottic inversion or incomplete inversion, than patients without vallecular residue.

VFE-2D. SCORING: HYOID-LARYNGEAL ELEVATION

The hyoid is described as the "skeleton" of the tongue and larynx. It is an omega-shaped bone situated superiorly to the thyroid carti-

lage and inferior to the mandible and is the only bone in the entire body that is not directly connected to another bone.

As the hyo-laryngeal complex elevates, the floor of the pharynx elevates with it resulting in a shortening of the pharynx (Figure 3–7). As discussed in Chapter 2, the principal function of laryngeal elevation is the opening of the upper esophageal sphincter (UES) by the application of traction to the anterior wall of the sphincter. The leading complex of laryngeal elevation is the anterior and superior movement of the hyoid bone. Elevation has two components: anterior movement and superior movement. The suprahyoid muscles contract after the mandible closes tightly. In a normal individual, this contraction from the immobile mandible allows for a vigorous movement and fixation at full contraction of the suprahyoid muscles. The fixation of the hyoid and mandible together offer a firm base for the elevation of the thyroid and cricoid cartilages. The laryngeal cartilages ascend as a result of thyrohyoid contraction. This final ascent by the cricoid opens the relaxed upper esophageal sphincter.

Objective measures of hyoid elevation have shown that the larynx moves approximately 2–2.5 centimeters from rest to maximum elevation (Dantas et al., 1990; Dengel, Robbins, & Rosenbek, 1991; Furukawa, 1983; Hamlet, Ezzell, & Aref, 1993; Kahrilas, Lin, Chen, & Logemann, 1996; Logemann, Kahri-

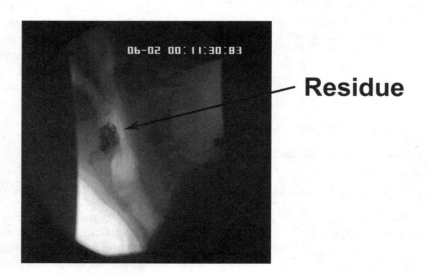

Figure 3-6. Residue in valleculae following the initial swallow.

Onset of elevation

Height of swallow

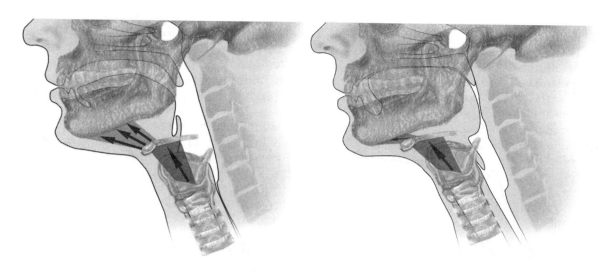

Figure 3-7. Superior and anterior hyoid movement results from contraction of the suprahyoid muscles.

las, Kobara, & Vakil, 1989; Nilsson, Isacsson, Isberg, & Schiratzki, 1989; Sundgren, Maly, & Gullberg, 1993). It has been found, however, that visually tracking hyoid and laryngeal elevation and then applying a subjective judgement of adequacy of elevation is at best inexact. Perlman et al. (1995) performed a correlation analysis comparing subjective and objective assessments of hyoid movement and found that the correlation was not strong. It was determined that evaluators were more likely to judge hyoid elevation to be inadequate when the anterior movement component of elevation was reduced.

The effect of laryngeal elevation on pharyngeal shortening and UES opening is paramount. In a simultaneous manometric and videofluoroscopic study, Olsson, Castell, Johnston, Ekberg, and Castell (1997) found that the pharyngeal constrictors played less of a role in the conveyance of the bolus through the pharynx than did the effect of pharyngeal shortening. The authors went on to claim that pharyngeal shortening could be the most important mechanism in bolus transport. Patients with reduced pharyngeal shortening will be more likely to demonstrate residue in the pyriform sinuses (Dejaeger et al., 1997).

The exact minimum amount of hyoid and laryngeal elevation necessary to adequately promote epiglottic inversion and UES opening is not known. And, if it were known, it would very likely be difficult to determine the presence of a defect subjectively.

VFE-2E. SCORING: POSTERIOR PHARYNGEAL WALL/PHARYNGEAL CONSTRICTORS

The pharyngeal constrictors are comprised of three obliquely positioned muscles that are stacked and layered from the cranium to the cervical esophagus. These muscles—the superior (craniopharyngeus), middle (hyopharyngeus), and inferior (thyropharyngeus) constrictors—contract sequentially during the propulsion of the bolus through the pharynx. The role of the pharyngeal constrictors is not so much to propel the bolus as it is to create the rigid walls of the propulsion chamber against which the tongue base applies pressure (Feinberg 1993; McConnel, Hood, Jackson, & O'Connor, 1994). The pharyngeal walls and tongue base contact one another as the tail of the bolus continues along the margin of the tongue. As the bolus tail passes beyond the tongue to the level of the larynx, the inferior constrictor contracts and clears the bolus into the opened pharyngoesophageal segment.

The movement of the pharyngeal constrictors can be monitored in either the lateral or AP projections. In the lateral plane, the distance between the anterior surface of the cervical vertebral bodies and the posterior border of the barium column. This movement sometimes is difficult to discern. When visualized, the perceived anterior movement of the posterior pharyngeal wall is the result of the compounding of lateral tissue as it bunches along the cervical raphe. In the AP projection, a cross section and medial movement of the pharyngeal walls can be monitored in relation to each other. Ekberg and Borgstrom (1989) found that the AP projection was much more effective for observing how displacement of the pharyngeal walls occurs during the pharyngeal swallow. Figure 3–8 illustrates the locations of the pharyngeal constrictors.

The pharynx is said to move superiorly to trap the bolus and then to constrict sequentially to force it down to the open esophagus. Radio-opaque markers placed on the posterior pharyngeal wall have been observed to move superiorly early in the pharyngeal stage of the swallow and then move inferiorly once the bolus passes by (Palmer, Tanaka, & Sievens, 1988). This superior movement could be due to the constriction of the longitudinal muscles of the pharynx (salpingopharyngeus, palatopharyngeus and stylopharyngeus) These muscles, when contracted, contribute to the short-

ening of the pharynx. Figure 3–9 illustrates bulging of the wall of the pharynx during the swallow.

No specific numbers are available for the objective determination of impaired pharyngeal wall motion. The clinician must look at the bolus and the location of residuals to infer weakened propulsion. Tongue driving force and pharyngeal constrictor rigidity coexist in a symbiotic fashion. It is recommended that this symbiosis be inspected for compromise when laryngeal elevation appears adequate but residue remains in the pharynx after the initial swallow. Reposition the patient to the AP projection and examine the cross-sectional movement of the pharyngeal walls. Look for incomplete or reduced movement. If the residue appears unilaterally, look specifically for reduced movement on the side demonstrating the residue. Diffuse residue in the absence of impaired laryngeal elevation or cricopharyngeal dysfunction, often will result in a visualization of reduced pharyngeal wall movement bilaterally.

VFE-2F. SCORING: CRICOPHARYNGEUS/UPPER ESOPHAGEAL SPHINCTER

Just below the pharyngeal air column and posterior to the arytenoid cartilages, the clinician will find the border of the hypopharynx and upper esophagus. The hypopharynx and the smooth muscles of the esophageal body are

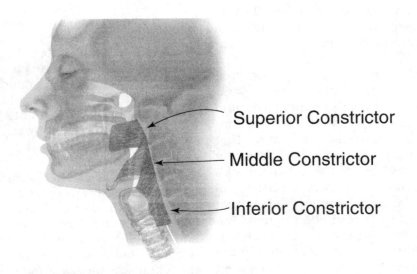

Superior Constrictor

Middle Constrictor

Inferior Constrictor

Figure 3-8. Location of pharyngeal constrictors.

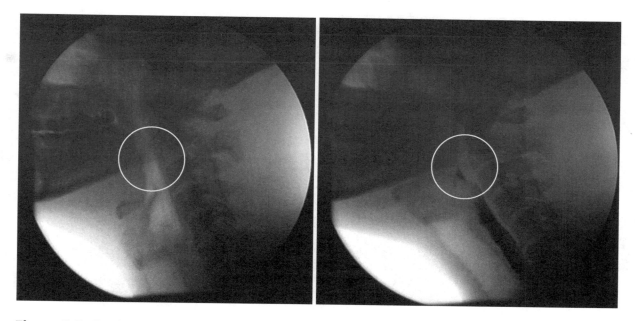

Figure 3-9. Posterior pharyngeal wall bulging during the pharyngeal swallow.

separated by a series of striated, skeletal muscles, comprised of the inferior pharyngeal constrictor (thyropharyngeus muscle and oblique fibers of the cricopharyngeus muscle), the horizontal fibers of the cricopharyngeus muscle, and the striated muscle of the upper esophagus. The entire high-pressure zone is approximately 3–4 cm in length (Goyal, 1984; Goyal, Martin, Shapiro, & Speckler, 1993) with the horizontal fibers of the cricopharyngeus making up approximately 1 cm of this length. The horizontal fibers of the cricopharyngeus insert into the lower lateral third of the cricoid cartilage and loop posteriorly in an arc that terminates on the opposite side of the cricoid.

The high-pressure zone of the upper esophageal sphincter is not well-visualized during fluoroscopy due to the tight contact of the mucosal walls. The best way to locate the UES is to identify structures that surround it. Locating the air columns of the trachea and hypopharynx are good starting points and will assist the clinician in distinguishing the superior and inferior latitudes of the high-pressure zone (Figure 3–10).

Kahrilas, Dodds, Dent, and Logemann (1988) suggested that the area of high pressure was approximately 1.5 cm distal to the pharyngeal air column. Cook and colleagues (1989) found that the area of high pressure was slightly lower, at a location approximately level with the middle and lower third of the

cricoid cartilage. Both Kahrilas et al. (1988) and Cook et al. (1989) assumed the area of high pressure to be at the level of the horizontal fibers of the cricopharyngeus. Goyal, Martin, Shapiro, and Speckler (1993), in a review of the role of the cricopharyngeal muscle, pointed out that both studies indicated a zone of high pressure that corresponds to an area just superior to the horizontal fibers of the cricopharyngeus. This area is approximately level with the middle of the cricoid cartilage and more likely is associated with pressure generated from the lower margin of the inferior pharyngeal constrictor muscle and not the horizontal muscles of the cricopharyngeus. Nevertheless, "cricopharyngeus" is widely used synonymously when medical professionals describe the UES (Figure 3–11).

The sphincter remains contracted until the pharyngeal swallow occurs at which time an inhibitory brainstem command causes the area of high pressure to become atonic. This allows for the traction being applied from laryngeal elevation to pull the front portion of the sphincter anteriorly and superiorly, effectively opening the UES and allowing for bolus transit into the upper esophagus.

The various parameters of UES opening can be affected by a number of variables. When bolus volume, for instance, is increased, progressive increases occur in UES diameter, cross-sectional area, and the duration of bo-

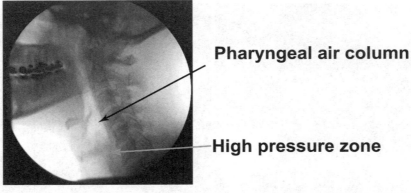

Figure 3-10. The high pressure zone of the UES is located between the inferior aspect of the pharyngeal airspace and the superior aspect of the tracheal air column.

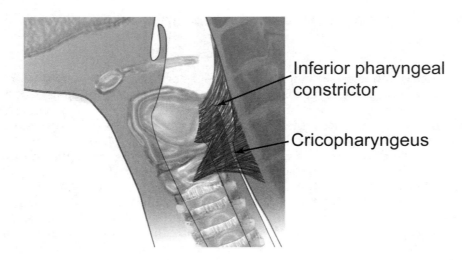

Figure 3-11. Configuration of cricopharyngeus and UES.

lus flow (Cook et al., 1989). Age-related changes in UES function have been observed in the elderly. Sphincter opening at the height of the pharyngeal swallow has been found to be significantly diminished in the elderly (Shaw et al., 1995). Lowered resting UES pressure and delayed UES relaxation also have been observed in the elderly (Fulp, Dalton, Castell, & Castell, 1990; Shaker et al., 1993).

Abnormal Cricopharyngeus/UES

Upper esophageal sphincter disorders can be due to structural or functional problems (Cook, 1993). Functional disorders are either a pri-

mary muscle dysfunction or secondary to impaired traction forces or incoordination of the application of the traction forces during the propulsion of the bolus. Structural disorders of the upper esophagus also will be discussed.

Primary UES Dysfunction

The safe and efficient transit of food from the pharynx to the esophagus requires an adequately patent path between the two passageways. In cases of cricopharyngeal achalasia, the muscles of the UES may fail to relax at the height of the pharyngeal swallow. This failure to relax can be due to a reduction in the inhibitory signals traveling from the brain-stem to the tonic UES. Hypertonic UES (elevated resting tonicity) has been described in patients with oculopharyngeal syndromes (O'Laughlin, Bredfeldt, & Gray, 1980), whereas incoordination of relaxation has been attributed to lateral medullary syndrome (Wallenberg's syndrome), syringobulbia, and Parkinson's disease (Cook, 1993). The incomplete relaxation of the UES results in reduced opening of the sphincter when traction is applied during laryngeal elevation. When the opening between the two passageways is incomplete, the transit of the bolus from the pharynx to the esophagus will be obstructed. This obstruction results in residue remaining in the pharynx, typically in the pyriform sinuses, after the swallow. This residual material may flow over the structural barriers and into the laryngeal inlet.

Patients who are suspected of having a primary dysfunction of the UES should receive a manometric examination in conjunction with the fluoroscopic evaluation. This will assist the care team in deciding whether treatment options should include myotomy, dilitation or strengthening exercise.

Secondary UES Dysfunction

Secondary UES dysfunction describes a set of conditions in which the muscles of the UES comply with medullary instructions to inhibit tonicity and are without the fibrosis or inelasticity discussed previously. The dysfunction occurs as the result of poor traction forces applied by the elevating larynx. During the fluoroscopic exam, this dysfunction will show findings similar to the primary UES dysfunction in that residue will appear in the lower pharynx after the swallow. The visual clue of poor laryngeal elevation may be due to the presence of the weakened suprahyoid muscles, or to tethering forces from tracheostomy tubes.

Structural UES Dysfunction

Postsurgery/Irradiation

Patients with irradiation to the UES may experience the fibrosis of the muscles with resulting reduced elasticity. Surgical procedures involving the musculature of the UES can result in scarring and similarly reduced elasticity. Even in the presence of appropriately timed inhibition of tonicity and adequate laryngeal elevation, the newly inelastic musculature may not open to the degree necessary to allow efficient passage of the bolus. Patients who are status postesophagectomy are particularly prone to dysphagia following surgery (Thomas et al., 1996), with one in four reporting solid food dysphagia (McLarty et al., 1997). Patients with postsurgical anastomotic leaks are more likely to develop fibrosis of the anastomotic site later during recovery (Bruns, Gawenda, Wolfgarten, & Walter, 1997).

Cricopharyngeal Bar

The horizontal fibers of the cricopharyngeus insert anteriorly along the lower third of the cricoid cartilage and course posteriorly at about the level of C5–C6. An anteriorly projecting "bar" or "cricopharyngeal bar (CP bar)" often is observed along the posterior pharyngeal wall at this level (Figure 3–12). This bar is found in approximately 5% of normal volunteers without dysphagia (Ekberg & Nylander, 1982) and often is confused with pathologic conditions. The CP bar is often identified as being representative of hypertrophy of the cricopharyngeus or is identified as achalasia, although the patient is without the typical manometric findings that would support these diagnoses (Cook, 1993). The cricopharyngeal bar sometimes is related to UES obstruction (Curtis, Cruess, & Bert, 1984) but more often is incidental.

Zenker's Diverticulum

Zenker's diverticulum is a herniation or outpouching of tissue in the striated portion of the upper esophagus resulting from reduced upper esophageal sphincter opening with normal pharyngeal propulsion and bolus flow (Shaw et al., 1996). It is thought that the tissue changes, specifically muscle fiber degeneration and the appearance of fat tissue in the cricopharyngeus, lead to reduced upper esophageal compliance during laryngeal elevation (Cook, Blumberg, Cash, Jamieson, & Shearman, 1992). This reduction in upper esophageal sphincter opening increases the hypopharyn-

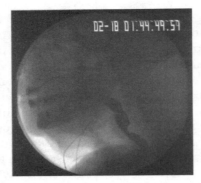

Figure 3-12. The prominent cricopharyngeus or cricopharyngeal "bar" is frequently observed in normal subjects and often is not indicative of pathology.

geal intrabolus pressure which results in the herniation of the tissue during bolus flow through the sphincter (Shaw et al., 1996) (Figure 3–13). Surgical removal of the pouch has been demonstrated to be ineffective in the treatment of the dysphagia associated with Zenker's diverticulum and has been widely replaced by cricopharyngeal myotomy (Konowitz & Biller, 1989; Skinner & Zuckerbraun, 1998).

Patients with documented Zenker's diverticulum may be referred due to worsening symptoms or for recurrence of symptoms following pouch removal or myotomy. Previous radiograms or fluoroscopic studies should be examined for location and size of the defect.

VFE-2G. SCORING: ESOPHAGUS

The esophagus is approximately 25 cm in length and courses from the inferior pharyngeal constrictor to the stomach below. The esophagus is not well-visualized under fluoroscopy until barium contrast material is introduced into the lumen. When viewed in the AP projection, the esophagus is observed to run downward from the pharyngeal airspace and deflect to the left as it passes around the heart (Figure 3–14). A depression on the left side of the esophagus is observed due to compression from the aortic arch. The esophagus terminates at the gastroesophageal junction where the lower esophageal sphincter (LES) is found.

The primary function of the esophagus is to carry food from the pharynx to the stomach. Once food enters the esophagus, a primary peristaltic wave is initiated that carries the bolus to the lower esophageal sphincter (LES), which relaxes, and allows the bolus to enter into the stomach. After the passage of the bolus, each respective sphincter contracts to its baseline tonic posture, illuminating the secondary function of the esophagus: to contain gastric contents within the stomach and prevent them from entering into the airway. Additionally, in the event of regurgitation, the esophagus functions to efficiently reject and propel material along a retrograde path out of the alimentary tract.

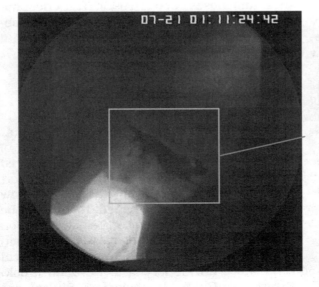

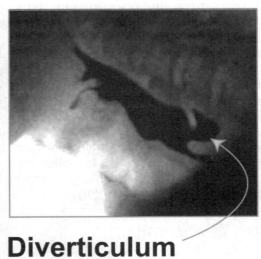

Diverticulum

Figure 3-13. An example of a diverticulum filling with barium contrast as the bolus flows through the striated portion of the esophagus.

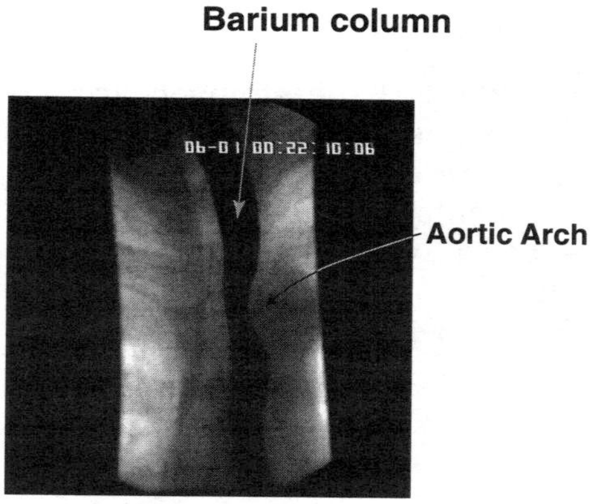

Barium column

Figure 3-14. The esophageal column filled with barium contrast. Note the small deviation in the path as the bolus passes around the aortic arch.

The superior 8 cm of the esophagus is surrounded by striated, skeletal muscle, whereas the lower 17 cm is made up of two layers of smooth muscle, an outer layer of longitudinal muscles and an inner layer of circular muscles. Contraction of the outer, longitudinal muscle layer, results in esophageal shortening, whereas contraction of the inner, circular muscle layer progressively squeezes the bolus in a peristaltic fashion to the LES.

The peristaltic wave that transports the bolus from the pharynx to the stomach has been described as a "peristaltic pump" (Brasseur, 1987) in which sinusoidal waves of first, relaxation, and then contraction, are projected along the length of the esophagus. The relaxation occurs in advance of the bolus head and the contraction follows along the tail. When occlusion of the lumen fails during contraction, often at the level of the aortic arch, some material may remain behind and should be considered a normal variant (Low & Rubesin, 1993). The portion of the esophagus adjacent to the aortic arch also is where the striated and smooth muscles interdigitate and often is the site where esophageal peristalsis is the least efficient. A secondary peristaltic wave often is observed to clear the residual bolus. Secondary peristaltic waves are reflexive waves that progress much like the primary peristaltic wave, except that they are not initiated by the swallowing of a new bolus. Distention of the esophagus propagates this reflexive secondary wave, which acts to propel whatev-

er material is causing the distention, usually refluxed gastric material or residuals, into the stomach.

The entire esophageal phase of the swallow lasts approximately 6–10 s (Margulis & Koehler, 1976) The inhibition of tonicity of the LES begins approximately 2 s after a swallow and continues to remain relaxed for approximately 7 s before tonicity returns.

There are predictable changes in the esophagus with aging. In the elderly, secondary esophageal peristalsis is either absent or is elicited less frequently after esophageal distension. LES relaxation in response to esophageal distension is less complete and less frequently elicited (Ren et al., 1995). The elderly also are more likely to demonstrate nonperistaltic "tertiary contractions" and delayed esophageal emptying. Tertiary contractions usually are found in the smooth muscle portion of the lower esophagus and appear fluoroscopically as an up-and-down movement of the bolus.

Abnormal Esophagus

Disorders of the esophagus can be divided into problems of motility and obstruction. The radiographic examination attempts to allow for the visualization of these anomalies through the judicious presentation of both liquid and solid boluses. Using solid food boluses in addition to liquid during the esophageal exam has proven to be beneficial for patients with unexplained dysphagia. Solid food boluses demonstrated significantly more frequent motor abnormalities than when the same patients were presented liquid to swallow (Mellow, 1983; Meshkinpour & Eckerling, 1996).

Disorders of the esophageal phase of the swallow are due to obstructions and/or motility disorders.

Obstruction

Obstructive narrowing of the esophagus can be due to intrinsic or extrinsic lesions. Patients may perceive an obstruction and report feelings of food "getting stuck." Patients appear to be most accurate in localizing proximal rather than distal obstructive lesions (Wilcox, Alexander, & Clark, 1995). Intrinsic distal lesions, such as a Schatzki ring, may develop as a result of gastroesophageal reflux. This mucosal narrowing is a thin, smooth stricture of the distal esophageal lumen that prevents the smooth transport of food through the LES (DeVault, 1996).

Patients with severe gastroesophageal reflux may undergo a surgical procedure, Nissen fundoplication, to improve the tonicity of the LES and reduce the escape of gastric contents into the esophagus. The procedure involves wrapping the upper portion the fundus (upper portion) of the stomach around the distal esophagus. Although this procedure is effective in preventing reflux in the vast majority of patients, side effects include obstructive dysphagia, typically experienced with solid food boluses (Hunter, Swanstrom, & Waring, 1996) (Figure 3–15).

A. Post Nissen Fundoplication

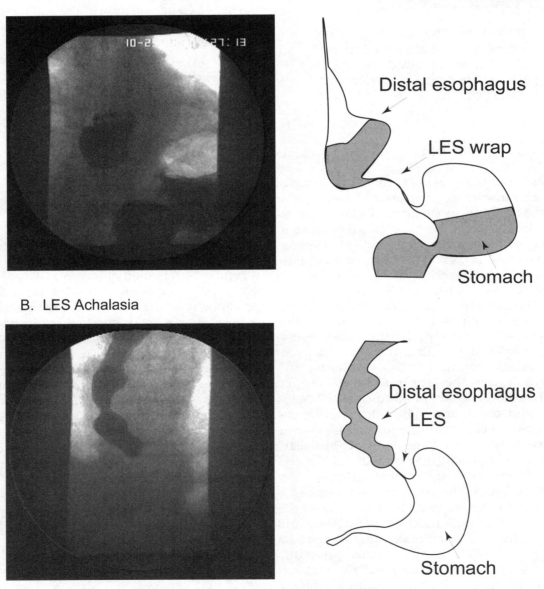

B. LES Achalasia

Figure 3-15. A. Hypertonic LES following Nissen Fundoplication. This patient experienced esophageal dysphagia immediately following the procedure. The esophagus is distended and full of contrast just proximal to the high pressure zone of the LES. **B.** In this patient with achalasia, the LES fails to open, resulting in a collection of the contrast material in the esophageal lumen. Tertiary contractions are observed.

Esophagitis can result in the narrowing of the esophageal lumen causing obstruction. This can result from gastroesophageal reflux, ingestion of chemicals, and candidial infection. Patients with poor esophageal motility may be unable to propel certain pills through the esophagus. When these pills rest against the esophageal mucosa, they may cause an ulceration and subsequent narrowing. These ulcerative lesions typically are observed in the mid esophagus near the aortic arch, where residuals typically are found (Low & Rubesin, 1993).

Esophageal webs causing dysphagia often are discovered in children and occur along the anterior wall of the cervical esophagus. They can cause considerable dysphagia. Cancerous tumors may occur intrinsically or cause compression on the esophagus from a location outside of the lumen. Intrinsic tumors may have the characteristic "lumpy, bumpy" appearance of a lobulated mass or may have a smooth contour. Extrinsic tumors may appear as smooth masses impinging on the lumen.

Motility Disorders

Achalasia is an esophageal motility disorder that is characterized by abnormal esophageal peristalsis and incomplete or absent opening of the LES. There is a characteristic beaklike narrowing of the distal esophagus. As the disease advances, the esophagus becomes dilated due to the constant stretching of the lumen above the noncompliant LES. Achalasia is thought to be due to a degeneration of the neurons that carry the inhibitory signal to the LES.

Patients with connective tissue disorders such as scleroderma, polymyositis, and rheumatoid arthritis, and patients with progressive neurological diseases also may have difficulties with esophageal motility.

VFE-2H. SCORING: AIRWAY PROTECTION

During the swallow, the pharynx is reconfigured from a respiratory to an alimentary tract (Kahrilas et al., 1996). The laryngeal airway can be compromised at any time before, during, or after this alimentary reconfiguration and return to respiration.

There are several components to airway protection associated with swallowing. They include laryngeal elevation, glottal closure, supraglottic closure, and epiglottic retroflexion over the airway. This discussion will be limited to closure of the laryngeal airway.

Glottic closure

Glottic closure is not well-visualized with fluoroscopy. The AP view gives a fair impression of true vocal fold and ventricular fold movement toward the mesial plane (Figure 3–16). The lateral projection allows the clinician to observe anterior tilting of the arytenoid cartilages, and contact of the arytenoids to the epiglottic base during laryngeal elevation. Unfortunately complete cord adduction is not well-visualized (Shaker, Dodds, Dantas, Hogan, & Arndorfer, 1990) and surety of the absence of tight closure is verifiable only when contrast material passes below the level of the cords when an event of aspiration is observed.

Airway protective reflexes can be observed during the oral stage of the swallow. It has been found that a brief partial adduction of the arytenoids and vocal cords occurs during the oral stage of the swallow when food or liquid enter into the pharynx. This transient adduction is not to be confused with the final movement of airway closure observed during the pharyngeal swallow (Dua, Ren, Bardan, Xie, & Shaker, 1997).

The final movement for airway closure seen during the pharyngeal stage of the swallow occurs just before UES opening and lasts for approximately 0.6–0.7 s (Dodds, Stewart, & Logemann, 1990). In the lateral projection, this closure is observed as a forward tilting of the arytenoids. At the apex of laryngeal elevation, the arytenoids will be observed to contact the base of the epiglottis with the retroverted epiglottis wrapping over the top of the tightly closed vestibule (Figure 3–17). The margins of the different tissues are identified variably during a swallow with bolus contrast. The clinician should be cued to the airspace separating the arytenoid shadow and the shadow representing the epiglottic base. The forward tilting movement of the arytenoid should occur prior to the entry of the bolus into the lower pharynx.

Abnormal Airway Closure

The coordination and timing of airway protection and bolus propulsion has been studied

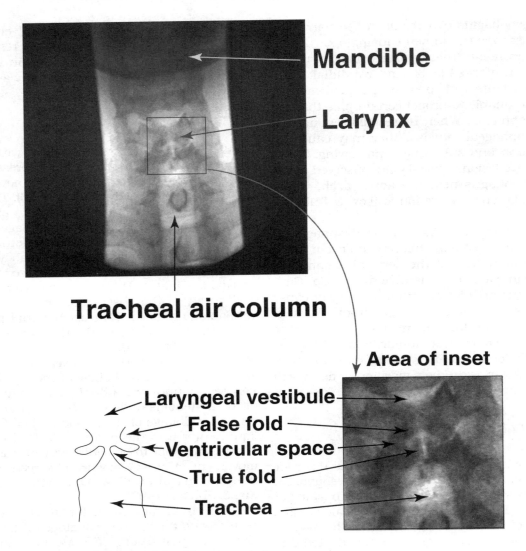

Mandible

Larynx

Tracheal air column

Area of inset

Laryngeal vestibule

False fold

Ventricular space

True fold

Trachea

Figure 3-16. AP view of laryngeal airway.

widely (Curtis, Cruess, Dachman, & Maso, 1984; Dua et al., 1997; Ren, Shaker, Zamir, Dodds, Hogan, & Hoffman, 1993; Shaker, Dodds, Dantas, Hogan, & Arndorfer, 1990; Zamir et al., 1996). As discussed earlier, the key to a successful and safe swallow is the rapid reconfiguration of the pharynx from respiratory tract to alimentary tract. It has been determined that the primary defect leading to the entry of food or liquid into the airway is the incoordination of this reconfiguration (Kahrilas, Rademaker, & Logemann, 1997). This incoordination often is related to poor CNS coordination due to reduced afferent input to the CNS and weakened or slowed responses to CNS motor commands.

Laryngeal paralysis will make an obvious contribution to the entry of food or liquid into the laryngeal airway. Review the discussion regarding recurrent laryngeal nerve damage in Chapter 2. Recurrent laryngeal nerve damage will lead to penetration of the airway during the pharyngeal stage of the swallow.

Flexible pharyngeal endoscopy allows for good visualization of airway protection patterns. Refer to Chapter 4 for further discussion of abnormal airway protection.

OBJECTIVE MEASURES

VFE-4. DURATION MEASURES

Calculating duration measures requires the employment of a time character generator

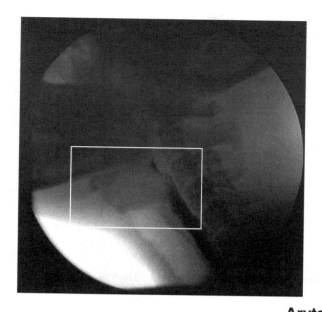

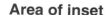
Area of inset

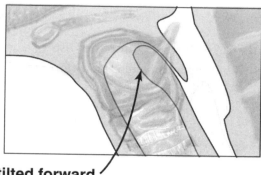

Arytenoid tilted forward

Figure 3-17. Arytenoid contact with epiglottal base.

during the recording of the fluoroscopic exam. With the time characters overlaid on the video signal, the clinician has the opportunity to pinpoint discrete anatomical movements and then determine the elapsed time between those movements and other events of interest. A number of researchers have employed duration measures to objectively compare and describe normal and abnormal biomechanical movements. The hopeful clinician expecting a rock-solid delineation between normal and abnormal swallows by employing duration measures will surely be disappointed. The within-subject and between-subject variability of duration measures is considerable and, as a rule of thumb, a number of trials should be averaged together to account for this variability (Lof & Robbins, 1990). The main purpose of employing these measures is to determine a baseline from which change can be measured after treatment and retesting.

In this text, the scoring and discussion will be limited to "duration of stage transition." This measure has, perhaps, attracted the most attention of any duration measure, and frequently is observed as being problematic in patients with varying diagnoses and across the age span. For the benefit of clinicians wishing to acquire other duration measures, a list of many duration measures and

the method for acquisition are listed in Tables 3–5 and 3–6.

Many clinicians will not have access to a time character generator during the recording process but still will be able to make a gross determination of these measures by counting frames of video. The clinician should attempt to review the tape on a deck that allows for frame-by-frame playback. Videotape records and plays back at 30 frames per second with each frame of video being roughly equal to 30 ms. The clinician can count the number of frames between the onset and offset of the event of interest and multiply that number of frames by 30 to arrive at the total number of milliseconds.

VFE-4C. SCORING: STAGE TRANSITION DURATION

The clinician must monitor the movement of the hyoid bone and bolus to acquire this measure. The onset of the measure occurs when the bolus head reaches the point where the ramus of the mandible intersects with the base of tongue. The endpoint occurs with the final anterior, superior moment of hyoid associated with the initiation of the pharyngeal stage of the swallow. The point at which the ramus of the mandible and the base of tongue

Table 3–5. Structures and events used in the evaluation of objective measures.

Event of Interest	Time at Which:
A. Beginning of posterior movement of the bolus	Bolus first begins posterior movement in the oral cavity
B. Enter the head of the bolus into the pharynx	Head of the bolus first reaches ramus of the mandible
C. Hyoid beginning maximum elevation	Hyoid bone begins movement toward its maximal upward excursion
D. Tail of the bolus into the UES	Tail of the bolus passes through the UES
E. Fist maximum velar elevation	Velum initially reaches its most elevated and retracted posistion
F. Last maximum velar elevation	Velum releases from its maximum position of elevation and retraction
G. Hyoid first maximum elevation	Hyoid first reaches its maximum elevation
H. Hyoid last maximum elevation	Hyoid releases from its maximum elevation
I. Hyoid first maximum anterior movement	Hyoid first reaches its most anterior position
J. Hyoid last maximum anterior movement	Hyoid releases from its most anterior position
K. Hyoid return to rest	Hyoid returns to its rest position
L. UES opening	UES begins to open
M. UES closing	UES begins to close

Source: Adapted from Lof, G. L., & Robbins, J. (1990). Test-retest variability in normal swallowing. *Dysphagia 4*, 236–242.

meet, when viewed in the lateral projection, is considered the division point between the oral and pharyngeal cavities (Figure 3–18).

This duration measure describes the amount of time elapsed between the moment of termination of the oral stage of the swallow and the moment of onset for the pharyngeal stage of the swallow. This is an important measure for examining the interaction between the propulsion of the bolus and the timeliness of airway protection. It is postulated that, the longer the delay in initiating the pharyngeal stage of the swallow after the arrival of the bolus into the pharynx, the greater the risk of aspirating the bolus into the lower airway (Perlman, Booth, & Grayhack, 1994).

The phenomenon of this delay in the transition between the oral and pharyngeal stages has been well-documented in the literature and has been given a number of different names including "delayed swallow reflex" (Lazarus & Logemann 1987; Veis & Logemann, 1985), "delayed pharyngeal response" (Robbins & Levin, 1988), "duration of stage transition" (Lof & Robbins, 1990; Robbins, Hamilton, Lof, & Kempster, 1992; Rosenbek, Roecker, Wood, & Robbins, 1996; Rosenbek et al., 1998), and "pharyngeal delay" (Langmore et al., 1998; Lazarus et al., 1993).

As a bolus becomes less viscous, the flow, or speed, with which it moves through the pharynx during the swallow increases. Normal subjects compensate for the faster flowing boluses by initiating the pharyngeal stage of the swallow in a more timely fashion. Research has indicated that thin liquid boluses are associated with more rapid onset of the pharyngeal stage of the swallow than more viscous materials. In normal subjects swallowing thin liquids, the pharyngeal stage of the swallow is initiated while the bolus head is still in the oral cavity, resulting in a negative

Table 3–6. Calculation of duration measures.

Abbreviation	Duration Measure	Events Used for Calculations	Calculation*
OTD	Oral transit duration	Enter head of the bolus in pharynx; beginning of posterior movement of the bolus	B-A=OTD
STD	Stage transition duration	Hyoid beginning maximum elevation; enter head of the bolus in the pharynx	C-B=STD
PTD	Pharyngeal transit duration	Tail of the bolus into UES; enter head of the bolus in pharynx	D-B=PTD
PRD	Pharyngeal response duration	Hyoid return to rest; hyoid beginning maximum elevation	K-C=PRD
DOVE	Duration of velum excursion	Last maximum velar excursion; first maximum velar excursion	F-E=DOVE
DOHME	Duration of maximum hyoid elevation	Hyoid last maximum elevation; hyoid first maximum elevation	H-G=DOHME
DOHMA	Duration of hyoid maximum anterior	Hyoid last maximum anterior movement hyoid first maximum anterior movement	J-I=DOHMA
DOOUES	Duration of open UES	UES Close; UES open	M-L=DOOUES
DTOUES	Duration to opening UES	UES open; beginning posterior movement of the bolus	L-A=DTOUES
OPTD	Oropharyngeal transit duration	Beginning of posterior movement of the bolus; Tail of the bolus into UES	D-A=OPTD

Refer to Table 3–5 for letters describing the structural movements necessary to obtain this calculation.
Source: Adapted from Lof, G. L., and Robbins, J. (1990). Test-retest variability in normal swallowing. *Dysphagia 4,* 236–242.

transition time. See Table 3–7 for typical pharyngeal delay times for liquid boluses.

Puree or solid food boluses, on the other hand, have a greater viscosity and flow much more slowly through the pharynx. Most viscous food materials also are fairly cohesive and, once prepared and formed into a bolus, will not break up readily. Because of this, the delicate and precise reconfiguration of the airway is not as urgent with the slower moving bolus. The normal individual will allow the bolus to traverse through the pharynx to the level of the vallecula prior to the initiation of the pharyngeal stage of the swallow. With solid food or puree boluses, it is not uncommon for a normal subject to continue mastication while preparing and advancing several small portions of the bolus to the level of the valleculae before initiating a single pharyngeal swallow.

Thin liquids offer a different challenge to both normals and dysphagic patients. Thin liquids are not cohesive and, once flowing, follow a path of least resistance. The liquid bolus will fill whatever cavity or channel is in that flow path until it overflows and another path is followed. Because thin liquids move so rapidly when falling through the pharynx, the relative risk of aspiration increases as the duration of the transition increases. Once the bolus exits the oral cavity and falls into the lower pharynx, it will fill and overflow each structural barrier until the airway is either penetrated or a swallow occurs (Figure 3–19). For this reason, the clinician should always limit the initial presentations to amounts that are not likely to overcome the structural barriers to laryngeal penetration.

There are no benchmarks for STD that will allow the clinician to make a binary determination of normalcy or pathology. The position of the bolus at the onset of the swallow may reveal more about the relative risk of lower airway penetration than the length of the delay. Both liquid and solid food boluses can remain high in the pharynx (i.e., in the vallec-

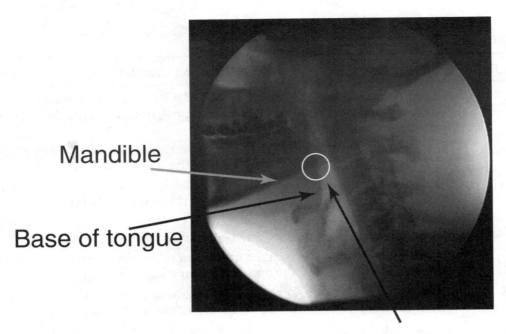

Mandible

Base of tongue

Point of intersection

Figure 3-18. Location of the intersection of the shadows of the tongue base and mandible.

Table 3–7. Normal pharyngeal delay times for liquid boluses.

Source	Bolus	Age Range	"Delay"
Robbins et al. (1992)	2 ml	65 years	−.07 s
Lazarus et al. (1993)	5 ml	18–80 years	−.06 s
Langmore and Murray (1994)	5 ml	60–80 years	−.19 s

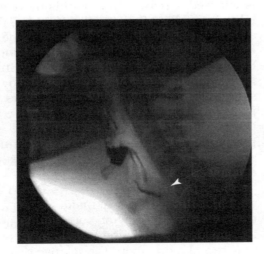

Bolus in pyriform sinus

Figure 3-19. This thin liquid bolus has spilled to the level of the pyriform sinuses before the initiation of the pharyngeal swallow.

ular space) for any length of time without putting the patient at risk of aspiration. Only when the bolus exits the vallecular space and travels into the area of the laryngeal inlet does the relative risk increase (Figure 3–20).

The phenomenon of the entry of a bolus into the pharynx prior to the initiation of the swallow is a highly variable event both within and across subjects. Rosenbek et al. (1996) reported wide variations within subjects. A single subject in that study demonstrated STDs of 0.03–6.60 s with 3 ml paste swallows. Perlman et al. suggested that a time period of greater than 1 but less than 2 s be considered a mild delay and that a delay of greater than 5 s be considered a severe delay.

The overall duration of the transition has been found to increase with age (Tracy et al., 1989). Robbins et al. (1992) reported that swallowing begins to slow after 45 years of age and that, by age 70 years, swallowing is significantly slower than in younger individuals.

The common problem of coordinating the reconfiguration of the pharynx from airway to

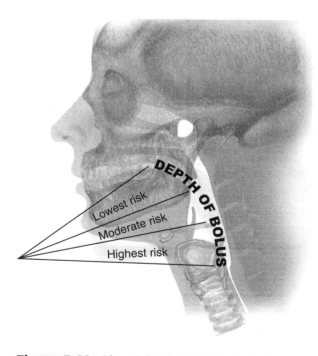

Figure 3-20. The risk of aspiration increases as the duration of the transition between the oral and pharyngeal stages increases. The risk also increases as the bolus head travels more deeply into the pharynx before the swallow.

alimentary tract is problematic for dysphagic patients regardless of etiology. Pharyngeal delay is seen in patients with tracheostomy and COPD (Coelho, 1987) patients that are status postendotracheal tube placement (deLarminat, Dureuil, Montravers, & Desmonts, 1992), head injury (Lazarus et al., 1987), Parkinson's disease (Bird, Woodward, Gibson, Phyland, & Fonda, 1994), and CVA (Bisch, Logemann, Radimaker, Kahrilas, & Lazarus, 1994; Lazarus et al., 1993; Rosenbek et al., 1996; Veis & Logemann, 1985).

VFE-4D. SCORING: OROPHARYNGEAL SWALLOWING EFFICIENCY

The clinician first should determine oropharyngeal transit duration (Tables 3–6 and 3–7). This is calculated by determining the time elapsed between the beginning of posterior movement of the bolus and the moment the tail of the bolus enters the UES. The clinician then must estimate the percentage of the bolus that is propelled into the esophagus following the first swallow. To obtain this number, the clincian must take into account the amount aspirated, if any, and the amount of residue left over in the pharynx following the initial swallow attempt. Once OPTD and the percentage swallowed has been determined the numbers can be plugged into the formula presented in Table 3–8.

OPSE is an overall measure of swallowing function that describes the interaction of the quickness of the movement of the bolus and the efficiency of the swallowing mechanism in clearing material from the oropharynx (Lazarus et al., 1996). According to Logemann et al. (1989), normal subjects swallowed 98% to 100% of a 1-cc liquid bolus on the initial swallow attempt. If a slight coating of barium contrast was observed after the initial swallow, the individual was estimated to have swallowed 98% of the bolus. Scores for normal subjects are dependent on the consistency used, with lower scores for more viscous materials. Rademaker, Pauloski, Logemann, and Shanahan (1994) found average scores for normals to be 85 for liquid swallows, 72 for paste swallows, and 61 for cookie swallows. Lazarus et al. (1996) found that normal subjects swallowing 1 ml liquid boluses obtained scores of 89.7 ± 8.4 (Table 3–9).

One element necessary for obtaining this measure is the estimation of the percentage of

Table 3–8. Calculating OPSE.

$$\text{OPSE} = \frac{100 - (\% \text{ residue} + \% \text{ aspiration before or during the swallow})}{\text{Oropharyngeal transit duration}}$$

Another way of calculating OPSE:

$$\text{OPSE} = \frac{\% \text{ Bolus transported into the esophagus}}{\text{OTD} + \text{PTD}}$$

Example: This patient swallows a liquid bolus and aspirates 5% of the bolus while 20% remains in the valleculae and pyriform sinuses. Oral transit duration lasted 0.70 s and pharyngeal transit time lasted 1.3 s.

$$\text{OPSE} = \frac{100 - (25)}{0.70 + 1.30}$$

$$\text{OPSE} = \frac{75}{2}$$

$$\text{OPSE} = 37.5$$

Table 3–9. Mean OPSE values for differing bolus consistencies, sizes, and etiology.

	Liquid	Paste	Cookie
Logemann et al. (1989)			
Normal	82 (67–128)	N/A	N/A
Brain-stem CVA	20 (5–51)	N/A	N/A
Rademaker et al. (1994)			
Normal	85 (35–167)	72 (48–108)	61 (12–115)
Stroke	68 (8–146)	35 (12–76)	43 (5–107)
Cancer Laryngeal (Nonfunctional)	52 (0–148)	57 (0–123)	46 (1–113)
Lazarus et al. (1996)			
Normal	90 (± 8.4)	N/A	N/A
Cancer (H&N)	51 (± 12)	N/A	N/A

the bolus that is propelled successfully into the pharynx following the initial swallow. This requirement adds a subjective element to an otherwise objective rating, in that the clinician must "guess" the volume of material by visually inspecting the two-dimensional shadow cast by the bolus. Although overall interjudge and intrajudge reliability for the OPSE measure were reported to be good by Logemann et al. (1989), Rademaker et al. (1994), and Lazarus et al. (1996), reliability for bolus size estimation independent of the other measures was never reported.

This number may give the clinician an impression of the overall efficiency of the initial swallow attempt but should not be used as a binary identifier of normalcy or impairment. The measure is highly variable between even normal subjects (Table 3–9). The proper use for this measure is as a marker for baseline and retest performance. For example, the measurement could be calculated before the initiation of radiation treatments and again after treatments are discontinued to determine, or monitor, decrements in performance. In the same manner, baseline performance could be estimated prior to the initiation of treatment and again after treatment trials.

If the estimation of oropharyngeal transit duration is not possible due to the lack of availability of slow-motion playback, the clinician may wish to perform a coarser estimation of efficiency. This can be done simply by counting the number of swallows necessary to clear the material from the pharynx or oral cavity. Most ordinary liquid and puree boluses (5 cc–30 cc) can be cleared in a single swallow and are generally followed by a second clearing swallow. Solid foods are a different matter. The harder the material the greater the amount of chewing to prepare it and the greater the number of swallows (Hiiemae et al., 1996).

VFE-5. SCORING: PENETRATION/ASPIRATION SCALE

Score the events associated with penetration or aspiration according to the 8-point scale developed by Rosenbek et al., (1996) (Table 3–10). The traditional description of penetration and aspiration will be used when employing this scale:

Penetration: The passage of material into the laryngeal inlet without passing below the level of the true vocal folds (Figure 3–21).

Aspiration: The passage of material below the level of the true vocal folds.

The event of penetration or aspiration is one of the principle findings of the videofluoroscopic examination. The detection of aspiration is often the single driving force that influences a physician to seek consultation on the behalf of a dysphagic patient. Frequently, the first question emanating from the consulting physician following the study is, "Did he aspirate?" Unfortunately, too many responses to this inquiry are answered in a binary (yes/no)

Table 3–10. Eight-Point penetration-aspiration scale.

Score	Description of Events
1	Material does not enter the airway.
2	Material enters the airway, remains above the vocal folds, and is ejected from the airway.
3	Material enters the airway, remains above the vocal folds, and is not ejected from the airway.
4	Material enters the airway, contacts the vocal folds, and is ejected from the airway.
5	Material enters the airway, contacts the vocal folds, and is not ejected from the airway.
6	Material enters the airway, passes below the vocal folds, and is ejected into the larynx or out of the airway.
7	Material enters the airway, passes below the vocal folds, and is not ejected from the trachea despite effort.
8	Material enters the airway, passes below the vocal folds, and no effort is made to eject.

Source: From Rosenbek, J. C., Robbins, J., Roecker, E. V., Coyle, J. L., & Woods, J. L. (1996). A penetration-aspiration scale. *Dysphagia.11*, 93–98. Reprinted with permission.

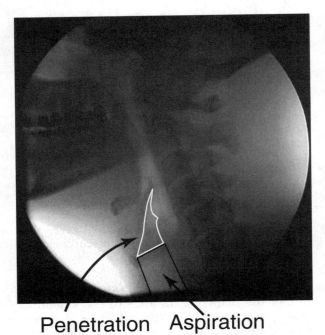

Penetration Aspiration

Figure 3-21. Penetration and aspiration boundaries as observed in the lateral projection.

fashion, without regard for events that surround the penetration or aspiration. As noted by the authors, a more precise description is available when two signs (aspiration or penetration) become eight.

The scale is multidimensional in that more than one type of behavior is being observed, judged, and reported. The scale accounts for the depth that the material travels and for the subject reaction to the material once penetrated or aspirated. The scale also attempts to define an ordinal "goodness" of the swallow. A score of 1 is the most benign and, as the score increases, so do the severity of the events observed. The most severe sign, a score of 8, is that of aspiration without effort to expel the material from the airway. The conventional term for this sign is "silent aspiration."

Although the aspiration-penetration scale allows the clinician to describe the events associated with aspiration or penetration more precisely, the clinician can enhance the description by characterizing the timing of the penetration or aspiration. Specifically, the clinician will want to describe whether the event occurs before, during, or after the initiation of the pharyngeal swallow. The timing of laryngeal penetration is strongly associated with specific impairments.

Penetration-Aspiration: Before the Swallow

This event almost always is due to a late airway protective response. One of the challenges presented to the clinician in this instance is to determine if the early release of the bolus was due to premature spillage or a delay in the pharyngeal response to an oncoming bolus. Premature spillage is due primarily to a compromised glosso-palatal seal with subsequent, involuntary, entry of material into the pharynx from the oral cavity. When this occurs the pharynx must accommodate the early arrival of the bolus fragment by generating a pharyngeal swallow, or by closing the airway and allowing the protective structural barriers and cavities to fill until a volitional propulsion of the bolus occurs. Shaker et al. (1994) and Shaker and Lang (1997) described a "secondary" pharyngeal swallow that occurs as a result of infusion of liquid into the pharynx or retrograde passage of material from the upper esophagus. This swallow was described as a "secondary pharyngeal swallow" because of its similarity to secondary peristalsis of the esophagus, in that the peristaltic action occurs at the level of the stimulus. The secondary pharyngeal swallow included laryngeal elevation and cricopharyngeal opening along with tongue contact to the posterior wall to propel the bolus through the UES. The element that is not included in this swallow is tongue contact to the hard palate and purposful propulsion of the bolus out of the oral cavity. These swallows were noted to occur when water was infused, via a transnasal catheter, toward the posterior wall.

When leakage does occur from the glosso-palatal seal, a co-occurring pharyngeal delay usually exists, in that some bolus material reaches the point where it enters the pharynx before the final superior and anterior movement of the hyoid bone. It is this co-occurrence that is the catalyst for so much confusion in terms, as many clinicians use the terms premature spillage, premature leakage, and pharyngeal delay interchangably. Pharyngeal delay describes the travel of a portion of the bolus into the pharynx before the initiation of the pharyngeal swallow, whether the travel of the bolus was volitional or the result of a poor seal. In many cases the clinician may be confused as to which behavior the patient is demonstrating. The clinician can circumvent this confusion by asking the patient to hold the bolus in his or her mouth until an instruction to swallow is given. In patients with a poor glosso-palatal seal, the loss of oral control of the bolus with subsequent premature spillage and co-occurring pharyngeal delay usually will occur. Patients with a good oral-palatal seal, but with a poorly organized pharyngeal response, when commanded to swallow, will volitionally propel the bolus into the pharynx before initiating the swallow.

Aspiration-Penetration: During the Swallow

Aspiration during the swallow is defined as material entering the airway after the final anterior and superior movement of the hyoid associated with the pharyngeal swallow and before the larynx returns to its resting position.

Material may enter the laryngeal inlet during the pharyngeal swallow under certain conditions. As the bolus is being propelled through the pharynx, the lower airways are subject to multiple, redundant, protective mechanisms, including true vocal fold closure, ventricular fold closure, anterior tilting of the arytenoids to the epiglottic base, and epiglottal retroflexion over the tightly closed laryngeal vestibule. If any of these protective functions is compromised, through weakness or incoordination, the laryngeal inlet can be penetrated.

Recurrent laryngeal nerve damage affects the ability of the intrinsic laryngeal muscles to contract fully. When the muscles of abduction do not act to close the airway, there is a risk of material entering the partially opened airway.

Patients with postsurgical scarring or irradiation of the UES and patients with tracheostomy tubes in place may suffer from a "tethering" effect during laryngeal elevation. The hyoid may elevate at the appropriate time and with adequate amplitude, but thyroid and cricoid elevation may lag behind, due to the tethering, resulting in late or incomplete approximation of the arytenoids to the epiglottic base. It is during laryngeal elevation that material enters this sometimes transiently opened airway.

As has been discussed previously, patients with poor hyoid elevation may not achieve epiglottic retroflexion. This may allow material to enter the laryngeal vestibule during laryngeal elevation. It should be noted that patients with adequate sphincteric laryngeal closure may allow penetration, but should be able to protect against aspiration, even following epiglottectomy.

Patients with other postsurgical changes that affect airway closure, such as hemilaryngectomy, may suffer penetration and aspiration during the swallow.

Penetration-Aspiration: After the Swallow

This event of aspiration occurs after the bolus has been propelled into the UES and the larynx comes back to rest.

Aspiration after the swallow typically is due to residuals left over in the pharynx following the initial swallow attempt. These residuals overcome the protective structures and cavities by overfilling and fall by gravity into the laryngeal vestibule (Figure 3–22). Residuals in the pharynx can be due to low propulsion forces in the pharynx, inadequate laryngeal elevation/pharyngeal shortening that results in poor UES opening, or a hypertonic or inelastic UES.

Other factors that can contribute to aspiration after the swallow are the retrograde passage of material from the lower ailementary tract back into the pharynx. This can be due to poor esophageal peristalsis, LES achalasia, or esophageal stricture, in which material may fill the esohagus to the point at which its capacity is reached and material flows back into the pharynx and penetrates the unprotected airway. Another scenario for aspiration after the swallow is the escape of material from a diverticulum back into the pharynx.

Conclusions

By precisely characterizing the event of penetration-aspiration and examining the temporal events surrounding penetration-aspiration, decisions regarding the implementation of specific interventions can more easily be made.

VFE-6. SCORING: INTERVENTION

Note the intervention techniques used for each consistency presented. Indicate their success

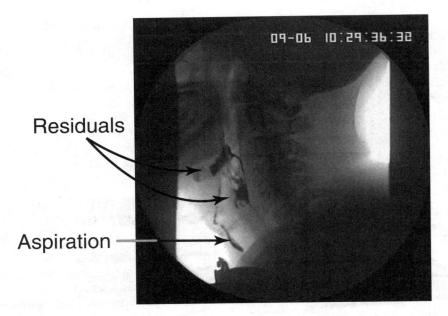

Figure 3-22. Residue remaining after the swallow falls into the laryngeal vestibule and passes into the trachea.

or failure by placing a "+" or "−" sign next to the notation. List modifications or additional information in the section reserved for notes.

As signs of dysphagia become evident during the fluoroscopic examination, attempts should be made to adjust elements that facilitate or compensate for the impaired swallow. As discussed in the clinical examination section, adjustments come in the form of :

Manipulations of bolus volume

Manipulation of bolus viscosity

Changes in means of delivery/use of devices

Application of postural changes

Application of behavioral maneuvers

Manipulation of Bolus Volume

This manipulation is enhanced greatly by the fine visualization of the bolus in the oral cavity and pharynx. Bolus volume control can assist patients with both coordination deficits and impaired propulsion. The key to the adjustment is in determining the capacity of the structural barriers to laryngeal penetration. Each structural barrier (i.e., vallecular space,

lateral channels, and pyriform sinuses) will have a "spillover" point that will have been probed as the graduated boluses were presented during the examination.

Patients with premature spillage may benefit from bolus volume adjustments by presenting amounts that are controlled more easily by the glossopalatal seal. When premature spillage and pharyngeal delay are found to co-occur, the capacity of the structural barriers of the pharynx should be considered, as this amount may be less than that which can be controlled orally.

Volume adjustments should be considered when pharyngeal propulsion forces are reduced and pharyngeal residuals remain after the initial swallow attempt. Again, the structural barriers of the pharynx should be capable of containing whatever residue remains. Further, the patient should not be stressed with every presentation. A slight decrement in the volume of a bolus can mean the difference between utilizing anxiety-provoking clearance maneuvers and a relaxed, though prolonged, meal.

Manipulation of Bolus Viscosity

The thinner the liquid, the more rapidly it will flow through the pharynx. When the duration of stage transition is extended, the flowing bolus can fill and quickly overflow into the laryngeal vestibule. If the speed of the onset of the pharyngeal stage of the swallow cannot be improved, the relative speed of the oncoming bolus *can* be adjusted. The key to viscosity adjustment of liquids is to slow the flow of the bolus just enough so that the pharyngeal stage of the swallow is initiated when the bolus is at or, preferably, above the vallecular space.

The clinician should have more than one, and preferably several, liquids of various viscosities available for presentation during the examination. Although true thin liquids are not likely to be emulated with liquid barium preparations, the clinician should attempt to prepare the thinnest possible solution without compromising the visualization of the bolus. The more viscous solutions should match the viscosity of foods and liquids that are easily prepared at home or are commercially available. Typical viscosity gradations would include thin liquids, nectar thick liquids, honey thick liquids, and pudding-thick liquids.

Changes in Delivery/Use of Devices

Fluoroscopy will allow for good visualization of oral stage impairments. The lateral projection also allows for excellent visualization of the effectiveness of customized feeding utensils. Patients who demonstrate difficulty in manipulating food in the anterior oral cavity should be viewed in the AP projection. Patients with consistent loss of oral control on one side of the oral cavity may benefit from presenting the food on the side with good control or intact sensation.

The clinician should anticipate the needs of these patients based on clinical findings and should have an array of utensils and delivery strategies in place before the initiation of the examination (Table 3–11).

Application of Postural Changes

Head Rotation

The patient is instructed to turn his or her head in the direction of the weakened side while keeping the shoulders squared. Once head rotation is accomplished, the instruction to swallow is given. The effect of this position change is observed best in the AP projection. Localization of bolus residue is not as well visualized in the lateral projection (see Figure 3–23).

Head rotation generally is used with patients who have unilateral pharyngeal weakness. Theoretically, head turn to the weakened side should effectively divert the bolus toward the intact side, allowing the muscular contraction of the intact lateral and posterior

Table 3–11. Examples of facilitations and indications for use.

Facilitation	Indications
Small volumes per swallow (e.g., 5 ml)	Severe and multiple pharyngeal/laryngeal abnormalities
Large volume per swallow (e.g., 10–20 ml)	Oral sensory deficits
Intake via spoon	Velopharyngeal incompetence that precludes sucking with a straw
Intake via straw	Signs suggesting that reflexive sucking/swallow is more efficient than volitional swallow
Intake via syringe or "glossectomy spoon"	Severe tongue preparation and bolus formation signs
Pudding consistency	Pharyngeal/laryngeal abnormalities
Liquid consistency	History suggesting isolated problem with opening of the pharyngoesophageal segment
Cold substance or hot substance	Sensation losses or reductions

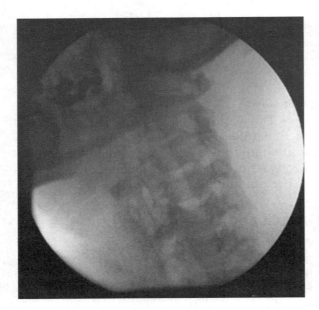

Figure 3-23. Fluoroscopic example of head rotation in the AP projection.

pharyngeal walls to support the pharyngeal propulsion of the bolus. The weakened side usually is effectively closed off when the head is rotated adequately. In a study of patients with Lateral medullary syndrome (LMS) and unilateral pharyngeal weakness, Logemann et al., (1989) found that head rotation improved OPSE. The LMS patients with head in the neutral position had a mean OPSE of 20. With head rotation to the weak side, OPSE scores increased to an average of 51. A mean score of 78 was recorded for control subjects. In the same study, Logemann et al. (1989) found that

an additional benefit of head rotation was the substantial reduction in UES resting pressure. With head rotation, UES resting pressure was reduced to 18 mm Hg, a 35% reduction from the resting pressure in the neutral position. The head rotation and resultant relaxed sphincter yielded significantly greater UES opening diameter in patients with LMS. In the neutral position, diameters of 7.7 mm were recorded and, with head rotation, this increased to 11.6 mm (normal = 13.8 mm).

Patients with bilateral weakness may benefit from turning their heads to the left and right while swallowing to take advantage of the beneficial effects of reduced UES sphincter tone.

Some patients with weakness or reduced sensation may not be able to generate a swallow with the head rotated. Others may not be able to rotate their heads fully, or to the point at which the facilitative effect is achieved. Probing for this possibility prior to the fluoroscopic examination will cue the clinician to the likelihood of successful implementation later in the exam. Table 3–12 provides a list of compensatory strategies, including head rotation.

Chin Tuck

The chin tuck is intended to reduce the likelihood of aspiration in the event of pharyngeal delay or premature spillage with co-occurring pharyngeal delay. When the chin is tucked toward the chest the AP dimensions of the pharynx are purported to be reduced in the AP dimension (Figure 3–24). For further discussion

Table 3–12. Examples of compensations and indications for use.

Compensation	Indications
Neck flexion (chin tuck)	Signs suggesting laryngeal protection problems
Neck rotation	Unilateral pharyngeal or laryngeal weakness signs
Supraglottic swallow	Laryngeal protection problems
Consecutive throat clear swallow	Intermittent wet hoarseness sign
Multiple swallow	Pharyngeal weakness signs
Nose occlusion	Signs of velopharyngeal incompetence
Rate of intake slowed	Cognitive limitations and/or sensory loss

Source: From Linden, P. (1989). Videofluoroscopy in the rehabilitation of swallowing dysfunction. *Dysphagia 3,* 189–191. Reprinted with permission.

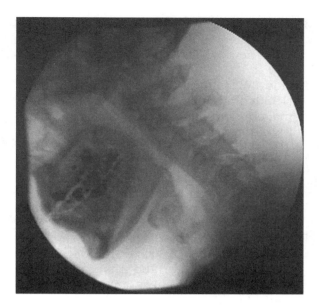

Figure 3-24. Chin tuck position in lateral projection.

regarding chin tuck, see the discussion regarding head positioning (clinical exam).

When implementing the chin tuck posture, the clinician will be monitoring the facilitative effect it may have on reducing pharyngeal delay and preventing penetration or aspiration. It would be expected that the bolus will remain in the oral cavity for a longer period of time, during which the pharyngeal stage of the swallow is initiated and the airway protected.

Mendelsohn Maneuver

This maneuver is designed to sustain the elevation of the larynx during the swallow. Sustained laryngeal elevation will, in turn, augment UES opening, which is the main objective of the maneuver.

To teach the maneuver, the patient is instructed to monitor laryngeal elevation during the swallow by holding his or her fingers against the thyroid cartilage. After a few swallows, the patient usually can identify the motion of the larynx elevating. The clinician then can demonstrate the maneuver to the patient by having the patient monitor the elevation of the clinician's larynx. The patient then should attempt to monitor his own elevation manually with the clinician monitoring and coaching the sustained elevation. When mastery is achieved, test swallows can be attempted.

This maneuver has a number of benefits. Cricopharyngeal opening duration and the duration of laryngeal elevation increases, as does the duration of closure of the laryngeal vestibule (Kahrilas, Logemann, Krugler, & Flanagan, 1991; Mendelsohn & McConnel, 1987; Miller, & Watkin, 1997). In a head and neck cancer patient, the Mendelsohn maneuver was found to improve coordination and timing of the various pharyngeal swallow events. These included timing of posterior movement of the tongue base to the pharyngeal wall in relation to airway closure and cricopharyngeal opening, with elimination of aspiration (Lazarus, Logemann, & Gibbons, 1993).

This maneuver may take some time to train. Performing this training in the fluoroscopic suite is usually not efficient if the patient is a "slow learner."

Superglottic and super supraglottic maneuvers will be discussed in Chapter 4.

VFE-7. NARRATIVE

This narrative section is not intended to serve as the final report. This section should be used to record miscellaneous procedural notes relating events that may have taken place during the session. An initial impression can be entered as well as the preliminary plan of action.

REFERENCES

Bird, M. R., Woodward, M. C., Gibson, E. M., Phyland, D. J., & Fonda, D. (1994). Asymptomatic swallowing disorders in elderly patients with Parkinson's disease: A description of findings on clinical examination and videofluoroscopy in sixteen patients. *Age and Ageing, 23*, 251–254.

Bisch, E. M., Logemann, J. A., Rademaker, A. W., Kahrilas, P. J., & Lazarus, C. L. (1994). Pharyngeal effects of bolus volume, viscosity, and temperature in patients with dysphagia resulting from neurologic impairment and in normal subjects. *Journal of Speech and Hearing Research, 37*, 1041–1059.

Brasseur, J. G. (1987). A fluid mechanical perspective on esophageal bolus transport. *Dysphagia, 2*, 32–39.

Bruns, C. J., Gawenda, M., Wolfgarten, B., & Walter, M. (1997). Cervical anastomotic stenosis after gastric tube reconstruction in esophageal carcinoma. *Langenbecks Archiv Fur Chirurgie, 382*, 145–148.

Coelho, C. A. (1987). Preliminary findings on the nature of dysphagia in patients with chronic obstructive pulmonary disease. *Dysphagia, 2*, 28–31.

Colangelo, L. A., Logemann, J. A., Pauloski, B., Pelzer, H., & Rademaker, A. (1996). T stage and functional outcome in oral and oropharyngeal cancer patients. *Head and Neck, 18*, 259–268.

Cook, I. J. (1993). Cricopharyngeal function and dysfunction. *Dysphagia, 8*, 244–251.

Cook, I. J., Blumberg, P., Cash, K., Jamieson, G. G., & Shearman, D. J. (1992). Structural abnormalities of the cricopharyngeus muscle in patients with pharyngeal (Zenker's) diverticulum. *Journal of Gastroenterology and Hepatology 7*, 556–562.

Cook, I., Dodds, W., Dantas, R., Massey, B., Kern, M., Lang, I., Brasseur, J., & Hogan, W. (1989). Opening mechanisms of the humans UES. *The American Journal of Physiology, 257*, G278–G759.

Curtis, D. J., Cruess, D. F., & Bert, T. (1984). The cricopharyngeal muscle: A videorecording review. *American Journal of Roentgenology, 142*, 497–500.

Curtis, D. J., Cruess, D. F., Dachman, A. M., & Maso, E. (1984). Timing in the normal pharyngeal swallow, prospective selection and evaluation of 16 normal asymptomatic patients. *Investigative Radiology, 19*, 523–529.

Dantas, R. O., Kern, M. K., Bassey, B. T., Dodds, W. J., Kahrilas, P. J., Brasseur, J. G., Cook, I. J., & Lang, I. M. (1990). Effect of swallowed bolus variables on oral and pharyngeal phases of swallowing. *The American Journal of Physiology, 258*, G675–G681.

Dejaeger, E., Pelemans, W., Ponette, E., & Joosten, E. (1997). Mechanisms involved in postdeglutition retention in the elderly. *Dysphagia, 12*, 63–67.

de Larminat, V., Dureuil, B., Montravers, P., & Desmonts, J. M. (1992). Impairment of deglutition reflex after prolonged intubation. *Anesthesie, Analgesie, Reanimation, 11*, 17–21.

Dengel, G., Robbins, J., & Rosenbek, J. C. (1991). Image processing in swallowing and speech research. *Dysphagia, 6*, 30–39.

DeVault, K. R. (1996). Lower esophageal (Schatzki's) ring: Pathogenesis, diagnosis and therapy. *Digestive Disease, 14*, 323–329.

Dodds, W., Stewart, E., & Logemann, J. (1990). Physiology and radiology of the normal oral and pharyngeal phases of swallowing. *American Journal of Roentgenology, 154*, 953–963.

Dodds, W. J., Taylor, A. J., Stewart, E. T., Kern, M. K., Logemann, J. A., & Cook, I. J. (1989). Tipper and dipper types of oral swallows. *American Journal of Roentgenology, 153*, 1197–1199.

Dua, K. S., Ren, J., Bardan, E., Xie, P., & Shaker, R. (1997). Coordination of deglutitive glottal function and pharyngeal bolus transit during normal eating. *Gastroenterology, 112*, 73–83.

Dua, K., Shaker, R., Ren, J., Arndorfer, R., & Hofmann, C. (1995). Mechanism and timing of nasopharyngeal closure during swallowing and belching. *American Journal of Physiology, 268*, G1037–G1042.

Ekberg, O., & Borgstrom, P. S. (1989). Graphic representation of pharyngeal wall motion during swallow: Technical note. *Dysphagia, 4*(1), 43–47.

Ekberg, O., & Nylander, G. (1982). Dysfunction of the cricopharyngeal muscle: A cineradiographic study of patients with dysphagia. *Radiology, 143*(2), 481–486.

Feinberg, J. (1993). Radiographic techniques and interpretation of abnormal swallowing in adult and elderly patients. *Dysphagia, 8*, 356–358.

Fulp, S. R., Dalton, C. B., Castell, J. A., & Castell, D. O. (1990). Aging-related alterations in human upper esophageal sphincter function. *American Journal of Gastroenterology, 85*, 1569–1572.

Furukawa, K. (1984). Cineradiographic analysis of laryngeal movement during deglutition. *Nippon Jibinkoka Gakkai Kaiho, 87*, 169–181.

Goyal, R. K. (1984). Disorders of the cricopharyngeus muscle. Symposium on the Larynx. *Otolaryngologic Clinics of North America, 17*, 115–130.

Goyal, R., Martin, S., Shapiro, J., & Speckler, S. J. (1993). The role of cricopharyngeus muscle in pharyngoesophageal disorders. *Dysphagia, 8*, 252–258.

Hiiemae, K., Heath, M. R., Heath, G., Kazazoglu, E., Murray, J., Sapper, D., & Hamblett, K. (1996). Natural bites, food consistency, and feeding behaviour in man. *Archives of Oral Biology, 41,* 175–189.

Hamlet, S., Ezzell, G., & Aref, A. (1993). Larynx motion associated with swallowing during radiation therapy. *International Journal of Radiation Oncology, 28,* 467–470.

Hunter, J. G., Swanstrom, L., & Waring, J. (1996). Dysphagia after laparoscopic antireflux surgery. *Annals of Surgery, 224,* 51–57.

Kahrilas, P., Dodds, W., Dent, J., & Logemann, J. (1988). Upper esophageal sphincter function during deglutition. *Gastroenterology, 95,* 52–62.

Kahrilas, P. J., Lin, S., Chen, J., & Logemann, J. A. (1996). Oropharyngeal accommodation to swallow volume. *Gastroenterology, 111,* 297–306.

Kahrilas, P. J., Lin, S., Rademaker, A. W., & Logemann, J. A. (1997). Impaired deglutitive airway protection: A videofluoroscopic analysis of severity and mechanism. *Gastroenterology, 113*(5), 1457–1464.

Kahrilas, P. J., Logemann, J. A., Krugler, C., & Flanagan, E. (1991). Volitional augmentation of upper esophageal sphincter opening during swallowing. *The American Journal of Physiology, 260,* G450–G456.

Konowitz, P. M., & Biller, H. F. (1989). Diverticulopexy and cricopharyngeal myotomy: Treatment for the high-risk patient with a pharyngoesophageal (Zenker's) diverticulum. *Otolaryngology—Head and Neck Surgery, 100,* 146–153.

Langmore, S. E., Terpenning, M. S., Schork, A., Chen, Y., Murray, J. T., Lopatin, D., & Loesche, W. J. (1988). Predictors of aspiration pneumonia: How important is dysphagia? *Dysphagia, 13,* 69–81.

Lazarus, C., & Logemann, J. A. (1987). Swallowing disorders in closed head trauma patients. *Archives of Physical Medicine and Rehabilitation, 68,* 79–84.

Lazarus, C., Logemann, J. A., & Gibbons, P. (1993). Effects of maneuvers on swallowing function in a dysphagic oral cancer patient. *Head & Neck, 15,* 419–424.

Lazarus, C. L., Logemann, J. A., Pauloski, B. R., Colangelo, L. A., Kahrilas, P. J., Mittal, B. B., & Pierce, M. (1996). Swallowing disorders in head and neck cancer patients treated with radiotherapy and adjuvant chemotherapy. *Laryngoscope, 106,* 1157–1166.

Lazarus, C. L., Logemann, J. A., Rademaker, A. W., Kahrilas, P. J., Pajak, T., Lazar, R., & Halper, A. (1993). Effects of bolus volume, viscosity, and repeated swallows in nonstroke subjects and stroke patients. *Archives of Physical Medicine and Rehabilitation, 74,* 1066–1070.

Lof, G. L., & Robbins, J. (1990). Test-retest variability in normal swallowing. *Dysphagia, 4,* 236–242.

Logemann, J. (1983). Anatomy and physiology of normal deglutition. In J. Logemann (Ed.), *Evaluation and treatment of swallowing disorders* (pp. 9–36). San Diego: College-Hill Press.

Logemann, J. A., Kahrilas, P., Cheng, J., Roa, Pauloski, B., Gibbons, P. J., Rademaker, A., & Lin, Z. (1992). Closure mechanisms of laryngeal vestibule during swallow. *American Journal of Physiology, 262,* G338–G344.

Logemann, J., Kahrilas, P., Kobara, M., & Vakil, M. (1989). The benefit of head rotation on pharyngoesophageal dysphagia. *Archives of Physical Medicine and Rehabilitation, 70,* 767–771.

Low, V. & Rubesin, S. (1993). Contrast evaluation of the pharynx and esophagus. *Radiological Clinics of North America, 31,* 6.

Margulis, A. R., & Koehler, R. E. (1976). Radiologic diagnosis of disordered esophageal motility. *Radiological Clinics of North America, 14,* 429–438.

McConnel, F., Hood, D., Jackson, K., O'Connor, A. (1994). Analysis of intrabolus forces in patients with Zenker's diverticulum. *Laryngoscope, 104,* 571–580.

McLarty, A. J., Deschamps, C., Trastek, V. F., Allen, M. S., Pairolero, P. C., Harmsen, W. S. (1997). Esophageal resection for cancer of the esophagus: Long-term function and quality of life. *Annals of Thoracic Surgery, 63,* 1568–1572.

Mellow, M. H. (1983). Esophageal motility during food ingestion: A physiologic test of esophageal motor function. *Gastroenterology, 85,* 570–577.

Mendelsohn, M. S., & McConnel, F. M. (1987). Function in the pharyngoesophageal segment. *Laryngoscope, 4,* 483–489.

Meshkinpour, H., & Eckerling, G. (1996). Unexplained dysphagia: Viscous swallow-induced esophageal motility. *Dysphagia, 11,* 125–128.

Miller, J. L., & Watkin, K. L. (1997). Lateral pharyngeal wall motion during swallowing using real time ultrasound. *Dysphagia, 12,* 125–132.

Nilsson, M. E., Isacsson, G., Isberg, A., & Schiratzki, H. (1989). Mobility of the upper esophageal sphincter in relation to the cervical spine: A morphologic study. *Dysphagia 3*, 161–165.

O'Laughlin, J. C., Bredfeldt, J. E., & Gray, J. E. (1980). Hypertonic upper esophageal sphincter in the oculopharyngeal syndrome. *Journal of Clinical Gastroenterology, 2*, 93–98.

Olsson, R., Castell, J., Johnston, B., Ekberg, O., & Castell, D. O. (1997). Combined video-manometric identification of abnormalities related to pharyngeal retention. *Academic Radiology, 4*, 349–354.

Palmer, J. B., Hiiemae, K. M., & Liu, J. (1997). Tongue-jaw linkages in human feeding: A preliminary videofluorographic study. *Archives of Oral Biology, 42*(6), 429–441.

Palmer, J. B., Tanaka, E., & Sievens, A. (1988). Motions of the posterior pharyngeal wall in swallowing. *Laryngoscope, 98*, 414–417.

Panchal, J., Potterton, A. J., Scanlon, E., & McLean, N. R. (1996). An objective assessment of speech and swallowing following free-flap reconstruction for oral cavity cancers. *British Journal of Plastic Surgery, 49*, 363–369.

Perlman, A. L., Booth, B. M., & Grayhack, J. P. (1994). Bideofluoroscopic predictors of aspiration in patients with oropharyngeal dysphagia. *Dysphagia, 9*, 90–95.

Perlman, A. L., Grayhack, J. P., & Booth, B. M. (1992). The relationship of vallecular residue to oral involvement, reduced hyoid elevation, and epiglottic function. *Journal of Speech and Hearing Research, 35*, 734–741.

Perlman, A. L., Van Daele, D. J., & Ottervacher, M. S. (1995). Quantitative assessment of hyoid bone displacement from video images during swallowing. *Journal of Speech and Hearing Research, 38*, 579–585.

Rademaker, A. W., Pauloski, B. R., Logemann, J. A., & Shanahan, T. K. (1994). Oropharyngeal swallow efficiency as a representative measure of swallowing function. *Journal of Speech and Hearing Research, 37*, 314–325.

Ren, J., Shaker, R., Kusano, M., Podvrsan, B., Metwally, N., Dua, K. S., & Sui, D. (1995). Effect of aging on the secondary esophageal peristalsis: Presbyesophagus revisited. *The American Journal of Physiology, 268*, G772–G779.

Ren, J., Shaker, R., Zamir, Z., Dodds, W. J., Hogan, W. J., & Hoffmann, R. G. (1993). Effect of age and bolus variables on the coordination of the glottis and upper esophageal sphincter during swallowing. *American Journal of Gastroenterology, 88*, 665–669.

Robbins, J., Hamilton, J. W., Lof, G. L., & Kempster, G. B. (1992). Oropharyngeal swallowing in normal adults of different ages. *Gastroenterology, 103*, 823–829.

Robbins, J., & Levin, R. L. (1988). Swallowing after unilateral stroke of the cerebral cortex: Preliminary experience. *Dysphagia, 3*, 11–17.

Rosenbek, J. C., Robbins, J., Roecker, E.V., Coyle, J. L., & Woods, J. L. (1996). A penetration-aspiration scale. *Dysphagia, 11*, 93–98.

Rosenbek, J. C., Robbins, J., Willford, W. O., Kirg, G., Schiltz, A., Sowell, T. W., Deutsch, S. E., Milanti, F. J., Ashford, J., Gramigna, G. D., Fogarty, A., Dong, K., Rau, M. T., Prescott, T. E., Lloyd, A. M., Sterkel, M. T., & Hansen, J. E. (1998). Comparing treatment intensities of tactile-thermal application. *Dysphagia, 13*, 1–9.

Rosenbek, J. C., Roecker, E. B., Wood, J. L., & Robbins, J. (1996). Thermal application reduces the duration of stage transition in dysphagia after stroke. *Dysphagia, 11*, 225–33.

Rubesin, S. E., Jones, B., & Donner, M. W. (1987). Radiology of the adult soft palate *Dysphagia, 2*, 8–17.

Schneider, H. J. (1997). Gross dysarthric movement disorders of the velopharynx. *HNO, 45*, 460–465.

Shaker, R., Cook, I. J., Dodds, W. J., & Hogan, W. J. (1988). Pressure-flow dynamics of the oral phase of swallowing. *Dysphagia, 3*, 79–84.

Shaker, R., Dodds, W., Dantas, R., Hogan, W., & Arndorfer, R. (1990). Coordination of deglutitive glottic closure with oropharyngeal swallowing. *Gastroenterology, 98*, 1478–1484.

Shaker, R., Junlong, R., Zamir, Z., Sarna, A., Liu, J., & Sui, Z. (1994). Effect of aging, position, and temperature on the threshold volume triggering pharyngeal swallows. *Gastroenterology, 107*, 396–402.

Shaker, R., & Lang, I. (1997). Reflex mediated airway protective mechanisms against retrograde aspiration. *American Journal of Medicine, 103*, 64s–73s.

Shaker, R., Ren, J., Podvrsan, B., Dodds, W. J., Hogan, W. J., Kern, M., Hoffmann, R., & Hintz, J. (1993). Effect of aging and bolus variables on pharyngeal and upper esophageal sphincter motor function. *The American Journal of Physiology, 264,* G427–G432.

Shaw, D. W., Cook, I. J., Gabb, M., Holloway, R. H., Simula, M. E., Panagopoulos, V., & Dent, J. (1995). Influence of normal aging on oral-pharyngeal and upper esophageal sphincter function during swallowing. *The American Journal of Physiology, 268,* G389–G396.

Shaw, D. W., Cook, I. J., Jamieson, G. G., Gabb, M., & Simula, M. E., & Dent, J. (1996). Influence of surgery on deglutitive upper-oesophageal sphincter mechanics in Zenker's diverticulum. *Gut, 38,* 806–811.

Skinner, K. A., & Zuckerbraun, L. (1998). Recurrent Zenker's diverticulum: Treatment with crycopharyngeal myotomy. *American Surgeon, 64,* 192–195.

Stachler, R. J., Hamlet, S. L., Mathog, R. H., Jones, L., Heilbrun, L. K., Manov, L. J., & O'Campo, J. M. (1994). Swallowing of bolus types by postsurgical head and neck cancer patients. *Head & Neck, 16,* 413–419.

Sundgren, P., Maly, P., & Gullberg, B. (1993). Elevation of the larynx on normal and abnormal cineradiogram. *The British Journal of Radiology, 66,* 768–772.

Thomas, P., Doddoli, C., Neville, P., Pons, J., Lienne, P., Giudicelli, R., Giovannini, M., Seitz, J. F., & Fuentes, P. (1996). Esophageal cancer resection in the elderly. *European Journal of Cardiothoracic Surgery, 10,* 941–946.

Tracy, J. F., Logemann, J. A., Kahrilas, P. J., Jacob, P., Kobara, M., & Krugler, C. (1989). Preliminary observations on the effects of age on oropharyngeal deglutition. *Dysphagia, 4,* 90–94.

Van Daele, D. J., Perlman, A. L., & Cassell, M. D. (1995). Intrinsic fiber architecture and attachments of the human epiglottis and their contributions to the mechanism of deglutition. *Journal of Anatomy, 186,* 1–15.

Veis, S. L., & Logemann, J. A. (1985). Swallowing disorders in persons with cerebrovascular accident. *Archives of Physical Medicine and Rehabilitation, 66,* 372–375.

Wilcox, C. M., Alexander, L. N., & Clark, W. S. (1995). Localization of an obstructing esophageal lesion. Is the patient accurate? *Digestive Disease and Science, 40,* 2192–2196.

CHAPTER 4

The Laryngoscopic Evaluation of Swallowing or FEES

"Come forth into the light of things."
William Wordsworth (1770–1850)
or

"Looking before and after, gave us not that capability. . ."
Sc. 4. Hamlet, William Shakespeare

INTRODUCTION

Flexible fiberoptics have been employed for a number of years by the various medical professions to visualize the nasal, pharyngeal, and laryngeal airways. In 1988, Langmore, Schatz, and Olsen published the first description of a comprehensive assessment of swallowing safety using flexible laryngoscopy. The examination, titled "FEES," or Fiberoptic Endoscopic Evaluation of Swallowing, required the transnasal passage of a flexible laryngoscope into the hypopharynx whereupon food and liquid were presented, the ensuing events observed, and therapeutic intervention applied. The FEES examination was purported to have the advantage of being portable, allowing the clinician to assess swallow function at the patient's bedside (Figure 4–1). An additional advantage was that there is no limitation to the amount of time available for ob-

serving swallow function, as there is no exposure to radiation.

IMAGING WITH FLEXIBLE ENDOSCOPY

The field of view of the endoscope includes only a fraction of the area that can be viewed with the fluoroscope. A typical fluoroscopic image will include the oral cavity, pharynx, and portions of the striated esophagus. At any given time, the endoscopist will visualize only the anatomy and biomechanical movements immediately in front of the objective lens of the endoscope. The oral, upper esophageal, and esophageal stages of the swallow will not be visualized during this procedure. Further, there is a period during which the image is obliterated due to the apposition of tissue,

153

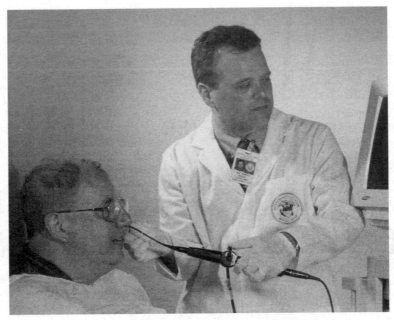

Figure 4–1. The patient is seated in a wheelchair as the endoscopist stands during the procedure.

usually base of tongue or velum to posterior pharyngeal wall, during the height of the pharyngeal stage of the swallow. In exchange for these disadvantages, the skilled endoscopist will be rewarded with an unequaled view of airway protective patterns, a very sensitive tool for detecting aspiration and an invaluable mechanism for biofeedback and patient education.

The elements to be considered when choosing the instrumental assessment should be considered carefully. The field of view should determine the instrumentation. If questions regarding oral stage impairments cannot be answered following the clinical examination, a fluoroscopic evaluation should be performed. Patients being seen for the first time with longstanding dysphagia or vague complaints and confounding signs during the clinical examination should receive a fluoroscopic examination. Patients with complaints of food being "stuck" at the level of the thyroid notch or below and patients with obvious signs of upper esophageal or esophageal dysphagia also should receive a fluoroscopic examination. The endoscopic evaluation serves well the patient with a sudden onset of pharyngeal dysphagia. Patients with pharyngeal signs who are in the acute phase after stroke, head injury, or surgery are good candidates for endoscopy. Additionally, patients that have received an initial fluoroscopic examination with confirmed pha-

ryngeal dysphagia could be re-tested via endoscopy to avoid the radiation and expense of the fluoroscopic battery. These and other indications for instrumental examinations are listed in Table 4–1.

ENDOSCOPIC MECHANICS

The flexible laryngoscope is configured to cast a "cold" light delivered from a xenon or halogen light source. Although both xenon and halogen light sources provide adequate light to assess swallow function, the xenon will provide a more natural color cast to the mucosal surface. Halogen light sources are considerably less expensive, but yield a bluish hue to the mucosal surface. The light is conducted along a fiberoptic bundle, which traverses the length of the scope. Depending on the configuration, the light is diffused through one or two lenses on the distal end of the scope to illuminate the cavity of interest. A separate lens on the distal end of the scope collects the reflected image and projects it along another bundle of light fibers to the eyepiece of the endoscope. The endoscopist can visualize the image by looking directly through the eyepiece or by utilizing a chip camera, which converts the image to a video signal, allowing the image to be viewed on a monitor and recorded on a video recorder.

Table 4–1. Indications for instrumental examinations.

Unresolved Clinical Condition	Fluoroscopy	Endoscopy
Oral stage dysphagia	X	
Upper esophageal or esophageal stage dysphagia	X	
Vague complaints	X	
Clinically inexplicable weight loss	X	
Initial exam for long-standing dysphagia	X	
Food stuck at thyroid notch or lower	X	
Sudden onset of pharyngeal dysphagia	X	X
Food "stuck" above thyroid notch	X	X
Retest, pharyngeal dysphagia	X	X
Biofeedback, pharyngeal dysphagia	X	X
Aspiration of secretions		X
Anatomic anomalies		X
Assess airway protection patterns		X
Fluoroscopy unavailable		X

The flexible insertion shaft of a typical laryngoscope is approximately 40 cm long and has a diameter of 3.2–4.0 mm (Figure 4–2). The tip of the flexible portion of the scope angulates upward and downward to allow dynamic control of the image being viewed. Manipulation of the angulation lever on the control portion of the scope adjusts the degree of the angulation of the tip. The typical laryngoscope has a 90° field of view and, depending on the configuration, a working depth of approximately 50 mm from the distal end of the scope.

The modern laryngoscope and chip camera provide a good, indirect visualization of structures from the nasal cavity to the anterior tracheal wall. Although the image is much improved, distortion in the lens system still occurs. The distortion is of two types: distance distortion and radial distortion.

Distance distortion is a loss of image resolution due to increasing distance between the object and the laryngoscope. As the laryngoscope moves further away from the image, light disperses and fewer of the objective fibers contribute to the visualization of the image at the eyepiece, resulting in a reduction in resolution. The *radial distortion* is inherent to the flexible endoscope. This distortion is related to the lens system and results in a progressive reduction in image size from the center to the peripheral field of view. Only the inner 50% of the image is represented symmetrically through the eyepiece (Figure 4–3). Further, a parallax effect occurs as the angle of the endoscope changes in relation to the plane of the object being viewed. Because of these distortion effects, it becomes very difficult to judge the size of an object or, without careful placement, to judge the symmetry of structures or their movements.

HANDLING THE ENDOSCOPE

The endoscope is designed to be viewed with the naked eye. The control portion of the scope typically is held in a manner so that the angulation control lever is positioned inferiorly and is manipulated by the thumb of the dominant hand. The opposite hand is used to control the insertion tube at the patient's nares during the procedure. Maintaining control of the depth of the insertion of the flexible portion of the tube is of great importance during the examination. By applying a light grip, the endoscopist can prevent inadvertent mucosal laceration or perforation caused by sudden patient movement. The control portion of the scope is rotated by the dominant hand and the angulation control lever manipulated by the thumb to pan precisely across the cavity and gain the optimal field of view.

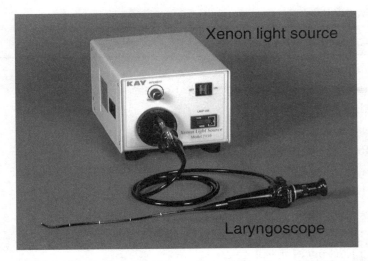

Figure 4–2. Illustration of endoscope and light source.

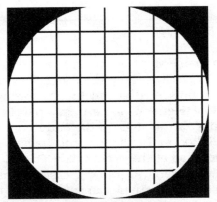 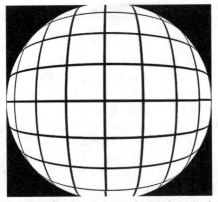

Symetrical grid without distortion   Radial distortion applied to grid

Figure 4–3. A radial distortion is observed when a symmetrical grid is visualized through the lens of a flexible laryngoscope. An item on the periphery of the image will appear smaller than an item of the same size in the middle of the image.

PATIENT POSITIONING

When performing the laryngoscopic swallowing examination, the endoscopist should, ideally, be utilizing a chip camera, which allows for viewing of the image on a video monitor. With the chip camera in place, patient positioning becomes less restrictive as close proximity of patient and clinician is no longer a necessity. The patient can be sitting in a chair or wheelchair or can be positioned to sit in bed. The endoscopist may either sit or stand during the procedure (Figure 4–4), but likely will find that standing allows for greater mobility when the bedside examination is performed.

When performing the examination, it is important to anticipate the need for repositioning later in the examination. If the patient is likely to benefit from biofeedback, space should be made available for unencumbered repositioning of the patient. If the session is to be dedicated to biofeedback, the patient may be positioned to face the screen prior to the placement of the endoscope (Figure 4–5).

TOPICAL ANESTHETIC

Although most patients tolerate the procedure well, some patients may find transnasal en-

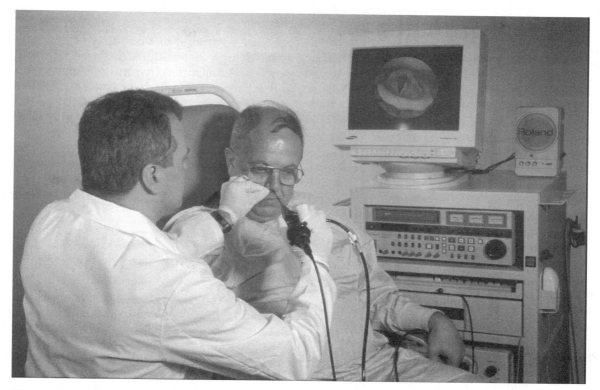

Figure 4–4. The endoscopist in the sitting position. The chair and monitor are situated to allow for easy visualization of the patient and projected image.

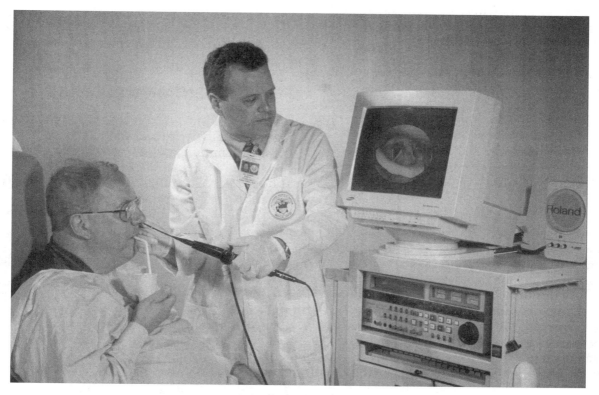

Figure 4–5. The endoscopist and monitor are positioned so that the patient can easily view the projected image for biofeedback and patient education.

doscopy uncomfortable. For those patients, a topical anesthetic (such as 2% viscous Lidocaine HCL) or a nasal vasoconstrictor may be necessary for the untroubled administration of the examination. Many practitioners claim that comfortable administration, without the use of anesthetic or vasoconstriction, is possible with careful insertion. Leder, Ross, Briskin, and Sasaki (1997) compared patient comfort levels following administration of a topical anesthetic, vasoconstrictor, placebo, or nothing to the nasal mucosa prior to transnasal endoscopy. The authors found no significant differences in patient comfort level among the four variables.

Singh, Brockbank, and Todd (1997) found no significant difference in comfort level between the application of 5% cocaine and the application of a saline solution in 60 patients undergoing transnasal endoscopy. It was found that contact with the inferior turbinate during insertion facilitated the most comfortable passage. This was contrasted with contact with the nasal septum, which was most likely to elicit discomfort. Both areas are supplied by branches of the pterygo-palatine ganglion of CN VII. The authors concluded that the cause of the discomfort may be that the septum is rigid, whereas the mucosa overlying the inferior turbinate can be compressed.

If anesthetic is to be used, the clinician should be warned against the use of aerosolized anesthetic preparations for this procedure, as the aerosol can travel to the pharyngeal mucosa and compromise afferent input to the swallow mechanism.

ENDOSCOPIC IMAGING OF OROPHARYNGEAL SWALLOWING

Much like in the fluoroscopic examination, the clinician must strive to integrate all of the elements that contribute to a viable oropharyngeal swallow. The components of the endoscopic assessment include the items listed in Table 4–2.

The integration of the components listed in Table 4–2 allows the clinician to estimate efficiency and ensure safety. As in the fluoroscopic examination, the clinician will be provided with detailed information that, when appropriately examined, will allow for the realization of the biomechanical basis of impairment. With this information, appropriate treatment goals can be formulated. The endoscopist should be careful to note the difference between a screening examination of dysphagia, which simply determines the presence or absence of penetration, aspiration, and residue, and a full endoscopic assessment of dysphagia. Langmore (1996) developed a full protocol that attends to the realization of the biomechanical basis of impairment and the effectiveness of interventions when employing laryngoscopy to assess the pharyngeal swallow. This full protocol is tradmarked and is described as a Fiberoptic® Endoscopic Evaluation of Swallowing® (FEES®).

LARYNGOSCOPIC PROTOCOL

The clinician will elicit swallows by presenting food and liquid of varying volumes and consistencies to the patient. The food and liquid should be light in color and sparsely tinted with blue or green food dye to enhance visibility. Foods that are dark or colored red or brown should be avoided, as they will blend in with the pharyngeal mucosa. Milk and many of the liquid nutrition formulas are light in color and reflect light well. Transparent liquids, such as water and many juices, will not reflect light and will be difficult to visualize at a distance or under lowered light conditions (i.e., in the trachea). Equipment needed is listed in Table 4–3.

FOOD PRESENTATION GUIDELINES

Food and liquid are presented in the same manner as they were in the clinical swallowing examination and fluoroscopic examinations. The objective of the examination is to show ability as well as disability. As always, the initial careful presentation of measured amounts limits the amount of penetration and/or aspiration early in the examination and reduces the likelihood of an aborted examination due to patient distress. As in the fluoroscopic examination, the laryngoscopic examination should not be aborted when a small amount of aspiration occurs. Aborting the examination prevents the implementation of the various adjustments that may alleviate future events of aspiration.

PLACEMENT OF THE ENDOSCOPE

The scope is placed transnasally along the path of least resistance. This is generally

Table 4–2. Components of the endoscopic assessment.

Identification of:

Normal and abnormal anatomy
Discrete structural movements
Temporal coordination of anatomic movements relative to bolus advancement
Trajectory of the bolus through the pharynx

Evaluation of the efficacy for:

Adjustments to the bolus volume, consistency, and rate of delivery
Adjustments in positioning
Implementation of maneuvers

Table 4–3. Material used for conducting the FEES.

Equipment Needed	Optional Equipment
Spoons/cups/straws	Time/date character generator
Puree/solids	Surface electromyography
Premixed liquids of varying viscosity	Pharyngeal manometry
Placebo tablet or capsule	
Videotape recorder	
Microphone	
Two percent viscous lidocaine	
Cotton tipped applicators	

the floor of the nose or in between the inferior and middle turbinates (Figure 4–6). Once a passage has been determined, the scope is inserted continuously until the nasopharyngeal vault is visualized. The clinician should position the scope just anterior to the vomer bone, which demarcates the point where the hard and soft palate articulate. It is at this point that velar function should initially be assessed. The superior path (between the inferior and middle turbinates or between the middle and superior turbinates) usually yields an improved view of nasopharyngeal function (Muntz, 1992).

After instructing the patient to breathe through his or her nose or "hum," the angulation control lever is depressed to angle the scope downward to allow insertion into the nasopharynx. As the scope is inserted further, the base of tongue and larynx come into view. The endoscopist now must exercise dynamic control of the endoscope, by rotating, inserting, and retracting, to optimize the view of the endolarynx. For the observation of general swallowing function, the distal end of the scope ideally is placed at the level of the uvula (Figure 4–7). When in this position, the field of view includes the base of tongue, posterior pharyngeal wall, lateral pharyngeal walls, and endolarynx. As the scope is advanced, fewer structures peripheral to the endolarynx are included in the field of view. The scope may be advanced to the tip of the epiglottis for optimal viewing of the pyriform sinuses and endolarynx prior to and during the initiation of the pharyngeal swallow. This is the ideal position to observe airway closure patterns during the swallow. The scope can be advanced further into the endolarynx to look into the subglottic region.

During the pharyngeal swallow, the velum elevates to close off the nasal port. Because of the transnasal placement, velar elevation causes the scope to be lifted superiorly during the swallow. Given adequate velar elevation and careful placement of the scope at the tip of the epiglottis, this lifting of the scope prevents mucosal damage due to inadvertent contact of

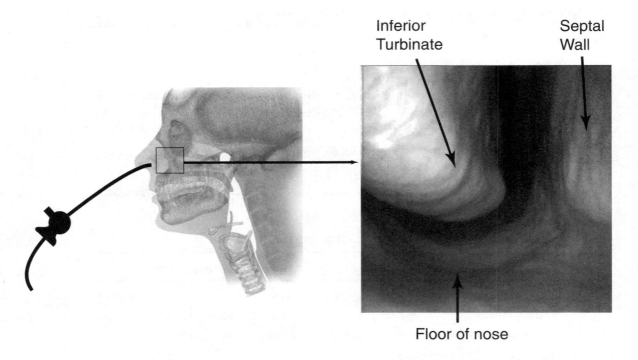

Figure 4–6. The view of the anterior nasal cavity shows the path of least resistance to the nasopharynx. In this case, along the floor of the nose.

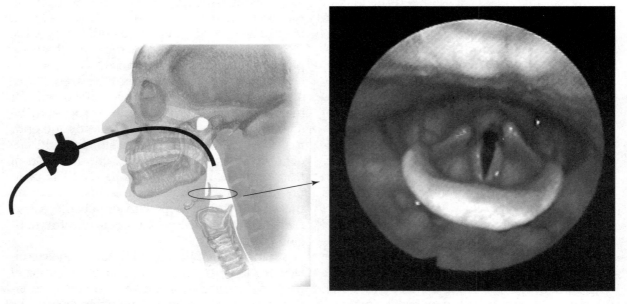

Figure 4–7. The endoscope is placed through the nasopharynx with the distal tip at the level of the uvula. With this positioning the field of view should include the posterior wall, base of tongue, lateral walls, and endolarynx.

distal end of the scope to the elevating laryngeal structures.

MAINTAINING THE FIELD OF VIEW

It is essential to sustain discipline in positioning before and after the swallow to maximize findings. Because the field of view is limited, findings must actively be pursued through the dynamic placement of the scope. Prior to each presentation of food or liquid, the endoscopist must strive to position the scope to include the area of interest. After each swallow, the scope should be inserted quickly into the laryngeal vestibule to scan the endolarynx and subglottic region for signs of penetration or aspiration that may have occurred during the period of obliteration (Figure 4–8).

The objective lens of the endoscope will become "gunked" during the examination due to contact with oropharyngeal secretions or food and liquid. This is inevitable during the examination, but the period of clear viewing can be prolonged with a few simple adjustments. When "gunking" occurs, retracting the scope by a few centimeters sometimes releases the material from the scope tip. If this does not clear the lens, angulating the tip of the scope to contact the posterior pharyngeal wall generally will wipe away the residue. If these techniques fail to clear the lens, the scope can be retracted into the nasopharynx and the subject can be requested to swallow. The elevating velum will trap the distal end of the scope against the posterior wall and scour the lens. If all of these methods fail, the scope must be retracted and cleaned before continuing with the examination. In the event of "gunking," it is important to remember to retract the scope initially by a few centimeters to avoid contact with the structures of the endolarynx and then to incorporate the cleansing procedures described above.

SCORING/PROTOCOL

The examination is broken into two sections. The observation section occurs during the initial passage of the endoscope and is reserved for the survey of anatomy, elicitation of anatomic movements, observation of secretion management, and the monitoring of spontaneous swallows. After the elements of the observation section are satisfied, food and liquid are presented and interventions attempted. The FEES scoring form is presented in Form 4–1.

OBSERVATION

❶ ANATOMIC NOTES

Write a short narrative account describing normalcy or deviations in the anatomic structures.

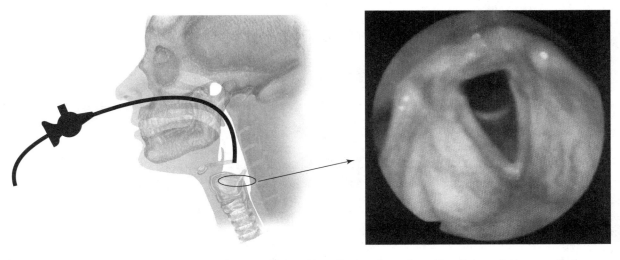

Figure 4–8. Low placement of the endoscope allows for visualization of the endolarynx and trachea.

Form 4–1
Fiberoptic Endoscopic Evaluation of Swallowing Scoring Form

OBSERVATION SECTION

❶ ANATOMIC NOTES:

_____

_____

❷ SECRETIONS RATING: _____

❸ SPONTANEOUS SWALLOWS: _____

❹ BREATH-HOLD: _____

❺ SENSATION: _____

❻ COUGH: _____

PRESENTATION OF FOOD AND LIQUID

Material	Ice	Puree	Soft	Solid	Liquids	
					THIN	THICK
❼ MAX AMOUNT:	____	____	____	____	____	____
❽ DST:	____	____	____	____	____	____
❾ ASP/PEN:>	____	____	____	____	____	____
❿ NO. SWALLOWS:	____	____	____	____	____	____
⓫ INTERVENTION:	____	____	____	____	____	____

BIOMECHANICAL OBSERVATIONS

⓬ VELUM: _____

⓭ EPIGLOTTIS: _____

⓮ AIRWAY CLOSURE:

⓯ _____

NARRATIVE:

_____

_____

The endoscope provides an excellent view of the surface mucosa of the nasopharynx, pharynx, and larynx. The initial scan with the endoscope should include a survey of the anatomy. The normal anatomy for the nasopharynx and pharynx are illustrated in Figures 4–9 and 4–10.

The patient should be positioned so that the head is in the neutral position. Careful inspection of the structural barriers to the laryngeal airway should be made. Symmetry of the structures and cavities should be noted with special attention to the natural flow path of the bolus (Figure 4–11). If asymmetry of the structures is observed, changes in head position can be elicited to determine any potential positive effect. The resting position of the epiglottis should be noted. Is the vallecular space available, or does the epiglottis obscure the vallecula by resting against the base of the tongue? Edema, and any detrimental effects that may be engendered by the edema to the protective barriers should be noted (Figure 4–12). Likewise, surgical changes and the effect on protective barriers should be described. The appearance of lesions, tumor, or mass effects should trigger a consultation for verification by otolaryngology (Figure 4–13).

❷ SECRETIONS

Characterize the appearance of oropharyngeal secretions as they become visible upon entry into the hypopharynx according to the Secretion Severity Rating Scale (Table 4–4 and Figure 4–14).

In normal subjects, oropharyngeal secretions are cleared from the hypopharynx by periodic spontaneous swallows throughout the day. The collection of oropharyngeal secretions in the laryngeal vestibule causes a change in voice quality known as "wet dysphonia" and traditionally has been thought to reflect an impairment of the efficiency of laryngopharyngeal clearance (Linden & Siebens, 1983). Among the factors contributing to the accumulation of secretions are a reduction in the frequency of swallowing, a reduction in the amplitude of the pharyngeal swallow, or a combination of reduced frequency and weakness.

The accumulation of oropharyngeal secretions within the laryngeal vestibule is highly predictive of aspiration of food and liquid later in the examination (Murray, Langmore, Ginsberg, & Dotsie, 1996). In that study, secretion ratings for normal subjects and hospitalized patients at risk for dysphagia were found to be significantly different. None of the young normals or age-matched elderly normals was found to have secretions resting within the bounds of the laryngeal vestibule during the observation segment of the examination, and the majority (68%) of the normals were rated as "0." Only hospitalized patients were observed to have secretions within the laryngeal vestibule and 70% had a rating of "1" or greater. Among the hospitalized patients, the secretion ratings for those who did aspirate were significantly different than those who did not. Further, all of the patients with a rating of "2" or higher were observed to aspirate food or liquid later, during the portion of the examination in which boluses were presented.

The finding of secretions in the vestibule should be an immediate visual marker for potential poor performance during the examination. With patients demonstrating this sign, it is suggested that 1 cc of ice chips be presented first in lieu of food or liquid. In patients who have been without oral feeding for extended periods of time, this small bolus presentation may "wake up" the system and generate spontaneous swallows that otherwise would not occur. Very small ice chip presentations are more likely to melt slowly and fill the protective cavities without overflow, giving the slow or incoordinated patient time to generate the pharyngeal swallow. Other patients may continue to perform poorly after several ice chips, alerting the clinician to halt the examination before catastrophic presentations of food or liquid.

❸ SWALLOW FREQUENCY

Dry swallows are identified by looking for events of "white out," or screen obliterations (Figure 4–15). Count the number of dry swallows observed during the first few minutes after the placement of the endoscope and before the offering of food or liquid.

During the swallow, the tongue and velum contact the posterior pharyngeal wall. When placed transnasally, the distal tip of the endoscope will be trapped transiently against the posterior pharyngeal wall by the velum or

A. Fluoroscopic view

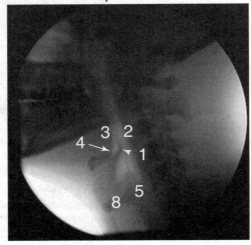

1- Epiglottis
2- Posterior pharyngeal wall
3- Base of tongue
4- Vallecular space

B. Laryngoscopic view

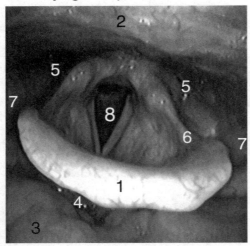

5- Pyriform sinus
6- Aryepiglottic fold*
7- Lateral pharyngeal wall*
8- Glottis

*Not well visualized fluoroscopically

Figure 4–9. Anatomy of pharynx as viewed with the laryngoscope.

A. **Anterior view of pharynx including base of tongue a vallecular space**

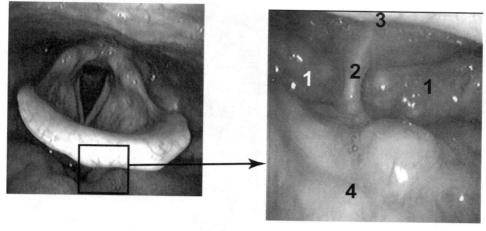

1- Vallecular space
2- Glosso-epiglottic band
3- Tip of epiglottis
4- Base of tongue

B. Endoscopic view of the endolarynx.

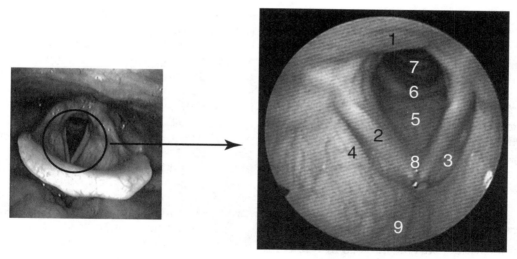

1- Inter-arytenoid space
2- True vocal fold
3- Ventricular space
4- Ventricular (false) fold
5- Crico-thyroid membrane
   (sub-glottic shelf)
6- Cricoid cartilage
7- Tracheal rings
8- Anterior commisure
9- Petiole of epiglottis

Figure 4–10. Anatomy of the endolarynx. *(continued)*

C.   View of the posterior pharynx and cricopharyngeal prominence

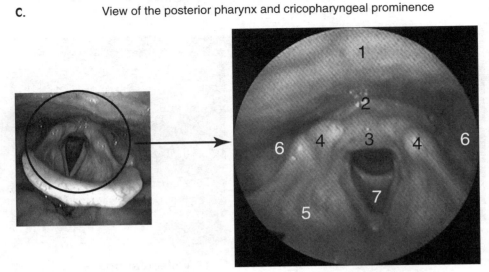

1- Posterior pharyngeal wall
2- Cricopharyngeal prominence
3- Inter-arytenoid space
4- Arytenoid
5- Endolarynx
6- Pyriform sinus

Figure 4–10. *(continued)*

base of tongue. This causes the light being emitted from the light delivery bundle to reflect off of the tissue it is in contact with. This appears as a flash of light that lasts approximately one half of a second in normal subjects (Perlman & Van Daele, 1993).

Swallowing is an activity that occurs throughout the waking hours at a rate of approximately 0.612 swallows/min and, during sleep, approximately 0.088 swallows/min (Lear, Flanagan, & Moorrees, 1965). Normal subjects swallow as often as they perceive the need to swallow. The urge to swallow is related generally to the accumulation of secretions in the pharynx. The transnasal placement of a catheter into the pharynx in normal subjects will result in an increase in salivary flow with a subsequent increase in the number of spontaneous swallows (Helm et al., 1982; Kapila Dodds, Helm, & Hogan, 1984). During the observation period of the examination, normal subjects were found to swallow approximately three times per minute, much higher than a normal subject without an endoscope placed transnasally (Murray et al., 1996). This may be related to increased saliva production resulting from irritation to nasal and pharyngeal mucosa. In that study, hospitalized patients were found to swallow less frequently

(0.89 swallows/min) than age-matched normals (2.82 swallows per min). Further, there was a significant difference in swallowing frequency among the aspirating and nonaspirating patients. Patients who aspirated were found to swallow 0.72 swallows/min while nonaspirating patients swallowed 1.16 swallows per min (*p*-value 0.047).

These findings could suggest several impairments. There may be a decline in sensation, in that the patient does not perceive the need to swallow the accumulated secretions. Another possibility is a decline in sensorium, resulting in a reduced drive to maintain swallow frequency. A synergistic combination of reduced sensorium and reduced sensation due to the effect of neurologic disease or medication could have a cumulative negative effect on the frequency of swallowing.

❹ BREATH-HOLDING

The patient should be requested to hold his or her breath. If laryngeal breath-holding is not observed, ask the patient to "bear down, as if lifting something heavy." Observe and then record the pattern of breath-holding according to the elements described in Table 4–5.

If the glottis does not close (Figure 4–16), visually monitor the presence of the biphasic

Anterior view of pharynx including base of tongue ai vallecular space

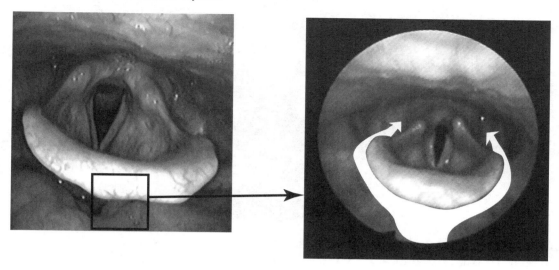

Figure 4–11. The peripheral anatomic borders of the larynx form barriers that protect against the entry of material into the trachea. Food, liquid, and secretions are guided around the endolarynx as they enter into the lower pharynx.

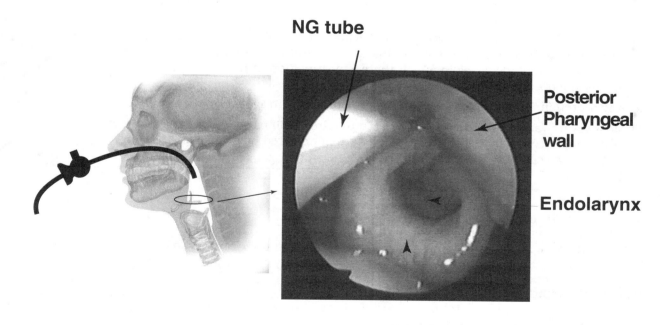

Figure 4–12. Edematous laryngeal structures reduce the effectiveness of the anatomic barriers.

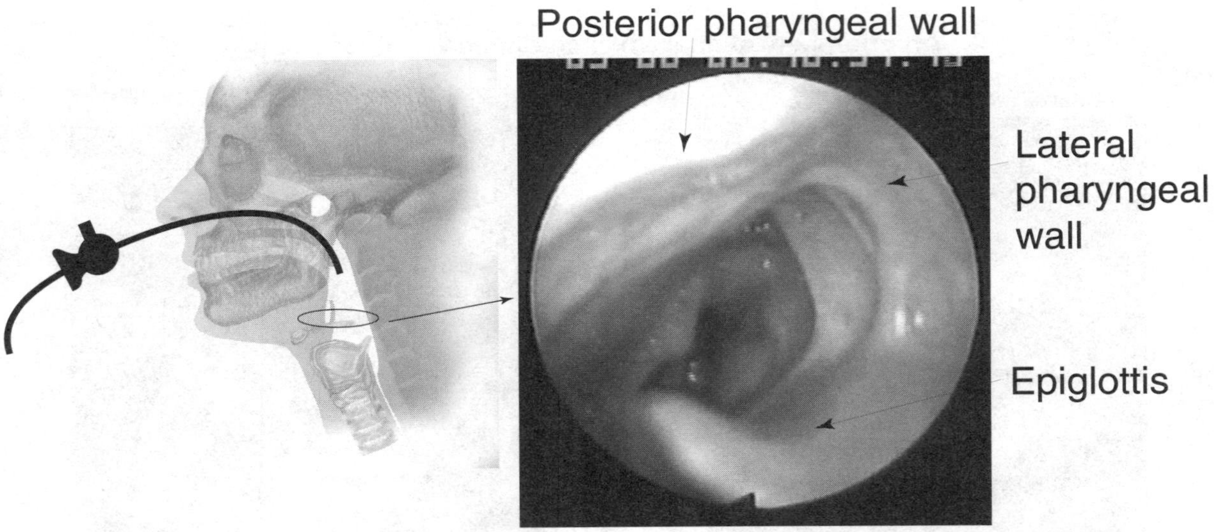

Posterior pharyngeal wall

Lateral pharyngeal wall

Epiglottis

Figure 4–13. The pharynx after surgical reconfiguration. In this patient the epiglottis has been sewn to the lateral pharyngeal wall, negating the natural protective barrier provided by the aryepiglottic fold on the patient's left side.

Table 4–4. Secretion severity rating scale.

0   Normal rating. Ranges from no visible secretions anywhere in the hypopharynx, to some transient secretions visible in the valleculae and pyriform sinuses. These secretions are not bilateral or deeply pooled.

1   Any secretions evident upon entry or following a dry swallow in the protective structures surrounding the laryngeal vestibule that are bilaterally represented or deeply pooled. This rating would include cases in which there is a transition in the accumulation of secretions during the observation segment.

2   Any secretions that change from a "1" rating to a "3" rating during the observation period.

3   Most severe rating. Any secretions seen in the area defined as the laryngeal vestibule. Pulmonary secretions are included if they are not cleared by swallowing or coughing by the close of the segment.

movement of the glottis associated with breathing. If the glottis remains open without the biphasic movement, breath-holding can be inferred. If the biphasic gesture toward abduction and adduction is present, it can be assumed that breath-holding was not achieved.

Much interest and energy has been expended on improving airway protection by facilitating breath-holding at the onset of the swallow. Flexible fiberoptics allow for verification of vocal fold closure by providing an excellent visualization of the different elements of airway valving; however, some very popular swallow maneuvers, such as the supraglottic swallow and super supraglottic swallow maneuvers, frequently are taught without the aid of glottic visualization.

Volitional breath-holding does not automatically result in laryngeal airway closure (Martin, Logemann, Shaker, & Dodds,1993; Mendelsohn & Martin, 1993). Mendelsohn and Martin (1993) reported that elicitation of "relaxed" breath-holding (breath-holding without special instruction) resulted in vocal fold closure in only 57% of the normal subjects tested. When Martin et al. (1993) asked patients to "hold your breath," optimum laryngeal valving was obtained in only 17%. When instructions were varied (i.e., "hold your breath hard"), the percentage of successful vocal fold

A. Normal "0"

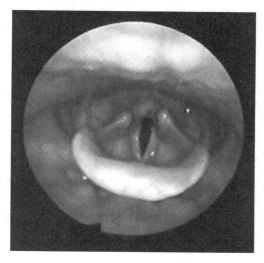

B. Sublogttic secretions "3"

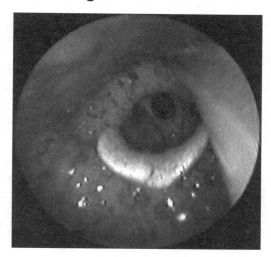

C. Secretions in vestibule "3"

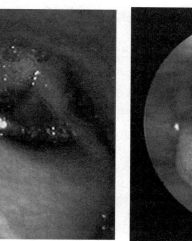

D. Dry secretions on pos. wall "2"

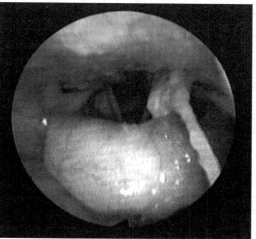

Figure 4–14. Examples of secretion collection in pharynx and scores.

approximation increased significantly. The fact that breath-holding was not attained consistently on command in normals was so dramatic a find that Mendelsohn and Martin (1993) suggested the following:

The high variability of laryngeal valving during breath-holding in normal subjects suggests that video nasolaryngoscopy should be undertaken in all patients who are taught the supraglottic swallow.

The apneic period that occurs during the height of the swallow has several components.

The first is inhibitory, in that the CNS transiently extinguishes the respiratory drive. The next several are obstructive, in that anatomic structures are positioned to prevent the exchange of gas. Two of the obstructive elements are the closure of the oral and nasal ports. Elements 4, 5, and 6 are true vocal fold closure, ventricular fold closure, and epiglottal retroflexion, respectively. Tight breath-holding should result in a sphinctericlike closure of the laryngeal vestibule. The true and false vocal folds should approximate and the arytenoids should tilt anteriorly, resulting in a "bunching" of tis-

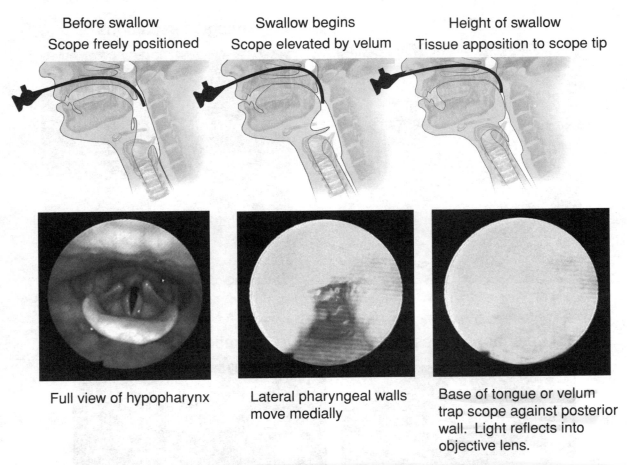

Before swallow
Scope freely positioned

Swallow begins
Scope elevated by velum

Height of swallow
Tissue apposition to scope tip

Full view of hypopharynx

Lateral pharyngeal walls move medially

Base of tongue or velum trap scope against posterior wall. Light reflects into objective lens.

Figure 4–15. White out is caused by the apposition of tissue against the distal end of the scope during the height of the swallow.

Table 4–5. Scoring guidelines for endoscopically observed breath holding patterns.

Breath holding not achieved

Transient breath holding with glottis open

Sustained breath holding with glottis open

Transient true fold closure

Sustained true fold closure

Transient true and ventricular fold closure

Sustained true and ventricular fold closure

sue within the vestibule. The lateral thyroarytenoid, with assistance from the vocalis, closes the vocal folds by contracting and drawing the arytenoid process toward the thyroid cartilage. The lateral cricoarytenoid rotates the arytenoid, bringing the vocal process medially and resulting in medial contact of both folds (Conrad et al., 1984).

McCulloch, Perlman, Palmer, and Van Daele (1996), using hook wire myography and simultaneous endoscopy, described the order of events as they occur during light breath-holding and tight airway closure. In light breath-holding, the true vocal folds adduct and the arytenoids contact simultaneously. This is followed by contraction of the true vocal folds, resulting in shortening of the folds and increased tension. In tight breath-holding, the order is the same, with ventricular fold adduction and forward tilting of the arytenoids quickly following true vocal fold adduction.

Certain patient populations, such as patients with severe chronic obstructive pulmonary disease (COPD), will have difficulty achieving closure of the cords for more than a few seconds before air hunger sets in. Other patients, such as those with stroke, will have

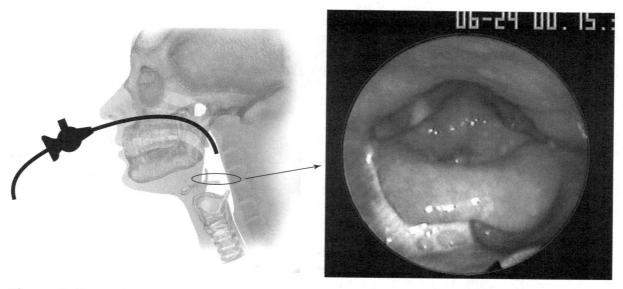

Figure 4–16. During tight breath holding the endolarynx closes in a sphincteric fashion, resulting in a tight seal.

difficulty coordinating any type of glottic closure. Others may be able to achieve closure transiently. In this group, using the image for immediate, "real-time" biofeedback is invaluable when attempting to train the super supraglottic swallow.

❺ SENSATION

Describe sensation in a narrative fashion according to the following criteria: Observe the patient's management of secretions within the layrngophayrnx. As material enters the laryngeal vestibule, there will be attempts to clear it in patients who perceive the need to clear. The clearance usually is performed by attempting to swallow, throat clearing, and "hawking" with expectoration. In other patients, whom we will infer to have reduced sensation, no clearance maneuver is attempted and secretions are seen to actively move in and out of the airway during rest breathing. Later during the examination, these findings can be compared to the aspiration-penetration scale to enhance the inference of "functional" sensation to penetrated or aspirated materials.

Sensation can be assessed objectively by incrementally applying precisely quantified puffs of air to the supraglottic laryngeal mucosa to determine a threshold for sensation (Aviv, Martin, Keen, Debell, & Blitzer, 1993). This is a relatively simple procedure, in which cali-brated air puffs are delivered through an instrument channel built into the shaft of the endoscope. One advantage to using this type of sensory testing is that an objective threshold for sensation is obtained prior to offering food or liquid. One of the disadvantages to this procedure is that light- and image-carrying fiber bundles in the endoscope are reduced in number to make room for the instrument channel, resulting in diminished picture size and definition. The user must consider whether this critical diminution in imaging is redeemed by the acquisition of the objective threshold, which, although of academic interest, does not fully describe the patient's "functional" sensation. Further, the puffs of air only test superior laryngeal nerve afferents found on the supraglottic larynx and not subglottic afferents supplied by the recurrent laryngeal nerve, which would activate the cough and clear response upon aspiration (Langmore, 1998). Conventional wisdom holds that aversive laryngeal stimulation generally results in airway closure (laryngeal adductory reflex), whereas aversive tracheal stimulation results in cough. The SLN does have some "irritant endings," which are said to contribute to generating the cough when the laryngeal mucosa is exposed to mechanical or chemical stimuli (Sant'Ambrogio & Sant'Ambrogio, 1996). Others feel that superior laryngeal nerve afferents do not play a necessary role in initiation of cough. Stockwell, Lang,

Zintel, White, and Gallagher (1993) found that there was no statistically significant difference between cough thresholds with and without superior laryngeal nerve blocks. More research relating impairment or disability to the objective data are expected and are of great interest.

For individuals without the apparatus to collect objective supraglottic sensory threshold, other, more primitive, observations and inferences regarding supralaryngeal sensation can be made. Start by observing resting respiration. The vocal folds should exhibit faint biphasic movements from abduction to adduction as the patient breathes in and out, respectively. This opening and closing of the larynx is said to make the airway more patent during inspiration and to act as a "brake" during expiration to slow the escape of gas from the lungs (Sant'Ambrogio & Mathew, 1986). This biphasic movement is the result of reflexogenic input from low-threshold myotatic mechanoreceptors located in the supralaryngeal mucosa (Wyke, 1973). When these mechanoreceptors are excited by positive or negative air pressures during the respiratory cycle, they evoke an afferent discharge in the superior laryngeal nerve that reflexively excites laryngeal motorneurons. At the onset of expiration, the thyroarytenoid and lateral cricoarytenoid muscles fire to abduct the folds slightly. During inspiration, the posterior cricoarytenoid displays a fluctuation in which activity begins to increase at the end of expiration and continues incrementally until the peak of inspiration, at which time it rapidly decreases. This biphasic opening and closing of the glottis is markedly reduced, but not completely extinguished in many patients with tracheostomy, which would suggest an additional sensory input based, possibly, on lung volume changes (Wyke, 1973).

In patients with vocal fold paralysis or intrinsic laryngeal muscular damage resulting in poor rotation of the arytenoids, this biphasic movement may be visible only on the unaffected side. For instance, patients with recurrent laryngeal nerve damage due to thoracic surgery will show arytenoid rotation only on the right side. If the movements are too slight to draw any conclusions about sensitivity or motor function, the patient can be asked to sniff in sharply. In normal subjects, this rapid inhalation results in a greater excitation of the mechanoreceptors and generally yields a more dramatic abduction. Poor abduction on the

sniff may be an indicator of poor sensation or reduced motor function.

⑥ COUGH

Instruct the patient to put forth his or her best effort in producing a cough:

"Take a breath and produce as great a cough as you possibly can." Characterize the cough or clearing maneuver according to the following components (Table 4–6):

Type of clearing maneuver:

Cough

Forced expiration

Throat clearing

Hawking

Effectiveness: If observable, comment on the effectiveness of the cough in clearing the airway of secretions or other debris.

For further description of the elements used in scoring the cough, refer to the discussion found in Chapter 2.

A functional volitional cough adds the essential element of safety to both the assessment and treatment processes. In patients with diminished sensation, the cued cough is elicited to clear the airway of material that has been penetrated or aspirated. As has been noted, the volitional cough is also an essential element of the supraglottic and super supraglottic swallow maneuvers.

Patients with motor coordination disorders or apraxia may be unable to generate an effective clearance maneuver. An ineffective volitional cough may not reflect the patient's ability to produce a strong and effective reflexive cough once stimulated. However, the patient with reduced sensation who cannot generate volitional clearance of the airway will not be a good candidate for therapeutic interventions that require this ability.

The effective volitional cough has several components (Figure 4–17). The first is inspiration, during which time the glottis abducts. The second is the tight supraglottic closure of the larynx, followed by increased tracheal air pressure and finally release of that pressure by the opening glottis.

After peak inspiration, the glottis closes down in a sphincterlike manner as the pharynx shortens. The lateral pharyngeal walls move medially to empty the pyriform sinuses

Table 4–6. Scoring guidelines for airway clearance.

Ineffective:	The effort does not clear material from the vestibule.
Mildly effective:	Material is expelled from the trachea and into the laryngeal vestibule.
Moderately effective:	Material is expelled from the laryngeal vestibule but not from the lower pharynx.
Effective:	Material is expelled from the vestibule and ejected from the lower pharynx.

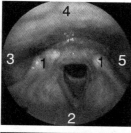

Glottis opens for inspiration.

1- Arytenoid
2- Epiglottis
3- Lateral pharyngeal wall
4- Posterior pharyngeal wall
5- Pyriform sinus

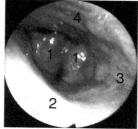

Supraglottic closure

The true and false folds form a tight seal as subglottic pressure rises. The lateral walls move medially as the pharynx shortens.

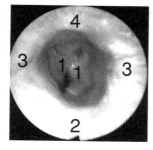

Tight pharyngeal squeeze with release of pressure

Material in the pyriforms and lateral pharyngeal channels are squeezed into the path of the flowing air and forced out of the airway.

Figure 4–17. Components of the cough. Inspiration (*top*). Supraglottic closure with increased tracheal pressure (*middle*). Release of pressure by glottis (*bottom*).

and lateral channels. This material then is pushed medially into the path of the airstream. The blast of air carries the debris to the oral cavity where it is expectorated or swallowed.

All of the components listed are desirable, but not essential, for the effective expulsion of material from the airway. Patients with tracheostomy, for instance, often expel material quite effectively without glottic closure to assist in the compression of pulmonary gases before the cough. Likewise, patients with recurrent laryngeal nerve damage will be unable to compress the supraglottic larynx but may be able to generate airflow great enough to clear the airway. The generation of the airflow is dependent on adequate inspiratory and expiratory efforts.

In conclusion, the clinician should monitor laryngeal abduction prior to the onset of the cough for an indication of inspiratory effort, laryngeal and pharyngeal compression as an indication of pressure-generating capability, and, finally, a forceful release of material from the airway to indicate effectiveness of the maneuver.

For a more thorough discussion of cough physiology see the clinical examination.

PRESENTATION OF FOOD AND LIQUID

❼ MAXIMUM AMOUNT/FOOD PRESENTATION GUIDELINES

Enter the size, in cc or functional units (spoonfuls, etc.), of the largest bolus presented to the patient in the space provided.

Food and liquid are presented in the same manner as they were in the clinical and fluoroscopic swallowing examinations. As always, the objective of the examination is to show ability as well as disability. The initial careful presentation of small, measured amounts will allow greater confidence when presenting larger boluses later in the examination. As in the clinical and fluoroscopic examinations, the examination should not be aborted when a small amount of aspiration occurs. Aborting the examination prevents the implementation of the various adjustments that may alleviate the event of aspiration.

❽ DURATION OF STAGE TRANSITION

If time characters have been recorded on the videotape, the following procedure can be used to calculate the duration of stage transition.

Onset: When the bolus head appears at the base of the tongue just superior to the vallecular space (Figure 4–18).

Endpoint: First frame of white out

If no time characters are imprinted on the tape, the duration can be calculated by counting single frames of video.

The measure of duration of stage transition was developed using moving fluoroscopic images. The conventional means for determining this duration required a determination of the elapsed time between the movement of the bolus into the pharyngeal cavity and the onset of the pharyngeal swallow. The fluoroscopic image afforded the clinician a view of the dynamic anterior and superior movement of the hyoid bone that is associated with the onset of the pharyngeal swallow. The movement of the

hyoid bone will not be visible to the endoscopist. For this reason, an endoscopically visible event must be employed as a surrogate to indicate the onset of the pharyngeal stage of the swallow.

As previously discussed, white out occurs as a result of either velar or tongue base tissue trapping the distal end of the laryngoscope against the posterior pharyngeal wall. This results in a flash of light back into the objective lens of the scope. The onset of white out has been shown to be closely timed with hyoid elevation (Logemann, 1995; Ohmae, Logemann, Kaiser, Hanson, & Kahrilas, 1995; Perlman & Van Daele, 1993) and, for this reason, serves as a good surrogate for hyoid elevation.

The second element necessary for determining this measure is bolus movement from the oral cavity into the pharynx. The fluoroscopic measure used the intersection point at which the shadow outlining the base of tongue meets the shadow outlining the ramus of the mandible.

Simultaneous laryngoscopic and fluoroscopic studies of swallowing performed at our laboratory have shown that careful placement of the endoscope within the lower nasopharynx will allow for visualization of a bolus as it passes from the oral cavity into the pharynx. Placement of the endoscope at the tip of the epiglottis, for instance, allows for excellent observation of vocal fold movement, but virtually eliminates the visualization of bolus transit through the upper pharynx (Figure 4–19).

The attainment of this measure requires the endoscopist to achieve appropriate placement of the endoscope, with clear visualization of the base of tongue, prior to the presentation of food or liquid to the patient. This may require the cooperation of the patient, if the patient is self-feeding, or of the assistant during the examination. It is always advisable to ensure that the lens is clear and that positioning is achieved before the bolus is presented to the patient.

Calculating this measure via endoscopy is not an exact analog of the fluoroscopic measure. The elapsed time invariably will be a few frames longer than the fluoroscopic measure due to the relatively later occurrence of white out. In patients with poor base of tongue or velar contact with the posterior pharyngeal wall, an even longer period of visualization will occur, resulting in a subsequently longer duration measure.

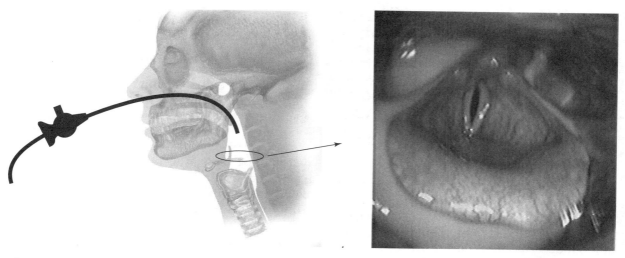

Figure 4–18. High scope position allows for visualization of the base of tongue and the oncoming bolus prior to the pharyngeal swallow.

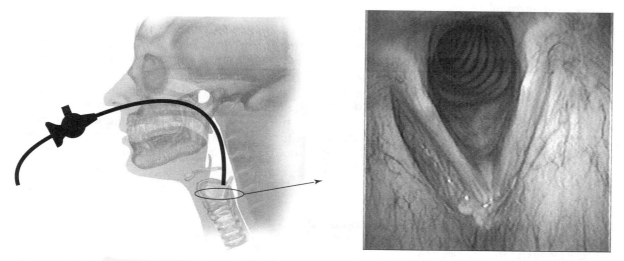

Figure 4–19. Low placement of the endoscope does not allow for visualization of bolus movement before the onset of the swallow.

Although the laryngoscopic measure of DST will not match up exactly with the fluoroscopic measure, it will describe the relative risk that accompanies the early arrival of a bolus into the pharynx as well as does fluoroscopy.

The flow pattern of the falling bolus is well-visualized as it moves through the pharynx prior to the initiation of the swallow. This is particularly important in patients with poorly configured structural barriers to penetration of the airway (i.e., epiglottis, vallecular space, aryepiglottic folds, or pyriform sinuses). In these patients, the effect of changes in head positioning are often well-visualized when employing the laryngoscope.

The pattern of airway protection also is well-visualized during the transition. When properly positioned, the laryngoscope allows for the visualization of the vocal folds and the falling bolus simultaneously. This gives the endoscopist an invaluable tool for determining the effectiveness of certain maneuvers that require tight glottal closure prior to the onset of the swallow, such as the supraglottic or super supraglottic maneuvers.

The DST measure is highly variable by nature (Rosenbek, Robbins, Roecker, Coyle, & Woods, 1996) both between and within patients. This would suggest that a difference of a few frames in the laryngoscopic and fluoroscopic measures should not make much difference when attempting to characterize the pattern of extended duration in a single subject. The difference would only be an issue if the two tools were being used for research, or to show changes in patient performance, without making clear the distinction between the measures.

➒ PENETRATION-ASPIRATION

As in the fluroscopic examination, score the events associated with penetration or aspiration according to the 8-point scale developed by Rosenbek et al. (1996) (Table 4-7). The traditional description of penetration and aspiration is used when employing this scale:

> *Penetration:* The passage of material into the laryngeal inlet without passing below the level of the true vocal folds.

> *Aspiration:* The passage of material below the level of the true vocal folds (Figure 4–20).

The timing of the event of aspiration or penetration is of great importance in determining the nature of the impairment and in planning for treatment. For further discussion regarding the use of this scale and the timing of aspiration, review the text in section VFE-5 in Chapter 3.

Aspiration Before the Swallow

With attention to careful placement of the laryngoscope, the endoscopist should be able to track the bolus reliably prior to the initiation of white out. In many cases, the event of aspiration will occur just at the onset of the pharyngeal swallow as the larynx begins to elevate and the bolus passes by the open airway. Given this, the penetration-aspiration event technically can occur "during" the swallow and still be observed before white out, in that hyoid elevation already is transpiring when the bolus enters the airway. This is strictly an academic question, as treatment for this impairment may be identical to that of a truly delayed swallow.

Events of penetration-aspiration before the swallow can be observed in either the high or low position. The lower position will afford less information regarding the timing and path of the bolus, but will provide a much more detailed view of airway protection. Positioning will depend on the clinician's sense of what should be treated and how that treatment will be enacted.

As a rule of thumb, for patients with timing and coordination problems or poorly functioning structural barriers, higher placement is indicated. In patients with laryngeal valving impairments, a lower position is indicated.

Making the judgment between penetration and aspiration before the swallow is diffi-

Table 4–7. Eight-point penetration-aspiration scale.

Score	Description of Events
1	Material does not enter the airway.
2	Material enters the airway, remains above the vocal folds, and is ejected from the airway.
3	Material enters the airway, remains above the vocal folds, and is not ejected from the airway.
4	Material enters the airway, contacts the vocal folds, and is ejected from the airway.
5	Material enters the airway, contacts the vocal folds, and is not ejected from the airway.
6	Material enters the airway, passes below the vocal folds, and is ejected into the larynx or out of the airway.
7	Material enters the airway, passes below the vocal folds, and is not ejected from the trachea despite effort.
8	Material enters the airway, passes below the vocal folds, and no effort is made to eject.

Source: From Rosenbek, J. C., Robbins, J., Roecker, E. V., Coyle, J.L., & Woods, J. L. (1996). A penetration-aspiration scale. *Dysphagia, 11,* 93–98. Reprinted with permission.

Penetration

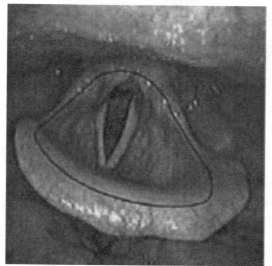

Within the black ring, but remaining above the vocal folds.

Aspiration

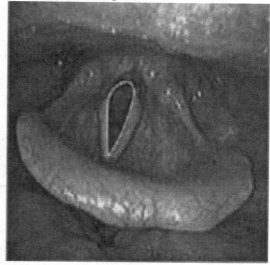

Within the white ring and below the vocal folds.

Figure 4–20. Anatomic boundaries for determining penetration and aspiration.

cult at times. Material may be observed clearly to fall within the glottis (Figure 4–21) in which case aspiration is determined and the following events are noted and judged according to the penetration-aspiration scale. However, when the glottis is closed before the event of penetration, material can be seen to enter the laryngeal vestibule and pool (Figure 4–22).

If material enters the vestibule and covers the glottis, it will be unclear as to whether penetration continues, or whether the laryngeal vestibule is being filled at a faster rate than material is escaping through the glottis and into the trachea. When this event occurs, the laryngeal vestibule and trachea must be inspected quickly and thoroughly for evidence of residuals, after white out when the view returns. The clinician again is warned not to use material that is clear or dark, as it will be poorly visualized under these circumstances. Milk and other lightly colored materials will leave a reflective film after contacting the mucosa, furnishing a useful "trail" for inspection.

Aspiration During the Swallow

This is perhaps the most difficult pharyngeal stage finding to determine when employing laryngoscopy. The period of obliteration will prevent direct viewing of penetration or aspiration.

The laryngeal vestibule and subglottic shelf (cricothyroid membrane) sometimes will hold clues as to the path of the bolus during the period of obliteration. Occurrences of laryngeal penetration, with resulting endolaryngeal residue, during the swallow are fairly easy to identify after the epiglottis returns to rest and the larynx opens up for inspection. Events of aspiration during the swallow are more problematic. Tracheal residue is fairly easy to visually locate if it is placed along the anterior wall of the trachea (Figure 4–23). However, the field of view of the endoscope will very rarely include the posterior wall of the trachea (Figure 4–24). The only evidence available that would point to an event of aspiration along the posterior tracheal wall would be residual reflective material in the area of the interarytenoid space. Should no evidence present itself, but aspiration during the swallow is suspected, the endoscopist should position the scope and wait for coughing or clearing attempts. If these do occur, the clinician should scan the vestibule for evidence of dye in the sputum. If the patient is suspected of being a silent aspirator, the clinician can request him or her to cough and then monitor the sputum, if produced, for evidence of dye. If all signs are negative but aspiration still is suspected, repeat the presentation.

Aspiration during the period of white out will not be observed directly as it occurs. Many

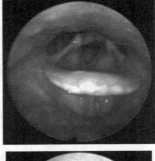

Head position turned left closes off left lateral channel and pyriform sinus

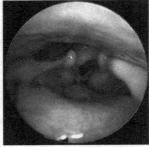

Material enters vestibule over left aryepiglottic fold

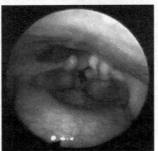

Material passes below the vocal folds and is directly aspirated before the onset of the swallow

Figure 4–21. Material is observed to fall into the glottis prior to the initiation of the swallow.

individuals dismiss the entire procedure, often citing this single weakness as the reason. This *would* appear to be a dramatic flaw in the examination for individuals who require direct observation of events as they occur. It has been my experience that when the experienced clinician employs deliberate endolaryngeal and tracheal inspection following each swallow, and combines this with sensible inferential skills, sensitivity for this finding is strongly enhanced and, often but not always, resolute.

Aspiration After the Swallow

This event generally is well-observed with endoscopy and should be detected reliably. Material can be observed to fall into the laryngeal vestibule as soon as the pharynx opens and the larynx is still descending.

The most likely time for the lens to become fogged or "gunked" is following the swal-

low. Care should be taken immediately to clear the objective lens of the scope if "gunking" occurs so that no salient events will be missed.

⑩ EFFICIENCY/NUMBER OF SWALLOWS

Count the number of swallows taken to clear a single bolus. The number of swallows can be determined by counting the occurrences of white out.

A single swallow should completely clear small boluses. Often, a second swallow accompanies the primary swallow even when no residual bolus is apparent. Patients with weakened bolus propulsion forces or with poor UES opening will demonstrate residuals in the pharynx following the swallow. When residuals remain after the swallow, the patient with intact sensation will attempt to clear the material with successive swallows. There are no

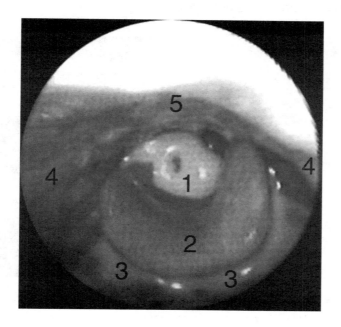

1- Pooled material in laryngeal vestibule
2- Epiglottis
3- Vallecula
4- Lateral pharyngeal walls
5- Posterior pharyngeal wall

Figure 4–22. Material is seen to pool on top of closed glottis before the initiation of the swallow. In the event of glottal opening, aspiration would occur.

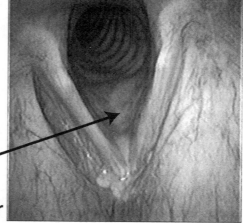

Aspirated material flowing down anterior tracheal wall.

Figure 4–23. Material is observed to rest along the anterior tracheal wall after an event of aspiration.

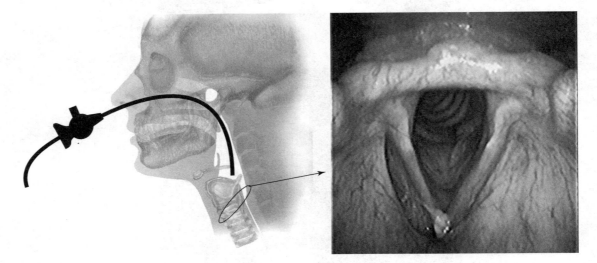

Figure 4–24. Aspirated puree food descending along the anterior tracheal wall. The forward tilt of the trachea allows for good visualization of aspirated material along the anterior tracheal wall but poor visualization of the posterior tracheal wall.

clear-cut data to suggest that a certain number of swallows will identify impairment or normalcy. An impression of weakness or mechanical noncompliance should be tangible when more than a few swallows are necessary to clear boluses as large as 25 cc. The number of swallows can be used to establish a baseline for performance and can be used to compare performance after intervention or spontaneous recovery.

The impression of weakness or poor UES opening should be compared and contrasted with findings from the clinical swallowing examination, the location of the residue, and other biomechanical findings that are observable using laryngoscopy.

⓫ SCORING: INTERVENTIONS

Note the intervention techniques used for each consistency presented. Indicate their success or failure by placing a "+" or "−" sign next to the notation. List modifications or additional information in the section reserved for notes.

As in the fluoroscopic examination, when signs of dysphagia become evident, attempts should be made to adjust elements that facilitate or compensate for the impaired swallow. Adjustments come in the same form as they would for the clinical or fluoroscopic exam. They are:

Manipulations of bolus volume

Manipulation of bolus viscosity

Changes in means of delivery/use of devices

Application of postural changes

Application of behavioral maneuvers

The success or failure of the intervention is judged by the effect it has on the transport of the bolus through the pharynx. Most of the intervention techniques are well-observed with laryngoscopy and have been described in VFE-6 in Chapter 3.

Some anatomic regions will not be viewed during laryngoscopy. Clinicians wishing to view oral stage impairments directly should use fluoroscopy or the clinical examination. Likewise, upper esophageal sphincter opening can only be viewed directly via fluoroscopy. Although one cannot view directly either the oral cavity or the UES via laryngoscopy, the effect of positioning and maneuvers on the bolus can be observed with laryngoscopy.

An example of this paradigm would be a case of oral leakage with co-occurring pharyngeal delay. Oral leakage occurs as a result of failure of the glossopalatal seal to contain a bolus within the oral cavity prior to the initiation of the pharyngeal swallow. It usually is accompanied by pharyngeal delay. This impairment becomes pathological only when the delay is of such duration that the bolus enters into the airway and penetration or aspiration occurs. The goal of any intervention should be to contain the bolus in the oral cavity until the swallow is initiated. This would mean that the successful implementation of positioning, chin-tuck, for instance, would result in a swallow without the early arrival of a portion of the bolus within the field of view of the endoscope prior to the initiation of the pharyngeal swallow. The successful maneuver therefore would present itself visually, endoscopically, as a lack of pharyngeal delay. Although the oral cavity and glossopalatal seal were not observed directly, the beneficial effect of the positioning can be verified.

Another example of this paradigm is observed in patients with residue that is located consistently in the pyriform sinuses. According to Dejaeger, Pelemans, Ponette, and Joosten (1997), residue in the pyriform sinuses is related to reduced pharyngeal shortening. Reduced pharyngeal shortening results in diminished UES opening, which prevents material from easily passing from the pharynx into the esophagus. Whether the cause of the residue is reduced laryngeal elevation or a hypertonic UES, the aim of any maneuver would be to augment UES opening to allow free passage of the bolus to the esophagus. In these cases, the Mendelsohn maneuver (Kahrilas, Logemann, Krugler, & Flanagan, 1991; Mendelsohn & McConnel, 1987; Miller & Watkin, 1997) or head rotation (Logemann, Kahrilas, Kobara, & Vakil, 1989) may be employed to augment UES opening during the pharyngeal swallow. Again, the success or failure of the maneuver is judged by the effect on the bolus. If less of the bolus is visible in the pyriform sinuses after the swallow using one of these maneuvers or if fewer swallows are necessary to completely clear the bolus, then the maneuver is considered a success. The effect of UES augmentation is not directly observed, but it is inferred with some surety.

One maneuver, the super supraglottic maneuver, is particularly well-viewed endoscopically.

The Super Supraglottic Maneuver

The super supraglottic maneuver is designed to minimize aspiration by producing volitional airway protection before, during, and after the swallow (Ohmae, Logemann, Kaiser, Hanson, & Kahrilas, 1996). This maneuver requires patients to tightly hold their breath before the swallow, to continue to hold their breath into the swallow, and to cough at the completion of the swallow.

This single maneuver can benefit the patient in a number of ways: It effectively prevents the aspiration of penetrated material before the swallow, aspiration during the swallow, and aspiration of penetrated material after the swallow. The super supraglottic maneuver is also said to produce earlier cricopharyngeal opening, prolong the pharyngeal swallow, and change the extent of vertical laryngeal position before the swallow (Ohmae et al., 1996), all of which promote the transit of the bolus through the UES.

As discussed in the volitional breath-holding section, laryngeal valving is not guaranteed when the subject is asked to hold his or her breath. By using endoscopy to visualize the breath-holding pattern, it is more likely that the maneuver will be appropriately implemented.

BIOMECHANICAL OBSERVATIONS

The astute observer can inspect the discrete movement of structures in the nasopharynx and pharynx and infer the underlying biomechanical actions necessary to support that movement. These movements can be observed during dry swallows or while presenting food and liquid to the patient. The endoscopist will be blessed with substantially greater visualization of airway protective patterns and, in turn, will be afflicted by the lack of visual information relating traction forces. The movements will be probed and discussed in terms of maximizing visualization, by the appropriate placement of the endoscope, and in terms of the underlying biomechanics where necessary.

OBSERVATION NOTATION FOR ALL BIOMECHANICAL OBSERVATIONS

Enter, in narrative form, information regarding impaired movement in the Biomechanical Notation section of the score sheet.

⑫ OBSERVING VELAR ELEVATION

When the interview and/or clinical examination yield findings of nasoregurgitation or the presentation of signs such as hypernasality, the clinician should be cued to investigate velar function thoroughly as it relates to swallowing during the endoscopic assessment.

The first movement to be observed after placement of the endoscope is that of the velum. Screening for velopharyngeal insufficiency can be performed on the first passage through the nasopharynx. After swallowing safety and risk of aspiration are assessed, the laryngoscope can be retracted into the nasopharynx again to probe for nasoregurgitation. Surprisingly, many patients with dysarthria who present with severe hypernasality and poor velopharyngeal closure during connected speech can achieve adequate velar elevation during the swallow. As a new or worsening symptom, nasoregurgitation in dysar- thric patients is quite dramatic and not often overlooked or unreported. In patients without complaints of nasoregurgitation, the following screening can be performed.

To maximize the observation of function, the initial position of the scope should include a view of the mucosa covering the vomer bone at the left or right periphery. This view will allow for observation of the superior surface of the velum and also allows for observation of the extent of elevation of the velum. To determine contact of the velum with the posterior wall, or to observe lateral defects in the velar sphincter, a more superior view is desired. This is achieved by placing the endoscope closer to the posterior wall and deflecting the tip inferiorly to look down through the nasopharyngeal port. The best view is obtained when the initial insertion of the laryngoscope follows a path between the middle and superior turbinate. This allows for a vantage point well above the tissue, preventing contact of the velum to the objective lens of the endoscope, and includes the entire nasopharyngeal seal during maximum elevation.

During the screening, nasopharyngeal function can be assessed by having the patient phonate nonsense syllables that alternate between nasally resonant sounds and oral plosives (/dunna, dunna, dunna/). Eliciting these syllables allows the clinician to observe the elevation and depression of the velum and gives an initial impression of strength and symmetry of the velum and the range of velar movement during speech. Once completed, the patient should be requested to swallow, to compare velar elevation during speech to velar elevation during the swallow. Some patients will present with hypernasality but will demonstrate an adequate velar seal during dry swallows. In these cases, a thorough probing for nasoregurgitation can be omitted if no evidence of nasal penetration or residue is evident when retracting the scope.

After the pharyngeal swallowing assessment is complete and a determination of safety is made, the scope can be retracted into the nasopharynx to probe for nasoregurgitation. The scope initially is positioned at the entrance to the nasopharynx with the vomer bone in the periphery. If the patient reports symptoms of nasoregurgitation, he or she should be presented with material that is of a consistency and volume consistent with the triggering of the event. Observe the symmetry of the leakage of material. Reposition the scope more superiorly if this assists in locating the area of weakness or defect. If nasal regurgitation is observed, a palatal lift prosthesis may be considered. Be sure to obtain good video recordings of both speech and nasoregurgitation for review by the prosthodontist. These recordings may assist in the design and fabrication of the prosthesis.

Velar elevation during the swallow is slightly different than that during speech. The excursion of the elevation is higher and the muscular components and timing are slightly different. For a complete review of velar elevation, refer to the discussion in the clinical examination (section CSE-13) and the fluoroscopic examination (VFE-2b).

⑬ EPIGLOTTIS

As previously discussed, the epiglottis provides protection to the laryngeal inlet in a manner that is both active and static. It functions primarily as a structural barrier that prevents the entry of secretions, food, liquid, and refluxed material from entering the lower airway.

Static Observation

The laryngoscope provides an excellent visualization of the epiglottis and allows the clinician to observe its static protective functions. The morphology of the epiglottis will predict its ability to act as a barrier. The normally configured epiglottis should rise above the base of the tongue and form a plow-shaped shield, which directs the advancing bolus laterally to channels formed by the aryepiglottic folds and lateral pharyngeal walls that terminate at the pyriform sinuses. At the lingual base of the epiglottis is the vallecular space, a space that serves as a temporary reservoir for the early arrival of the bolus prior to a swallow or as a storage space for residue following the swallow.

The passive protective function of these structures can be assessed in the early stages of the evaluation, when the initial small boluses or ice chips are being presented. In patients with a significantly delayed swallow or in patients who are unable to initiate a pharyngeal swallow, the melting ice chip will be seen to flow down the base of the tongue to the vallecular space where it is divided by the epiglottis into symmetrical rivulets that flow around the airway to the pyriforms below. Some patients may present with an anatomic configuration that compromises this protective function. The epiglottis may rest against the base of the tongue, negating the anterior and superior shield that it provides to the airway. Surgical restructuring also can affect the sheilding of the airway.

The supraglottic laryngectomy includes resection of the epiglottis and false vocal folds, leaving the patient with no structural barrier to airway penetration other than the true vocal folds. An edematous epiglottis can obliterate the channels lateral to the airway and direct bolus material to spill directly into the endolarynx.

Active Observation

During the pharyngeal swallow, the epiglottis is retroflexed over the larynx to provide a redundant layer of protection to the airway. The initial movement of the epiglottis to horizontal often is transiently visible for a few video frames during the period just prior to white out. Perlman and Van Daele (1993), in a study of simultaneous ultrasound and laryngoscopy, reported that the initial movement of the epiglottis to horizontal was observed an average of 136 ms before the appearance of the bolus on the base of tongue. Interestingly, in the same study, initial hyoid elevation, the mechanism principally responsible epiglottal retroflexion, was not observed until, on average, 75 ms before the appearance of the bolus on the base of tongue. This curious fact could be explained by the configuration of the tongue base before the passage of the bolus from the oral cavity. The base of tongue is seen to move

anteriorly to form a chute to accept the oncoming bolus (Dodds, Stewart, & Logemann, 1990). This anterior movement of the tongue, when viewed relative to a stationary epiglottis, could be interpreted incorrectly as the posterior movement of the epiglottis. This almost certainly is the case, as in later studies (Logemann, et al., 1992; Perlman, Van Daele, & Otterbacher, 1995; Van Daele, Perlman, & Cassell, 1995), hyoid movement was identified as the action that provided the necessary traction to initiate epiglottal movement to horizontal. For further discussion regarding the physiology of epiglottal retroflexion, refer to section VFE- 2c of the fluoroscopic examination.

Although the initial movement to horizontal can be observed, the period of white out obscures the remaining portion of epiglottal movement to full horizontal and further movement beyond horizontal. At the end of the period of white out, the tongue base falls away from the posterior wall, allowing for visualization of the pharyngeal space as the larynx descends. It is at this point that the retroflexed epiglottis is well visualized. Although not available for inspection on every single swallow, in normal subjects, the retroverted epiglottis is observed more frequently at the end of white out than not (Figure 4–25). The clinician should be alert for this finding during the observation section of the examination during nonbolus, spontaneous swallows.

At the end of white out, in the normal subject, the fully retroflexed epiglottis should be positioned so that the tip is tucked between the posterior pharyngeal wall and the cricopharyngeal opening. The larynx continues to descend to the resting position as the longitudinal muscles of the pharynx relax and the lateral walls fall away from midline. At this time the epiglottis is observed to flip back to its resting position. Perlman and Van Daele (1993) found that the average time of return of the epiglottis to rest after the opening of the pharynx was 106 ms. This equates to approximately three to four frames of video tape following white out.

During the initial period of familiarization with the procedure, the novice endoscopist may find it difficult to discern this movement in "real time." It is recommended that, if not observed during the examination, the tape be thoroughly reviewed for evidence of retroflexion. It is important to remember that epiglottal movement is passive, in that it is com-

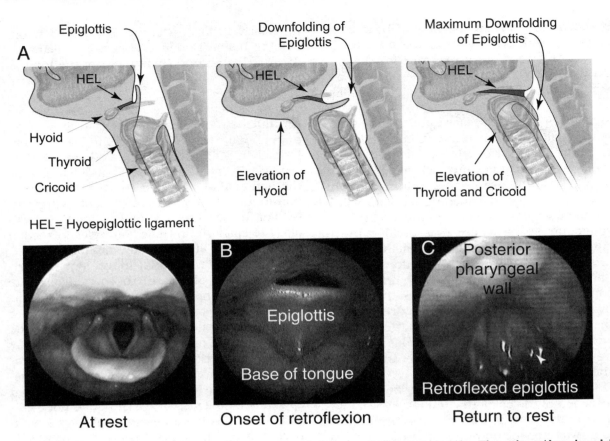

Figure 4–25. A. Mechanisms affecting downfolding of the epiglottis. The elevating hyoid applies anterior traction to the base of the epiglottis through the hyoepiglottic ligament resulting in the downfolding of the epiglottis to horizontal. Laryngeal cartilage elevation and base of tongue pressure contribute to the completion of the downfolding. **B.** The epiglottis is sometimes observed to move to horizontal before the swallow is initiated. **C.** The retroflexed epiglottis is frequently observed immediately following whiteout.

pletely dependent on a combination of hyoid elevation, laryngeal elevation, and, to a lesser degree, tongue base retraction. Because of this dependency, retroflexion is one of the few solid determinants of adequate hyoid and laryngeal elevation available to the endoscopist.

When epiglottal retroflexion is absent, the epiglottis can be observed to have remained upright with the lateral margins of the epiglottis vertically folded between the lateral pharyngeal walls (Figure 4–26). As the pharyngeal walls fall away from one another, the lateral margins of the epiglottis are spread apart to the resting position. When hyoid and laryngeal elevation is poor, UES opening is compromised, resulting in residue remaining in the pyriform sinuses (Dejager et al., 1997). If epiglottal retroflexion is observed consistently to be incomplete at the end of white out and residue is observed in the pyriform sinuses

following swallows, the clinician can strongly infer that hyoid and laryngeal elevation are impaired and confidently proceed with the appropriate intervention.

The detection of epiglottal retroflexion at the end of the swallow is dependent on the sensitivity of the chip camera to adjust to the rapidly expanding pharynx as it returns to rest. Many modern chip cameras employ an "auto-iris" function that attenuates the brightness of the video image to avoid the bright "flare" associated with close approximation of the light beam to tissue. The advantage of the auto-iris function is that it allows for the very close inspection of pharyngeal mucosa without direct adjustment of the light source, as the image is automatically attenuated. The drawback is that the attenuation often requires a few frames of video before the proper brightness is achieved. During the period of

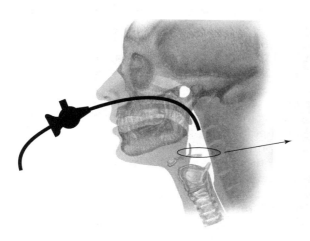
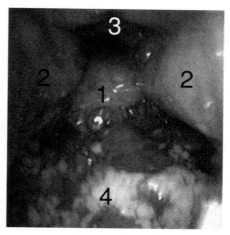

1- Tip of epiglottis
2- Lateral pharyngeal walls
3- Posterior pharyngeal wall
4- Base of tongue

Figure 4–26. In this patient with poor epiglottal retroflexion, the epiglottis remains upright and is squeezed between the lateral pharyngeal walls during the pharyngeal stage of the swallow.

white out, chip cameras equipped with the auto-iris will, appropriately, attenuate the brightness by dimming the "flare" associated with the close approximation of the tissue to the tip of the scope. As the tissue falls away at the close of the pharyngeal swallow, the auto-iris attempts to adjust to the rapidly expanding pharyngeal lumen. The result is a few frames of "dark" video that coincide exactly with the period during which epiglottal retroflexion is observed. It therefore is advisable that, before purchasing a chip camera, information regarding auto-iris function is reviewed. Some newer cameras allow for the selective enabling and disabling of this function.

Careful inspection of the static epiglottis will allow the clinician to observe the adequacy of structural barriers as well as the capacity of pharyngeal cavities and to set the pace for the presentation of food or liquid during the examination. The observation of the dynamic epiglottis will provide the endoscopist with insight as to the robustness of laryngeal elevation and, when combined with patterns of bolus residue, allow for some gross estimation of UES function.

⑭ AIRWAY CLOSURE

Laryngoscopy is the ideal medium for observing the complex series of movements involved in airway closure. To follow the pattern of airway protection, proper positioning of the endoscope is necessary. The endoscope can be jostled by the movement of the velum during speech and will be pulled superiorly, away from the endolarynx, when the velum elevates during the swallow. In most cases, the scope will need to be advanced to the level of tip of the epiglottis to fully observe airway protective patterns.

During the swallow, the pharynx makes a rapid change in configuration from airway to propulsive chamber for the alimentary tract. The coordination and timing of this rapid transition requires functional afferent and efferent mechanisms that adapt quickly to changes in the viscosity and volume of the material presented. Any compromise during the reconfiguration can lead to the penetration of airway.

During chewing, the pharynx maintains the configuration of an airway with vocal fold motion limited to the biphasic motion of abduction and adduction associated with inspiration and expiration. When saliva is produced during mastication, it falls freely into the pharynx to rest in the valleculae or pyriform sinuses. Food also is propelled into the pharynx to rest in the vallecula prior to the initiation of the swallow. When either of these events occurs, the glottis is seen to make a brief partial adduction (Dua, Ren, Bardan, Xie, & Shaker, 1997). This partial adduction is referred to as the pharyngoglottal closure reflex and is thought to prevent the aspiration of oral contents during the oral preparatory stage of the swallow (Ren et al., 1994).

During the swallow, vocal fold closure is highly variable both within subjects and between subjects. Shaker, Dodds, Dantas, Hogan, & Arndorfer, (1990), using concurrent fluoroscopy and laryngoscopy, found that three types of patterns of vocal fold adduction (Figure 4–27) occurred in all normal subjects during the swallow (Table 4–8).

Although Type 3 swallows were observed to remain open during laryngeal elevation and continued to appear to be open at the onset of white out, the other two types of swallows were, at times, observed to convert to Type 3 swallows during the peak of laryngeal elevation. The fact that laryngeal valving was not maintained from the onset of the swallow in normal subjects was a stunning discovery.

Ohmae et al. (1996) also found that arytenoid adduction and subsequent arytenoid closure were the initial events during normal swallowing and that true vocal fold closure occurred later in the swallow after the onset of laryngeal elevation. Further, the authors found that the bolus often was visible endoscopically at the level of the pyriform sinuses before true vocal fold closure had been achieved.

The combination of tenuous surety of breath-holding (Martin et al., 1993; Mendelsohn & Martin, 1993) and the discovery of later-than-expected laryngeal valving in normal subjects challenged the popular supraglottic maneuver intervention. Ohmae et al. (1996) found that, with appropriate instructions, tight breath-holding prior to the swallow yielded tight valving before the swallow and that the tight valving continued, unabated, throughout the pharyngeal stage of the swallow.

The timing and order of muscular contraction for airway closure in swallowing, breath-holding, and phonation are somewhat different. McCulloch, Perlman, Palmer, and Van Daele (1996), using hook wire electrodes with simultaneous laryngoscopy, looked at the ordered events contributing to airway closure during the swallow. The first movement is arytenoid medial contact. The true folds (thyroarytenoids) were found to move passively to midline without contraction. As in Shaker et al. (1990), true folds were not always observed to contact each other. The arytenoids are then observed to tilt forward until they contact the base of the epiglottis. At this time the true folds may reopen at the beginning of laryngeal elevation. This is followed by epiglottal retroflexion as the larynx continues to elevate. At the initiation of the period of white out, the true vocal folds were noted to be opened 94% of the time. The true thryroarytenoid was noted to contract actively an average of 0.063 s after white out, a moment well after the initation of the swallow and concurrent with the passage of the bolus through the cricopharyngeus.

Much like Ohmae et al. (1996), McCulloch et al. (1996) found that, when tight breath-holding is enacted before the swallow, the pattern is quite different. The thyroarytenoid and arytenoids make firm medial contact. The arytenoids tilt forward to the base of the epiglottis with tight laryngeal valving. The swallow then commences with epiglottal retroflexion and continuous tight laryngeal valving.

⑮ NARRATIVE/CLOSING THE EXAMINATION

After all of the salient findings have been determined and interventions attempted, the clinician is able to withdraw the scope and report the findings. This narrative section is not intended to serve as the final report. This section should be used to record miscellaneous procedural notes relating events that may

Table 4–8. Glottal closure patterns associated with swallowing.

Type 1:	Observed in 58% of the swallows. The vocal folds are observed to remain in contact along their entire length after laryngeal elevation is initiated.
Type 2:	Observed in 7% of the swallows. The vocal folds are in contact in the anterior half of their length but slightly separated in the posterior portion, leaving a small gap.
Type 3:	Observed in 35% of the swallows. The vocal folds are not in contact with each other, leaving a small, elongated triangular opening between the folds.

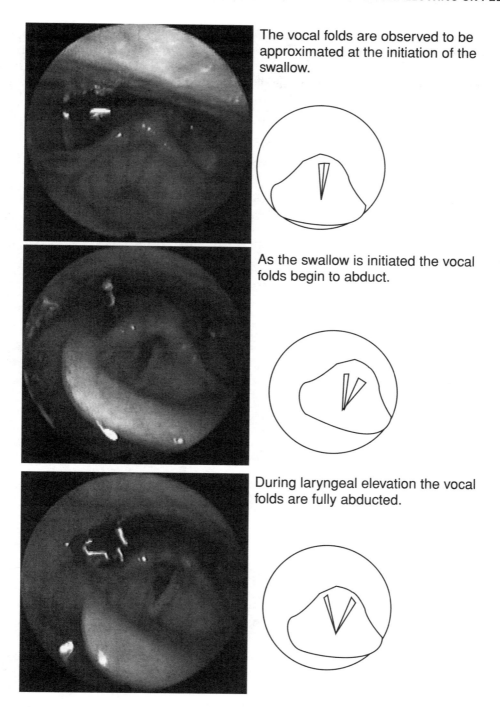

The vocal folds are observed to be approximated at the initiation of the swallow.

As the swallow is initiated the vocal folds begin to abduct.

During laryngeal elevation the vocal folds are fully abducted.

Figure 4–27. Opening of the glottis during laryngeal elevation is frequently observed in normal subjects.

have taken place during the session. An initial impression can be entered as well as the preliminary plan of action.

If the patient was unable to observe the examination in real time, the clinician may wish to review the tape with the patient. Use the audio portion of the examination at this time to give the patient some sense of connection with the moving image on the screen. The important findings can be shown and the success or failure of intervention demonstrated to the patient and family members or direct caretakers.

Once the patient is satisfied with the review, the initial findings can be generated (see completed sample scoring form in Form 4–2). For details regarding the final report, see Chapter 5. Even when using the FEES® moniker, it is useful to identify the procedure as a laryngoscopic examination somewhere in the narrative as, often, many health professionals will confuse this examination with transoral esophageal endoscopy.

Form 4–2.
Completed Fiberoptic endoscopic evaluation of swallowing scoring form.

OBSERVATION SECTION

❶ ANATOMIC NOTES:

Arytenoids and post cricoid area erythatous and edematous. Left aryepiglottic fold edematous and bruised.

❷ SECRETIONS RATING: 2

❸ SPONTANEOUS SWALLOWS: 8/minute

❹ BREATH-HOLD   Tight valving when asked to "bear down"

❺ SENSATION   Inferred to be good. Noted to clear secretions from the laryngeal vestibule and swallow or expectorate repeatedly.

❻ COUGH   Cough on command was strong and effective. Cleared laryngeal vestibule and pharynx of collected material.

PRESENTATION OF FOOD AND LIQUID

Material	Ice	Puree	Soft	Solid	Liquids THIN	THICK
❼ MAX AMOUNT	2 chips	10cc's	5cc's	5cc's	10cc's	none
❽ DST	2 sec.	8 sec.	8 sec.	5 sec.	2 sec.	Na
❾ ASP/PEN	2	4	4	2	1	na
❿ # SWALLOWS	4	4	6	8	4	na
⓫ INTERVENTION	none	none	mend	mend	none	na

BIOMECHANICAL OBSERVATIONS

⓬ VELUM   Elevation within normal limits. No compromise of nasopharyngeal seal.

⓭ EPIGLOTTIS   Not observed to fully retroflex. Squeezed between lateral walls during swallow.

⓮ AIRWAY CLOSURE   Full tight closure before arrival of bolus into vestibule.

(continued)

---

⑮ NARRATIVE:

Seated upright. Dobhoff tube in right nares. Placed scope transnasally through left nares without event. Secretions copious and throughout pharynx. Patient able to clear secretions from airway. Hyoid and laryngeal elevation inferred to be poor given absence of epiglottal retroflexion. This finding matches poor elevation on clinical exam. Moderate residue in vallecula following each initial swallow attempt. Repeated penetration of residue without aspiration due to vigilant airway protection.

Mendelsohn maneuver implemented with success. Fewer swallows necessary to clear. Patient fatigued quickly using maneuver.

Impression: Moderate dysphagia characterized by poor laryngeal elevation, with subsequent poor UES opening resulting in residue which is penetrated following initial swallow attempt. Patient with good sensation protects airway and swallows until pharynx is clear.

Plan: Recommend PO puree and liquids for pleasure/supplementation to tube feeding. Initiate therapy to train Mendelsohn. Monitor for improved strength and upgrade as appropriate.

REFERENCES

Aviv, J. E., Martin, J. H., Keen, M. S., Debell, M., & Blitzer, A. (1993). Air pulse quantification of supraglottic and pharyngeal sensation: A new technique. *Annals of Otology, Rhinology and Laryngology, 102,* 777–780.

Conrad, H., Rattenborg, C., Klain, M., Barton, M., Logan, W., & Holaday, D. (1984). Opening and closing mechanisms of the larynx. *Otolaryngology—Head and Neck Surgery, 92,* 402–405.

Dejaeger, E., Pelemans, W., Ponette, E., & Joosten, E. (1997). Mechanisms involved in post-deglutition retention in the elderly. *Dysphagia, 12,* 63–67.

Dodds, W., Stewart, E., & Logemann, J. (1990). Physiology and radiology of the normal oral and pharyngeal phases of swallowing. *American Journal of Radiology, 154,* 953–963.

Dua, K., Ren, J., Bardan, E., Xie, P., & Shaker, R. (1997). Coordination of deglutitive glottal function and pharyngeal bolus transit during normal eating. *Gastroenterology, 112,* 73–83.

Helm, J. F., Dodds, W. J., Hogan, W. J., Soergel, K. H., Egide, M. S., & Wood, C. M. (1982). Acid neutralizing capacity of human saliva. *Gastroenterology, 83,* 69–74.

Kahrilas, P. J., Logemann, J. A., Krugler, C., & Flanagan, E. (1991). Volitional augmentation of upper esophageal sphincter opening during swallowing. *The American Journal of Physiology, 260,* G450–G456.

Kapila, Y. V., Dodds, W. J., Helm, J. F., & Hogan, W. J. (1984). Relationship between swallow rate and salivary flow. *Digestive Diseases and Science, 29,* 528–533.

Langmore, S. E. (1998). Laryngeal sensation: A touchy subject. *Dysphagia, 13,* 93–94.

Langmore, S. E., Schatz, K., & Olsen, N. (1988). Fiberoptic endoscopic examination of swallowing safety: A new procedure. *Dysphagia, 2,* 216–219.

Lear, C. S. C., Flanagan, J. B., Jr., & Moorrees, C. F. A. (1965). The frequency of deglutition in man. *Archives of Oral Biology, 10,* 83–99.

Leder, S. B., Ross, D. A., Briskin, K. B., & Sasaki, C. T. (1997). A prospective, double-blind, randomized study on the use of a topical anesthetic, vasoconstrictor, and placebo during transnasal flexible fiberoptic endoscopy. *Journal of Speech-Language-Hearing Research, 40,* 1352–1357.

Linden, P., Siebens, A. A. (1983). Dysphagia preceding laryngeal penetration. *Archives of Physical Medicine and Rehabilitation, 64,* 281–284.

Logemann, J. A. (1995). Dysphagia: Evaluation and treatment. *Folia Phoniatrica and Logopaedics, 47,* 140–164.

Logemann, J. A., Kahrilas, P. J., Cheng, J., Pauloski, B. R., Gibbons, P. J., Rademaker, A. W., Lin, S. (1992). Closure mechanisms of laryngeal vestibule during swallow. *American Journal of Physiology, 262,* G338–G334.

Logemann, J., Kahrilas, P., Kobara, M., & Vakil, M. (1989). The benefit of head rotation on pharyngoesophageal dysphagia. *Archives of Physical Medicine and Rehabilitation, 70,* 767–771.

Martin, B., Logemann, K. J., Shaker, R., & Dodds, W. (1993). Normal laryngeal valving patterns during three breath-holding maneuvers: A pilot investigation. *Dysphagia, 8,* 11–20.

McCulloch, T. M., Perlman, A. L., Palmer, P. M., & Van Daele, D. J. (1996). Laryngeal activity during swallow, phonation, and the Valsalva maneuver: An electromyographic analysis. *Laryngoscope, 106,* 1351–1358.

Mendelsohn, M. S., & McConnel, F. M. (1987). Function in the pharyngoesophageal segment. *Laryngoscope, 4,* 483–489.

Mendelsohn, M. S., & Martin, R. E. (1993). Airway protection during breath-holding. *Annals of Otology, Rhinology and Laryngology, 102,* 941–944.

Miller, J. L., & Watkin, K. L. (1997). Lateral pharyngeal wall motion during swallowing using real time ultrasound. *Dysphagia, 12,* 125–132.

Muntz, H. (1992). Navigation of the nose with flexible fiberoptic endoscopy. *Cleft Palate Craniofacial Journal, 29,* 507–510.

Murray, J., Langmore, S. E., Ginsberg, S., & Dostie, A. (1996). The significance of accumulated oropharyngeal secretions and swallowing frequency in predicting aspiration. *Dysphagia, 11,* 99–103.

Ohmae, Y., Logemann, J., Kaiser, P., Hanson, D., & Kahrilas, P. (1995). Timing of glottic closure during normal swallow. *Head & Neck, 17,* 394–402.

Ohmae, Y., Logemann, J. A., Kaiser, P., Hanson, D. G., & Kahrilas, P. J. (1996). Effects of two breath-holding maneuvers on oropharyngeal swallow. *Annals of Otology, Rhinology and Laryngology, 105,* 123–131.

Perlman, A., & Van Daele, D. (1993). Simultaneous videoendoscopic and ultrasound measures of swallowing. *Journal of Medical Speech-Language Pathology, 1,* 223–232.

Perlman, A. L., VanDaele, D. J., & Otterbacker, M. S. (1995). Quantitative assessment of hyoid bone displacement from video images during swallowing. *Journal of Speech and Hearing Research, 38,* 579–585.

Ren, J., Shaker, R., Dua, K., Trifan, A., Pdvrsan, B., & Sul, Z. (1994). Glottal adduction response to pharyngeal water stimulation: Evidence for a pharyngoglottal closure reflex. [Abstract]. *Gastroenterology, 106,* 558.

Rosenbek, J. C., Robbins, J., Roecker, E. V., Coyle, J. L., & Woods, J. L. (1996). A penetration-aspiration scale. *Dysphagia, 11,* 93–98.

Sant'Ambrogio, G., & Mathew, O. (1986). Laryngeal receptors and their reflex responses. *Clinics in Chest and Medicine, 7*(2), 211–222.

Sant'Ambrogio, G., & Sant'Ambrogio, F. B. (1996). Role of laryngeal afferents in cough. *Pulmonary Pharmacology, 9,* 309–314.

Shaker, R., Dodds, W. J., Dantas, R. O., Hogan, W. J., & Arndorfer, R. C. (1990). Coordination of deglutitive glottic closure with oropharyngeal swallowing. *Gastroenterology, 98,* 1478–1484.

Singh, V., Brockbank, M., & Todd, G. (1997). Flexible transnasal endoscopy: Is local anaesthetic necessary? *Journal of Laryngology and Otology, 111,* 616–618.

Stockwell, M., Lang, S., Yip, R., Zintel, T., White, C., & Gallagher, C. G. (1993). Lack of importance of the superior laryngeal nerves in critic acid cough in humans. *Journal of Applied Physiology, 75,* 613–617.

VanDaele, D. J., Perlman, A. L., & Cassell, M. D. (1995). Intrinsic fibre architecture and attachments of the human epiglottis and their contributions to the mechanism of human deglutition. *Journal of Anatomy, 186,* 1–15.

Wyke, B. D. (1973). Myotatic reflexogenic systems in the larynx. *Folia Morphologica (Praha), 21,* 113–117.

CHAPTER 5

Reporting the Findings/ Communication/ Patient Education

"Write the vision, and make it plain upon tables, that he may run that readeth it."

Habakkuk ii. 2.

or

"It may well wait a century for a reader."

John Kepler (1571–1630)

The narrative section of the score form is provided for the summation of findings and the declaration of impressions and recommendations. Many clinicians use checklists to reports and archive findings from the instrumental examinations. Although these forms may appear to be time-savers, the imprecision of such a record often does not match the wealth and complexity of the findings. The narrative should include the items listed in Table 5–1.

Table 5–1. Sections of the narrative report.

Introductory statement

Results

Impressions

Recommendations

Record of patient education

INTRODUCTORY STATEMENT

The narrative report should include an introductory statement describing the purpose of the examination and the patient's current subjective complaints. The consistencies and volume of consistencies presented should be mentioned as well as the projections employed (Table 5–2).

RESULTS SECTION

This section is reserved for objective statements only (Table 5–3). I have found it helpful to describe the events as they occur in sequence. In other words, oral events are reported first followed by pharyngeal events and, finally, upper esophageal and esophageal events.

Table 5–2. Introductory statement example.

Mr. Smith is a 58-year-old man, seven weeks status post CABG (coronary artery bypass graft) with postoperative tracheostomy placement and ventilatory support for four weeks. Mr. Smith has been weaned from ventilator, and is now fitted with a #8 metal trach tube. When plugged voicing is breathy, cough is weak. Blue dye test (ice chips) was negative for dye at trach site and after deep suctioning. Clinical signs of aspiration (coughing) consistently noted following thin liquid swallows. Primary nutrition is provided via Dobhoff tube. Labs indicate good hydration and nutrition parameters, no active pulmonary problems or infection.

The patient states it is "difficult to start a swallow." This assessment was performed to determine readiness for PO intake. The patient was seated upright and presented puree, thin liquids, thick liquids and solid foods in amounts ranging from 2–35 cc. A barium capsule was also presented. The subject was viewed in the lateral and AP projections.

Table 5–3. Results section example.

In the lateral projection, small cervical osteophytes were noted at the level of c3–4. In the AP projection, movement of the true and ventricular folds were noted to be asymmetric with incomplete adduction on breath holding and phonation. Movement of the vocal folds appeared reduced on the patient's left side.

The oral preparatory and oral stages of the swallow were unremarkable for all consistencies and volumes presented. The duration of the transition between the oral and pharyngeal stages of the swallow averaged 5 seconds and was noted with all consistencies presented. Puree and solid food boluses were noted to fall to the vallecular space prior to the initiation of the pharyngeal stage of the swallow. Liquid consistencies of all volumes were noted to fall to the level of the pyriform sinuses prior to the initiation of the swallow. Thin liquids presented in volumes greater than 20 cc were consistently noted to overflow the pyriform sinuses and fall into the laryngeal vestibule prior to the initiation of the pharyngeal stage of the swallow. Once initiated, the pharyngeal stage of the swallow was noted to be of adequate amplitude. There was no evidence of residue following the initial swallow attempt. The material falling below the vocal folds was completely cleared into the pharynx with spontaneous coughing. Chin-tuck positioning reduced the duration of the delay and consistently eliminated the penetration and aspiration of the liquids.

The upper esophageal and esophageal stages of the swallow were screened. Esophageal transit for liquid consistencies was unremarkable. Solid food transit was complete but significantly longer. Solid food residue was noted to accumulate at the aortic arch. The patient perceived this stasis and reported the food to be "stuck" at the suprasternal notch. The residual was easily cleared from the esophagus with thin liquid swallows.

The barium tablet was safely consumed and traveled through the alimentary tract without problems.

When a particular stage is completed without obvious impairment, it should be stated as being so.

This is the "just the facts" section in which events are described without attempts to interpret the findings. Statements such as, "Pharyngeal delay was severe" should be forfeited for statements such as, "The transition from oral to pharyngeal stages averaged 5 seconds for thin liquid swallows." The term "weakened" should not be used in this section. Although the clinician may infer force or pressure decrements from observing the effect of biomechanical movements on the bolus, only the biomechanical movements or duration measures, as they were observed, should be described.

The upper esophageal and esophageal phases of the swallow should be reviewed. In some settings, the traditional "Triple Phase Swallowing Study" or "Cookie Swallow" do not include the esophageal phase of the swallow. In many other settings, a screening of the esophageal stage of the swallow is performed using any of the consistencies presented during the oropharyngeal exam. A "solid food challenge" is of particular interest in patients with suspected esophageal motility problems. Often, only liquids are used during radiological examination of the esophagus or traditional barium swallow. Solid food, because of its high viscosity and cohesion, is less likely to allow visualization of the surface mucosa of the esophagus but is more likely to result in esophageal stasis than liquids. It is the solid food esophageal stasis that often leads to referred "phantom" sensation higher in the pharynx following the swallow.

It often is useful to add a barium tablet during the fluoroscopic examination, or a blue or green colored placebo capsule during the endoscopic examination, to determine readiness and/or safety for oral administration of medication.

A more thorough description of biomechanical interactions should follow. The patient's reaction to events of aspiration and any spontaneous compensation or facilitation always should be included. The success or failure of interventions should be noted as well as possible reasons for the failures. Finally, plans for the initiation or the discontinuation of therapeutic intervention should be reviewed.

There has been very little in the way of valid severity scales offered to the clinical practitioner in the dysphagia literature. A useful scale might combine both biomechanics and function and would consider the degree of impairment and the degree to which the patient is handicapped by the dysfunction.

Careful attention should be paid to the nutritional and hydration parameters of the patient in question. Often, the event of aspiration, because of its drama, will gain considerable management attention, obscuring the malnourished or dehydrated patient's needs.

IMPRESSIONS SECTION

This is the section reserved for tying together all of the findings from the examination (Table 5–4) . It is expected that the clinician will supply the consulting physician with the "how and why" of the dysphagia as it manifests itself in his or her patient. At this time, a collective initial statement that includes a severity rating usually is helpful. For example,

"Mr. X presents with moderate oropharyngeal dysphagia characterized by an incoordination of airway protection and bolus propulsion with subsequent aspiration of thin liquids."

RECOMMENDATIONS

The recommendation section should include the items listed in Table 5–5.

The recommendation section may be the only section that is thoroughly reviewed by anyone reading the narrative. The clinician may wish to print the recommendation section in bolder or larger type than the rest of the report for quick visual access (Table 5–6). It is important to remember that the clinician's role is that of a consultant. The recommendations are posed as suggestions, not orders, that should be considered in the light of all other circumstances that affect the patient's total care. An

Table 5–4. Impressions section example.

Mr. Smith presents with moderate pharyngeal dysphagia characterized by an incoordination of bolus propulsion and airway protection resulting in thin liquid aspiration. Mr. Smith appeared to be sensitive to the aspirated material and demonstrated consistent and successful expulsion of the aspirant from the airway with coughing. Employment of a chin-tuck position prior to the initiation of the swallow was successful in eliminating the aspiration events.

Airway protection likely is compromised due to recurrent laryngeal nerve damage secondary to the CABG. However, the presence of protective coughing and robust pharyngeal and esophageal stages of the swallow and absence of pulmonary pathology or infection would indicate oral feeding. Due to the length of NPO status, the patient likely will need close monitoring during trial feedings.

introductory statement that makes this clear should precede all recommendations.

After filing the report, the information should be communicated to the care team to ensure that the appropriate diet is ordered and that all other coordinated tasks are initiated.

COMMUNICATION/PATIENT EDUCATION

Once completed, the results of the examination should be reviewed with the patient. Although time is not always available, the patient should, at the very least, be shown the most salient snippets of the video recording. A well-informed patient is more likely to comply with recommendations and is likely to be more motivated, and less mystified, when asked to enact therapeutic measures.

The Joint Commission on the Accreditation of Healthcare Organizations (JCAHO) has created guidelines, to ensure that each element that might compromise the patient's education has been addressed fully. Table 5–7 provides a quick review of the guidelines with accompanying suggestions for attaining compliance.

Table 5–5. Items for inclusion in the recommendations section.

Per oral status (NPO, PO, PO with conditions, etc.)

Diet recommendations with consistency and viscosity descriptors

Feeding instructions

Other consultation or orders (calorie counts, dental consultation, etc.)

Follow-up schedule

Table 5–6. Recommendations section example.

Example Recommendations:

If consistent with overall plan of medical management the following recommendations should be considered:

Advance diet to soft solid foods with liquids thickened to a nectar consistency

Coordinate calorie count with dietitian to determine adequacy of PO intake

Allow water between meals

Initiate therapy to train chin tuck position

Will continue to follow daily

Table 5–7. Joint Commission on the Accreditation of Healthcare Organizations (JCAHO) guidelines for patient education.

JCAHO Guideline	Procedure for Ensuring Compliance
The patient's learning needs, abilities, preferences, and readiness to learn are assessed.	✓ Be certain that written instructions for any intervention (including: exercises, maneuvers, positioning, changes in viscosity or volume, and means of presentations) are optimized for the patient's cognition, language, and visual limitations.

Table 5–7. *(continued)*

JCAHO Guideline	Procedure for Ensuring Compliance
	✓ Keep the language simple ✓ Provide the instructions in the patient's native language if possible ✓ Use large type
Patients are educated about the safe and effective use of medical equipment.	✓ Fully demonstrate adaptive feeding equipment before issuing. ✓ Have the patient demonstrate the proper use of the equipment to you.
Patients are educated about potential drug/food interactions, and provided counseling on nutrition and modified diets.	✓ Review the diet modifications with the patient ✓ Show examples of different food consistencies ✓ Review measurements in functional terms i.e., use spoon or cupfuls and not milliliters or cubic centimeters in your description. ✓ Patients with restriction on thin liquids should be instructed on the appropriate means for maintaining hydration.
Patients are educated about rehabilitation techniques to help them adapt or function more independently in their environment.	✓ The interventions should be implemented with independent performance in mind where appropriate.
Patients are informed about access to additional resources in the community.	✓ Telephone numbers and addresses of associations and support groups for stroke, neuromuscular diseases, and cancer should be provided to the patient as appropriate.
Patients are informed about when and how to obtain any further treatment the patient may need.	✓ Any of the written material distributed to the patient regarding therapeutic intervention or community resources can also contain contact numbers for the department and other important numbers.
When the hospital gives discharge instructions to the patient or family, it also provides these instructions to the organization or individual responsible for the patient's continuing care.	✓ Effective compliance often is the result of effective instruction. Be sure to include multiple copies of material for the caregivers. ✓ The material should be written in a way that is easy to understand.
The hospital plans, supports, and coordinates activities and resources for patient and family education.	✓ A personal review of the videotaped studies should be provided for the patient's family if appropriate. ✓ Written material and instructions should be available through the institution.
The patient and family educational process is collaborative and interdisciplinary, as appropriate to the plan of care.	✓ All disciplines that effect the plan of care should provide input during the patient education process, either in person or by proxy. ✓ This should include making written or multimedia educational materials available through their service.

CHAPTER 6

Final Thoughts

"Not everything that counts can be counted, and not everything that can be counted counts."
(Sign hanging in Albert Einstein's office at Princeton)

The clinician assigned with the task of assessing the dysphagic patient forms a profile of risk and benefit by the light cast from a patient's unique health history and clinical condition. Although many patients appear abundantly similar, each may thrive or succumb due to the contribution of a single element, be it age, respiratory status, hydration parameters, or the myriad of other variables that can be combined and encountered. Given the large array of elements that can affect outcome, it is impossible to suggest all of the possibilities in this text. It is hoped that what has been suggested is a means for thinking about how the assessment process benefits the patient.

Not all swallow assessments are equal. Depending on the setting, the assessment process typically is initiated by a care team member who recognizes, and decides to act on, a risk for malnutrition/dehydration, pulmonary consequence, or compromised quality of life. The assessment process may require an intensive "lips to stomach" survey of the alimentary tract in a young patient with weight loss, or it may encompass a seemingly simple determination of the safety of water sips for a patient with end-stage disease under pallia-

tive care. Whatever the case, a management issue will be raised and forwarded in the form of a clinical question.

When the clinical question is raised in a modern medical facility, an array of tools can be employed to respond. Fluoroscopy and laryngoscopy are easily accessible to the majority of individuals working in acute care settings. Either examination can provide an accurate and reliable answer to the simple binary questions regarding the presence or absence of aspiration, penetration, and residue. However, neither tool, without additional instrumentation, will provide the examiner with information regarding pressure, the amplitude of muscular contraction, or the propagation of neuromuscular events. A narrow sampling of sensation can be assessed directly via endoscopy, but the clinical value of the actual objective measure remains elusive. There is no question that the measurement of movement and the timing of the duration of different events have contributed to our understanding of swallow biomechanics. In clinical practice, however, these measures are meager substitutes for function.

In this text, the clinician has been alerted to identify a number of findings of great importance that are easily and reliably identified, for example, aspiration or Zenker's diverticulum. Other findings, such as reduced laryngeal elevation, are equally important but of equivocal reliability due to the subjective nature of the judgment. That subjectivity can be reduced. Much time and effort has been expended by various researchers, using sophisticated digital imaging, to determine the precise extent of, for example, anterior and superior hyoid elevation during the swallow. However, the typical reader will be hard-pressed to apply these measurements without considerable investment in capital equipment and time spent learning the methods for acquiring the data. And, in the end, without the instrumentation, subjectively judging the adequacy of a biomechanical movement, such as laryngeal elevation, leaves even the most experienced clinicians in poor agreement (Perlman, Van Daele, & Ottervacher, 1995). Still, subjective measures are propagated. Clinicians are encouraged, at the hand of conventional wisdom, to use the two dimensions provided by fluoroscopy to make three-dimensional judgments regarding the percentage of bolus aspirated (Figure 6–1).

Without additional instrumentation, subjectivity is the bane of those attempting to judge the adequacy of physiologic movements and bolus percentages. But, even when the instrumentation is readily available, between-subject variability reduces the likelihood of linking a precise measure to poor performance. Variability is the plague of all swallowing measures. Even in normal subjects, the within- and between-subject variability of duration measures is such that the performance of a single swallow may not be a true representation of actual capabilities (Lof & Robbins, 1990). I do feel, however, that the clinician who is just beginning to use instrumentation to assess dysphagic patients should practice acquiring all of the duration measures possible. By doing so, the eye becomes accustomed to grouping the movements, and the single swallow observed in

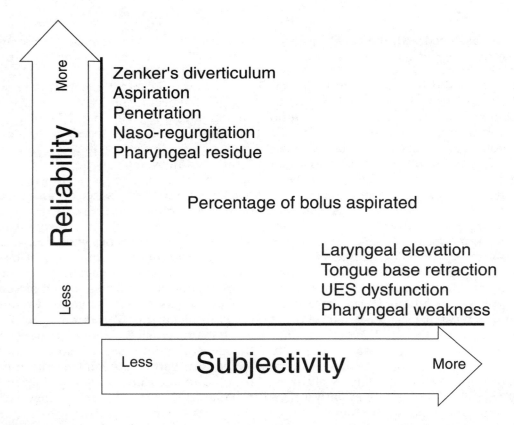

Figure 6–1. Subjectivity and reliability are often inversely related. Objective judgments, such as aspiration, are highly reliable, while estimates of laryngeal elevation are less objective and less reliable.

real time is no longer a blur of activity, promoting confidence and efficiency during the administration of the protocol.

"Early and provident fear is the mother of safety."
Edmund Burke (1729–1797)

or

"For every complex problem, there is a solution that is simple, neat, and wrong."
H. L. Mencken (1880–1956)

Perhaps because of its objectivity and, perhaps, due to the drama of the finding, aspiration has prevailed as the central event of many swallowing assessments. It is presumed, by many clinicians, that aspiration of food, liquid, secretions, or refluxed gastric contents will induce aspiration pneumonia. Yet, many clinicians will recount the patient who consistently aspirates but never suffers from aspiration pneumonia (Ekberg & Hilderfors, 1985; Horner, Masssey, Ris, Lathrop, & Chase, 1988; Martin et al., 1994). Still, the direction of NPO (nothing per oral) orders continues to be recommended reflexively in anticipation of preventing pneumonia in patients who aspirate even small amounts. Consideration often is not given to long-term "aspirators" without pneumonia who consistently demonstrate the ability to reflexively clear material from the airway. I have, unfortunately, followed up on many cases in which patients who have been safely maintaining nutrition and hydration for years, undergo videofluoroscopy or laryngoscopic examinations for the first time and are ordered to stop eating. This not only deprives the patient of the physical pleasure and relief of taking in food and liquid for sustenance but also requires the placement of an alternate form of nutritional support, such as feeding tubes or parenteral nutrition.

Langmore et al. (1998) concluded that dysphagia and aspiration are necessary, but not sufficient, conditions for the development of aspiration pneumonia. Other factors must be considered, including functional status and health status. Langmore et al. found that patients who were dependent for feeding had the greatest odds of acquiring aspiration pneumonia. This makes sense, in that patients who cannot feed themselves are at the mercy of others, frequently untrained but well-meaning caregivers, who may commence or continue the feeding when the patient is in a state of fatigue, lethargy, inattention, or sedation. Patients dependent for feeding also will likely be dependent for oral care. A reduction in the frequency of oral hygiene contributes to the promotion of oral flora that could be harmful if aspirated.

The sequelae to an event of aspiration is often the placement of a feeding tube, in the hopes that preventing the aspiration event will prevent aspiration pneumonia. In fact, the cure, tube feeding, is closely associated with aspiration pneumonia (Hasset, Sunby, & Flint, 1987; Langmore et al., 1998; Olivares, Segovia, & Revuelta, 1974; Peck, Cohen, & Mulvihill, 1990; Sitzmann, 1990). Langmore et al. (1998) suggested that patients with tube feeding continue to aspirate oropharyngeal secretions and that oropharyngeal secretions are more likely to be colonized in these patients because of a reduction in the perception of need to maintain oral hygiene in patients who do not eat. Further, aspiration of refluxed tube feedings is not uncommon.

"'Tis a little thing
To give a cup of water; yet its draught
Of cool refreshment, drained by fevered lips,
May give a shock of pleasure to the frame
(and) Renews the life of joy in happiest hours."
Thomas Noon Talfourd (1795–1854)

Finally, the quality of life of the patient should not be dismissed. Eating and drinking are fundamental and symbolic biological processes. Being denied this simple and basic drive to satisfy hunger and thirst can be both demeaning and demoralizing.

Although the state of dehydration can be controlled with IV therapy and tube feedings, the perception of thirst often remains in the acute phases of disease. In 19 end-stage cancer patients receiving IV therapy, little relationship was found between level of thirst and the amount of IV fluids received, blood urea nitrogen (BUN), or sodium blood levels. Of those 19 patients, six experienced mild thirst, eight moderate thirst, and four severe thirst (Musgrave, Bartal, & Opstad, 1995).

Thirst is governed by secretions of arginine vasopressin $[AVP]_p$. As $[AVP]_p$ increases, so does the perception of thirst. There is a linear relationship between the increase in plasma osmolality (increased osmolality is a sign of dehydration) and the increase in $[AVP]_p$. It has been hypothesized that the oropharyngeal stimuli that accompanies rehydration through swallowing has a great effect on relieving thirst. To test this hypothesis, Figaro and Mack (1997) rehydrated individuals under three conditions: through oral swallowing, infusion through a nasogastric tube, and swallowing with concurrent extraction of the swallowed material through a nasogastric tube while measuring the secretion of $[AVP]_p$. It was found that the subjects who swallowed the liquid and subjects who swallowed with concurrent extraction had a more immediate relief of thirst and inhibition of $[AVP]_p$ than those who were rehydrated with infusion through a tube. Although decreased thirst and inhibition of $[AVP]_p$ was observed in those with extraction, they did not show simultaneous improvements in osmolality, suggesting rehydration. It was concluded that oropharyngeal stimuli contribute to relief of the perception of thirst by inhibiting the secretion of $[AVP]_p$.

In addition to inhibiting secretion of $[AVP]_p$, colder water is judged to be more pleasant and has the beneficial effect of inducing an elevated rate of saliva flow that, consequently, leaves the mouth in a wetter state (Brunstrom, Macrae, & Roberts, 1997). This research supports the claims of McCann, Hall, and Groth-Juncker (1994). In that study of comfort care for terminally ill patients, it was found that complaints of thirst and dry mouth were relieved with mouth care and sips of liquids, in amounts far less than that needed to prevent dehydration.

And so, a small sip of cold water may bring great relief to a thirsty patient.

No rigid directives or "cookbook" fixes for dysphagia assessment have been offered in this text. It is hoped that clinicians will administer recommendations that suit the safety needs of the patient tempered with a healthy respect for the innumerable combinations of health status elements, including quality of life, that can affect positive and negative outcomes.

REFERENCES

Brunstrom, J. M., Macrae, A. W., & Roberts, B. (1997). Mouth-state dependent changes in the judged pleasantness of water at different temperatures. *Physiology and Behavior, 61,* 667–669.

Ekberg, O., & Hilderfors, H. (1985). Defective closure of the laryngeal vestibule: Frequency of pulmonary complications. *American Journal of Radiology, 145,* 1159–1164.

Figaro, M. K., & Mack, G. W. (1997). Regulation of fluid intake in dehydrated humans: Role of oropharyngeal stimulation. *American Journal of Physiology, 272,* R1740–R1746.

Hassett, J. M., Sunby, C., & Flint, L. M. (1987). No elimination of aspiration after percutaneous gastrostomy. *Journal of Clinical Gastroenterology 9,* 90–95.

Horner, J., Massey, E. W., Ris, J. E., Lathrop, D. L., & Chase, K. N. (1988). Aspiration following stroke: Clinical correlates and outcome. *Neurology, 38,* 1359–1362.

Langmore, S. E., Terpenning, M. S., Schork, A., Chen, Y., Murray, J. T., Lopatir, D., & Loesche, W. J. (1998). Predictors of aspiration pneumonia: How important is dysphagia? *Dysphagia, 13,* 30–39.

Lof, G. L., & Robbins, J. (1990). Test-retest variability in normal swallowing. *Dysphagia, 4,* 236–242.

Martin, B., Corlew, M., Wood, H., Olson, D., Golopol, L., Wingo, M., & Kirmani, N. (1994). The association of swallowing dysfunction and aspiration pneumonia. *Dysphagia, 9,* 1–6.

McCann, R. M., Hall, W. J., & Groth-Juncker, A. (1994). Comfort care for terminally ill patients. The appropriate use of nutrition and hydration. *Journal of the American Medical Association, 272,* 1263–1266.

Musgrave, C. F., Bartal, N., & Opstad, J. (1995). The sensation of thirst in dying patients receiving i.v. hydration. *Journal of Palliative Care, 11,* 17–21.

Olivares, L., Segovia, A., & Revuelta, R. (1974). Tube feeding and lethal aspiration in neurological patients: A review of 720 autopsy cases. *Stroke, 5,* 654–657.

Peck, A., Cohen, C., & Mulvihill, M. N. (1990). Long-term enteral feeding of aged demented nursing home patients. *Journal of the American Geriatrics Society, 38,* 1195–1198.

Perlman, A., Van Daele, D., & Ottervacher, M. (1995). Quantitative assessment of hyoid bone displacement from video images during swallowing. *Journal of Speech and Hearing Research, 38,* 579–585.

Sitzmann, J. V. (1990). Nutritional support of the dysphagic patient: Methods, risks, and complications of therapy. *Journal of Parenteral and Enteral Nutrition, 14,* 60–63.

Index